MW00654021

INTEGRATED HEALTH CARE FOR PEOPLE WITH AUTISM SPECTRUM DISORDER

INTEGRATED HEALTH CARE FOR PEOPLE WITH AUTISM SPECTRUM DISORDER

Edited by

ELLEN GIARELLI, EdD, RN, CRNP

and

KATHLEEN M. FISHER, PhD, RN, CRNP

(With 27 Other Contributors)

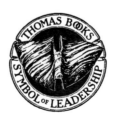

CHARLES C THOMAS • PUBLISHER, LTD.
Springfield • Illinois • U.S.A.

Published and Distributed Throughout the World by

CHARLES C THOMAS • PUBLISHER, LTD.
2600 South First Street
Springfield, Illinois 62704

This book is protected by copyright. No part of
it may be reproduced in any manner without written
permission from the publisher. All rights reserved.

© 2016 by CHARLES C THOMAS • PUBLISHER, LTD.

ISBN 978-0-398-09101-9 (paper)
ISBN 978-0-398-09102-6 (ebook)

Library of Congress Catalog Card Number: 201503188

With THOMAS BOOKS *careful attention is given to all details of manufacturing
and design. It is the Publisher's desire to present books that are satisfactory as to their
physical qualities and artistic possibilities and appropriate for their particular use.*
THOMAS BOOKS *will be true to those laws of quality that assure a good name
and good will.*

Printed in the United States of America
MM-R-3

Library of Congress Cataloging-in-Publication Data

Integrated health care for people with autism spectrum disorder / edited by Ellen Giarelli and Kathleen Fisher ; with 27 other contributors.
    p. ; cm.
  Includes bibliographical references and index.
  ISBN 978-0-398-09101-9 (paper) -- ISBN 978-0-398-09102-6 (ebook)
    I. Giarelli, Ellen. II. fisher, Kathleen, 1954–
    [DNLM: 1. Child Development Disorders, Pervasive–therapy.
2. Delivery of Health Care, Integrated. WS 350.8.P4]

  RC553.A88
  616.85′882–dc23
                                                201503188

This book is dedicated to all our families, our patients with autism spectrum disorder, their family caregivers, and the professionals who are committed to excellence in life-long care.

EDITORS

Ellen Giarelli, EdD, RN, CRNP

Ellen Giarelli is an associate professor in the Doctoral Nursing Program in the College of Nursing and Health Professions at Drexel University, Philadelphia. Dr Giarelli received a BS in nursing and a BS in biology from the State University of New York at Stony Brook, a masters degree in nursing from New York University, a Doctorate of Education from Rutgers, the State University of New Jersey, and post-doctoral education in psychosocial oncology and HIV/AIDS from the University of Pennsylvania School of Nursing. Dr. Giarelli is Co-I of the CDC funded Study of Epidemiology of Early Development (SEED) and was PI of an initiative funded by the Philadelphia Health Care Trust to integrate nursing into the care of people with ASD. She was research project director of the UPENN School of Nursing CDC funded Center for Autism and Developmental Disabilities Research and Epidemiology (CADDRE) and the director of the Pennsylvania Autism and Developmental Disabilities Surveillance Program (PADDSP). In addition to the awards from the CDC, her funded projects include an R21 from NIH/NINR to study self-management of genetic disorders. She is a Certified Registered Nurse Practitioner in Pennsylvania and principal investigator for several externally funded studies of autism spectrum disorders.

Kathleen M. Fisher, PhD, RN, CRNP

Kathleen Fisher is Professor of Nursing at Drexel University. She is a family nurse practitioner with a PhD in public administration and Health Policy from Penn State University. In 2001 with the collaboration of state and county agencies, she developed the South Central PA Health Care Quality Unit (HCQU), to oversee care and services for individuals with intellectual and developmental disability (I/DD) in nine counties in Pennsylvania. Dr Fisher has conducted a NINR funded study to describe decision making by proxy for those with I/DD also in Pennsylvania. Her research interests include intellectual disabilities (ID), proxy decision making, and exploring transitions with aging for those with ID.

CONTRIBUTORS

Joan Rosen Bloch, PhD, CRNP

Joan Rosen Bloch joined Drexel University as a full-time faculty member in 2005. She received her BSN from Thomas Jefferson University in 1978, MSN from the University of Pennsylvania in 1981, and PhD from the University of Pennsylvania in 2001. During her doctoral studies, she was awarded a two-year NIH pre-doctoral research fellowship in the Center for Vulnerable Women, Children and Families. Upon completion of her PhD, she was awarded a NIH post-doctoral research fellowship at the Center for Health Outcomes and Policy. Complementing her doctoral coursework at the University of Pennsylvania's School of Nursing was extensive coursework in both the School of Medicine and the Wharton Business School, enhancing her perinatal epidemiology and maternal-infant policy research abilities. As a certified Women's Health Nurse Practitioner since 1981, she has practiced in a variety of settings: City clinics, HMOs, and private practice. Her current practice in a Philadelphia federally-funded prenatal center informs her teaching and research. At Drexel University, she teaches women's health and research to BSN, MSN, and doctoral nursing students. She has received funding to investigate caregiver issues related to parenting children with neurodevelopmental disabilities throughout the life cycle.

Michael J. Brenner, BS, MPH

Michael Brenner graduated from the University of Vermont with a degree in microbiology and completed public health training at the University of Pennsylvania's Master of Public Health program. During his undergraduate career, Michael worked for a social services agency providing crisis intervention and residential services to the developmentally disabled in Vermont. After working in a specialized inpatient psychiatric unit for children with disabilities in Maine, he decided to pursue graduate training in public health in order to better understand the epidemiology of complex conditions like ASDs. Michael is currently a medical student and continues his research in the field of epidemiology.

James E. Connell, PhD

James Connell is a practicing psychologist, a nationally certified school psychologist, and a board certified behavior analyst conducting mental health, behavioral health, and educational research in community settings. Dr. Connell is an associate professor at Drexel University in the School of Education. Prior to Drexel, he was a research assistant professor in the Department of Psychiatry at the University of Pennsylvania and an assistant professor in the School Psychology Program at Temple University. For the past 10 years, his scholarship and clinical practice has focused on the conceptualization and implementation of evidence-based interventions in community settings, and the development and refinement of consultant-driven procedures to ensure program fidelity. He has more than 15 years of experience working in school systems and mental and behavioral health settings providing consultative support to direct care staff and educators on the implementation of evidence-based interventions. He has published numerous studies identifying external variables associated with the adult behavior change needed to ensure successful program implementation and has critiqued and edited numerous peer-reviewed papers on the same topic. He has taught graduate level courses in academic and behavioral interventions, and school and community-based consultation models and procedures.

Meghan N. Davignon, MD

Meghan Davignon received her MD from the University of Colorado Health Sciences Center and her pediatrics residency training through The Children's Hospital Colorado. She completed a fellowship in Developmental and Behavioral Pediatrics in 2014 at The Children's Hospital of Philadelphia and currently works as a developmental pediatrician at Kaiser Roseville Medical Center in Northern California. She specializes in the diagnosis and care of children with autism spectrum disorders and other neurodevelopment disabilities. Her research interests include improving the hospital experience for patients with ASD and determining predictors for successful outcomes for children with autism spectrum disorders who have been referred for behavioral therapy.

Leah I. Stein Duker, PhD, MA, OTR/L

Leah I. Stein Duker is a research assistant professor in the Mrs. T.H. Chan Division of Occupational Science and Occupational Therapy at the University of Southern California (USC). She earned her bachelor's degree in neuroscience and behavioral biology from Emory University, her master's degree in occupational therapy from USC, and her PhD in occupational science from USC. She has over 10 years of experience working with individuals with autism spectrum disorders and other developmental and physical disabilities, and her practice has focused on pediatrics in both the school and clinic settings. Her research interests include the impact of the physical, sensory, and social environment on patient and family experience during distressing health care procedures. Specifically, she is interested in the efficacy of environmental modifications to reduce physiological stress and anxiety, behavioral distress, and perception of pain in a variety of patient populations. She also has experience in the collection, analysis, and interpretation of both traditional wired and innovative wireless electrodermal activity data in the measurement of sympathetic stress and arousal. She has presented extensively, both locally and nationally, and has over ten publications in these areas of research.

Jennifer Harrison Elder, PhD, FAAN

Jennifer Harrison Elder is a professor and the associate dean for research at the University of Florida's College of Nursing. Prior to that, she served as Chair of the Department of Healthcare Environments and Systems. She has taught across all levels of the curriculum since her initial appointment in 1992 and currently focuses on directing the PhD program, teaching research methods courses for PhD students and providing research experiences for undergraduate honors students. Dr. Elder has spent 32 years studying autism and related child neuropsychiatric disorders, methods of educating families, and reducing caregiver stress of children with autism. Dr. Elder has been the primary investigator on four NIH/NINR grants and co-investigator on three others. She has given numerous international research presentations including an invited presentation in New Delhi by India's president. She is a fellow in the American Academy of Nursing and frequently reviews for NIH, and the American Nurses Foundation.

Marie Foley, PhD, RN

Marie Foley is the dean of the College of Nursing at Seton Hall University in South Orange, New Jersey. Dr. Foley has been a nurse educator since 1985. Her teaching experience includes most levels of nursing education, and programs. She has taught in BSN, RN to BSN, CNL, MSN and PhD programs at Seton Hall University, Kean University, the College of Saint Elizabeth, and NYU. She is a pediatric and school nurse and has taught courses in growth and development, pediatrics, research, and nursing theory. Her research interests include topics in school nursing, child temperament, ADHD, and parenting, mentoring school nurses and new faculty. She is a Certified Clinical Nurse Leader, and NJ-Certified School Nurse. She is a member of the National Association of School Nurses and the School Nurse Educator special interest group Sigma Theta Tau International, Eastern Nursing Research Society, and the Natioinal League for Nursing. She received her BSN from Fairleigh Dickinson University, her school nurse certification from Seton Hall University, her MA in nursing education and a PhD from New York University

Maria A. Fragala-Pinkham, PT, DPT, MS

Maria A. Fragala-Pinkham is a physical therapist and clinical researcher in the Research Center for Children with Special Health Care Needs at Franciscan Hospital for Children (FHC), Boston, MA. Dr. Fragala-Pinkham received her bachelor of science degree in physical therapy from Northeastern University, Boston, MA; a master of science degree in human movement science from the University of North Carolina–Chapel Hill; and a doctor of physical therapy degree from Massachusetts General Hospital Institute of Health Professions in Boston, MA. In her current position, Dr. Fragala-Pinkham conducts clinical research, provides PT intervention for outpatients, and directs the Adaptive Sports Program at the hospital. She has 30 years of clinical experience and has worked in a variety of clinical pediatric settings including early intervention, schools, home care, and hospital inpatient and outpatient programs. In addition, she has developed community-based adapted sports and fitness programs for children including an adapted ice skating program and an adaptive bicycle program. She is one of the senior authors of the Pediatric Evaluation of Disability-Computerized Adaptive Test, a pediatric functional outcome measure that was released in 2012. Dr. Fragala-Pinkham has published articles on the topics of pediatric outcome measures, effectiveness of therapeutic interventions and fitness for children with disabilities. She has presented on clinical topics and research findings for local, national, and international audiences.

Kathleen G. Freeman, PhD, RNC-NIC

Kathleen Freeman is adjunct faculty at the Drexel University, College of Nursing and Health Professions. She has been in nursing education for over 20 years and has taught at the University of Pennsylvania, Rutgers University, and the College of New Jersey. Within undergraduate, graduate, and RN-BSN education curriculums, she has taught human development, maternal-child health, community health, nursing foundations and theories, and autism. Certified in neonatal intensive care nursing and holding a Certificate in Applied Behavior Analysis from Rowan University, Dr. Freeman has a clinical background in the developmentally vulnerable and has expanded this expertise to include autism spectrum disorders (ASD) as a parent of an adult child with ASD. She contributed one of the first articles published on compliance with health procedures for the child with ASD in *Pediatric Nursing*, Dr. Freeman's passion for maternal-child health and improving the lives of those affected by ASD leads her to research and projects that include enhancing nursing ASD education, perinatal risks for ASD, developmental issues for the family with a child with a disability, family advocacy for services, and behavioral pediatrics. She received her BSN from the University of Pennsylvania, MS in maternal-child health nursing from the University of Delaware, and a PhD from the University of Maryland.

Eron Y. Friedlaender, MD, MPH

Eron Friedlaender is an associate professor of clinical pediatrics at the University of Pennsylvania School of Medicine and an attending physician in the emergency department at The Children's Hospital of Philadelphia. Dr. Friedlaender completed formal training in child advocacy and injury prevention through an NIH training grant, during which time she earned a masters in public health. She has investigated patterns of healthcare utilization by victims of child maltreatment, studied risk factors for injuries within the built environment, and served as principal investigator of the Injury Free Coalition for Kids in Philadelphia. She currently leads development of care initiatives and programming within the hospital to ensure access to and delivery of quality services to children with autism spectrum disorders.

Terisa P. Gabrielsen, PhD

Terisa Gabrielsen is a school psychologist specializing in interdisciplinary collaboration to improve care and treatment options for children with autism spectrum disorder. Following her doctoral training at the University of Utah and internships in Utah schools and The Children's Hospital of Philadelphia, she was a post-doctoral fellow at the Center for Autism Research in Philadelphia. She is now training school psychology students at Brigham Young University and continues her community outreach and interdisciplinary research on early intervention for toddlers and social skills training for teenagers.

Marcia R. Gardner, PhD, RN, CRNP, CPN

Marcia Gardner joined the faculty of the College of Nursing at Seton Hall University, South Orange, New Jersey, as an associate professor. She received a BSN from

Georgetown University, a master's in nursing from New York University, a post-master's certificate as a pediatric nurse practitioner from the State University of New York at Stony Brook, and a PhD in nursing science from the University of Pennsylvania. She was a clinical fellow in the Leadership in Neurodevelopmental Disabilities program at Children's Hospital of Philadelphia and a fellow in the AACN Academic Leadership Program. With an extensive background in high-risk neonatal care as well as in general pediatrics, she has taught pediatric nursing at both the undergraduate and graduate levels. She has been a department chair and assistant dean for both BSN and MSN programs. She is certified in pediatric nursing and as a pediatric nurse practitioner by the National Certification Board of Pediatric Nurse Practitioners and Nurses, and has research interests related to parenting of developmentally vulnerable infants and children.

Connor M. Kerns, PhD

Connor Kerns is trained in clinical psychology and Assistant Research Professor in the AJ Drexel Autism Institute and the Department of Psychology at Drexel University in Philadelphia, PA. Her clinical work and research focuses on the overlap, assessment, and treatment of emotional and stress-related disorders in individuals with ASD.

Paul A. Kettl, MD, MHA

Paul Kettl is currently Clinical Professor of Psychiatry at the Perelman School of Medicine of the University of Pennsylvania, and education director for behavioral health at the Philadelphia VA. Formerly, he served as chair of the Department of Psychiatry at Penn State's College of Medicine. He enjoys teaching, and last year, received the Dean's Award for Excellence in Clinical Teaching at an Affiliated Hospital, Perelman School of Medicine of the University of Pennsylvania, and received the Distinguished Educator Award from Penn State's College of Medicine along with other teaching awards from thirteen separate medical school classes from Penn State. He has served as a consultant in the past for seven pharmaceutical companies and has been named by his peers as one of the "Best Doctors in America" every year since 2003. He has a longstanding interest in public policy, and was the Democratic nominee for US Congress from his district in the past, losing to the republican incumbent in the general election.

David S. Mandell, DSc

David S. Mandell is an associate professor of psychiatry and pediatrics at the University of Pennsylvania's Perelman School of Medicine, where he directs the Center for Mental Health Policy and Services Research. He is the associate director of the Center for Autism Research at The Children's Hospital of Philadelphia. His research focuses on improving the quality of care individuals with autism receive in their communities and studying the best strategies to successfully implement proven-efficacious practices in community settings. Dr. Mandell is the author of more than 80 peer-reviewed scientific publications, many of which examine correlates of unmet need among children with psychiatric and developmental disabilities and strategies for reducing disparities. He co-chaired the Commonwealth of Pennsylvania's Autism Task Force from 2003 to 2006 and consults with the Department of Public Welfare to help them develop appropriate policies to meet the needs of families of children with autism. He currently serves as a member of the US Department of Health and Human Services Interagency Autism Coordinating Committee. Dr. Mandell holds a bachelor of arts in psychology from Columbia University and a doctorate of science from the Johns Hopkins Bloomberg School of Public Health.

Judith Miller, PhD

Judith Miller is assistant professor of psychology at the Perelman School of Medicine, University of Pennsylvania. She is a clinical psychologist with over 20 years of research and clinical experience with individuals with ASD, of all ages and levels of functioning. She directs the Research Assessment Clinic at the Center for Autism Research, the Children's Hospital of Philadelphia, and an ASD training program for psychology fellows, interns, and graduate students. Her research interests focus on identifying the essence of ASD to improve screening, diagnosis, and diagnosis of co-occurring conditions. She and her colleagues have worked closely with several units at The Children's Hospital of Philadelphia to improve the hospital experience for patients with ASD and their families.

Surabhi Mulchandani, MS

Surabhi Mulchandani is the manager of genomics education and outreach at the Division of Genomic Diagnostics at the Children's Hospital of Philadelphia (CHOP). Ms. Mulchandani is a board certified and licensed genetic counselor. She received a masters degree in molecular and human genetics from India and a masters degree in genetic counseling from California State University, Northridge. Ms. Mulchandani worked as a senior genetic counselor in the genetic testing lab at CHOP for five years before moving on to her current role. As a genetic counselor, Ms. Mulchandani interpreted complex data generated by genome wide array technology in context of patient's clinical information, provided genetic education, counseling, and risk assessment and served as a bridge between clinicians and the lab. In her current role, Ms Mulchandani manages various educational activities for the division including the fellowship program for future lab directors, and genetic testing rotations for genetic counseling student in addition to leading a project on genetic testing utilization for The Children's Hospital of Philadelphia. She has been involved in multiple research studies on genomic testing. Ms Mulchandani's interest lies in understanding the clinical, psychosocial, ethicolegal, and economical impact of genetic testing on patients, families, health care providers, and the society as whole.

Craig Newschaffer, PhD

Craig Newschaffer is founding director of the A.J. Drexel Autism Institute at Drexel University and a professor in the Department of Epidemiology and Biostatistics at the Drexel University School of Public Health. Dr. Newschaffer is an epidemiologist whose main research focus is the discovery of modifiable autism risk factors. He is principal investigator of an NIH Autism Centers of Excellence (ACE) research network that implements the Early Autism Risk Longitudinal Investigation (EARLI)–a large cohort study designed specifically to study pre, peri- and neonatal autism risk factors and biomarkers by following mothers of children with autism at the start of subsequent pregnancies. Dr. Newschaffer has also been a site PI for the ADDM Network and SEED Studies, and currently leads a project exploring innovative approaches to autism case confirmation for the National Children's Study (NCS). He is a fellow of the American College of Epidemiology and serves as an associate editor of the *American Journal of Epidemiology* and on the editorial boards of *Autism Research* and the *Journal of Neurodevelopmental Disorders.*

Romy Nocera, PhD

Romy Nocera is a research assistant professor and the director of clinical research in the Department of Emergency Medicine. She received her BS from the University of Pittsburgh, her MA and PhD from Bowling Green State University, and completed neuroscience fellowships at BGSU and Lankenau Institute for Medical Research. She has taught numerous courses in psychology, psychobiology, gerontology, and research methods and statistics, and was awarded the I.M. Freeburne Award for Excellence in Teaching at BGSU. She currently teaches in the annual Translational Medicine Research Course for fourth-year medical students and serves as a preceptor for their simulated research projects. In addition, Dr. Nocera heads the EM Resident Research Program, and serves as advisor to several pre-medical master's students in fulfilling their research requirements. She oversees multiple funded clinical trials and maintains her own program of research in the field of neuroscience. Her past research interests and experience included neuropsychological assessment of persons with Alzheimer's disease, caregiver stress, neuronal receptor expression in Alzheimer's and in normal aging, and stem cell treatment for ischemic stroke. She is currently conducting research focused on relationships between weather variables and stroke incidence, and in the relationship between aphasia at stroke onset and patient outcomes. She is a member of the Society for Neuroscience.

Margaret E. O'Neil PT, PhD, MPH

Margaret O'Neil is associate professor and research faculty member in the Department of Physical Therapy and Rehabilitation Sciences at Drexel University, Philadelphia, PA. She has a secondary appointment in Drexel's School of Public Health, Department of Community Health and Prevention. She received her bachelor of science degree in biology from Providence College, Providence, RI; her a master of science degree in physical therapy from Duke University, Durham, NC; her master of public health degree from the University of North Carolina– Chapel Hill and her PhD from Drexel University (formerly MCP Hahnemann University). Dr. O'Neil's research focuses on measuring physical activity and fitness in children and youth with physical disabilities (cerebral palsy) and chronic conditions (obesity). In addition she examines the effect of innovative interventions (i.e., active video gaming) to promote physical activity and fitness, and conducts both laboratory-based and community-based research studies to examine reliability and validity of physical activity measures and to examine the effect of activity-based interventions on physical activity and fitness in children. She has been the recipient of multiple grants including NIH and the Department of Education. Dr. O'Neil has published articles on the physical activity and fitness measures and outcomes for children with disabilities and obesity and she has done multiple local, national, and international presentations on these topics.

Elizabeth Pfeiffer, PhD, OTR/L, BCP

Beth Pfeiffer is an associate professor at Temple University where her primary responsibilities are teaching and research. Her research focuses on sensory processing, autism, and mental health across the lifespan. Dr. Pfeiffer has completed effectiveness studies on the use of sensory-based interventions in both children and adults. Her recent work focuses on developing a measure to assess the impact of the sensory environment on participation in daily activity for very young children with autism spectrum disorders. Additionally, she was recently funded to develop advocacy-based ecological interventions, and study the impact of the sensory environment on employment outcomes for adults with autism spectrum disorders.

Jennifer A. Pinto-Martin, PhD, MPH

Jennifer Pinto-Martin is the Viola MacInnes/Independence Professor and Chair of Biobehavioral Health Sciences in the University of Pennsylvania School of Nursing with a secondary appointment in the Department of Epidemiology in the School of Medicine. She is the director of the University of Pennsylvania's Masters of Public Health Program. Dr. Pinto-Martin began her career as an epidemiologist and as the project director for the Neonatal Brain Hemorrhage (NBH) Study, a longitudinal study of neonatal brain injury in low birthweight infants. The NBH Study has had continuous NIH support for this research since 1984 and has conducted five separate assessments of the cohort. Dr. Pinto-Martin's primary research focus is the epidemiology of autism spectrum disorder. She is currently the director and principal investigator of the Pennsylvania Center for Autism and Developmental Disabilities Research and Epidemiology (PA-CADDRE), one of six such centers funded by the Centers for Disease Control and Prevention to study the etiology of ASD. PA-CADDRE is currently involved in data collection for the Study to Explore Early Development (SEED), a multi-site, case-control study of the risk factors associated with ASD. In addition, Dr. Pinto-Martin just completed a study funded by NIH to assess the prevalence of ASD in the NBH cohort. Dr. Pinto-Martin is also working with the International Clinical Epidemiology Network on a study, funded by NIH- Fogarty, on the prevalence of ASD and other childhood disabilities.

Marian Reiff, PhD

Marian Reiff has a PhD from Columbia University in sociomedical sciences, specializing in medical anthropology and public health. She also has a master's degree in social work and social policy from the London School of Economics. She has taught medical anthropology, and has clinical experience as a social worker in medical, psychiatric and community settings. Dr. Reiff is a senior research investigator in the Division of Translational Medicine and Human Genetics at the Perelman School of Medicine, at the University of Pennsylvania. She was principal investigator on a research project funded by the National Institutes of Health that used mixed methods (including in-depth interviews and surveys) to examine the impact of uncertainty about the results of genomic testing on children with autism and their families. Dr. Reiff's research explores the psychosocial and cultural contexts of health behavior and health care. In addition to investigating the implications of genome-wide testing for families and healthcare providers she studies public attitudes regarding genetics and mental illness.

Lindsay Shea, DrPH

Lindsay Shea is the director of the Eastern Region Autism Services, Education, Resources and Training Collaborative (ASERT) Eastern Region at Drexel University and senior manager of the recently launched A.J. Drexel Autism Institute. Dr. Shea has led and managed autism-focused policy and research projects locally, in Pennsylvania and with a national scope for 10 years. Dr. Shea first-authored the Pennsylvania Autism Census Report and her research interests are based in creating and utilizing an evidence base in forming, evaluating, implementing, and modifying social and health policies.

Margaret C. Souders, PhD, CRNP, PNP

Margaret C. Souders is an assistant professor at the University of Pennsylvania, School of Nursing and a clinician educator. She has an appointment in the Clinical Genetics Department at The Children's Hospital of Philadelphia as a pediatric nurse practitioner. She has completed a two-year post-doctoral fellowship in the Center for Sleep and Respiratory Neurobiology at the University of Pennsylvania where she has a research program in sleep science. After conducting over 400 home visits and talking with individuals with autism spectrum disorder (ASD) and their caregivers, we identified that the environmental modifications, behavioral strategies and intensity of the sleep intervention needs to be tailored to the specific characteristics of the individual with ASD, the detailed needs of the family, and the complexity of the sleep problems. She is a member of a multi-disciplinary team of experts including a nurse practitioner and sleep scholar from the University of Pennsylvania, a behavioral psychologist and autism expert from Drexel University, an occupational therapist and sensory expert from Jefferson University and caregiver of a child with ASD and insomnia from Philadephia.

Renee Turchi, MD MPH, FAAP

Renee Turchi is the medical director of the PA Medical Home Program which is a statewide and state/federally funded medical home program for pediatric practices in the Commonwealth of Pennsylvania. As medical director of the Center for Children with Special Health Care Needs at St. Christopher's Hospital for Children, she delivers primary care for children and youth with special health care needs and has multiple grants supporting evaluation of health care delivery to this fragile population of children. She is an associate professor at Drexel University School of Public Health and College of Medicine.

Carl V. Tyler, Jr., MD, MS

Carl V. Tyler is the Geriatrics and Research Director for the Fairview Hospital/ Cleveland Clinic Family Medicine Residency Program and associate professor in Cleveland Clinic Lerner College of Medicine of Case Western Reserve University. After graduating from Northeastern Ohio Universities College of Medicine (now Northeast Ohio Medical University), he completed one year of post-graduate studies in psychiatry and human behavior at the University of California, Irvine, followed by a three-year residency in family practice at Fairview General Hospital. He is board-certified in family medicine and geriatric medicine. He completed two post-doctoral fellowships through Case Western Reserve University: the first, concentrating in aging and disability, leading to a master of science degree; the second, an NIH-sponsored fellowship in practice-based research design and methodology. Dr. Tyler joined the faculty at Fairview in 1995. He serves as director of the Developmental Disabilities-Practice Based Research Network, a multi-stakeholder research group with representatives from the advocacy, service, and health care communities. Dr. Tyler's clinical and research interests include the primary medical care of adults with developmental disabilities and practice-based health services research utilizing electronic health records. Dr. Tyler and his wife, Maca, have three daughters, Ana, Aleksandra, and Natalija.

Kate E. Wallis, MD

Kate E. Wallis is currently a resident physician in the Department of Pediatrics at New York University School of Medicine. Dr. Wallis received her MD and MPH degrees from Stony Brook University School of Medicine. She earned her BA from the University of Pennsylvania. She has been working with individuals with autism spectrum disorder for 15 years. Dr. Wallis's major research interests include the epidemiology of autism, the history of medicine, and improving care for individuals with chronic medical problems. She has published in the field of developmental disabilities, writing about the difficulties of screening for autism spectrum disorder across different cultures and the diagnosis and management of enuresis and encopresis in typically and atypically developing children. Dr. Wallis will be starting a fellowship in behavioral and developmental pediatrics at The Children's Hospital of Philadelphia.

FOREWORD

Every one of us depends on health care providers for essential preventative, treatment, and emergency care for ourselves or our loved ones. This continuum of care ideally includes personalized, evidence-based support for prevention and wellness, maintenance, and in illness and crisis. For routine care, we trust our healthcare providers to check up on us and tell us if things are going well or if something about our health has gone awry. We make calls, wait for our appointments, fill out checklists, answer questions, and participate in exams. These encounters might be routine or life-changing. Having that care is something we often take for granted when we go to the doctor's office. Most of us can count on being able to report our history and symptoms and trust the people we encounter are there to help us.

Now, what if you were one of the 1–2% of people who has autism spectrum disorder (ASD)? How would that change your healthcare encounter? From early on, your parents may have a nagging feeling that something is different. They may question if you can hear and wonder why you do not turn around when they call your name in that sweet baby voice they use to get your attention. At the 18-month well-baby check-up, your mother might keep a close eye on the nurse and doctor for any sign that something is different or wrong. She might apologize when you cry and arch your back as you are examined. She might be anxious and relieved at the same time when asked to answer questions about how many words you are using, if you smile when others smile at you, if you point out objects, if you pretend to talk on the phone. You may be frustrated that you cannot say you are hungry, bothered when people interrupt your close inspection of a toy to get you to look at them, and distracted by the hums and whirls of the machines and sounds in the background.

From the earliest age, when the social communication and interaction and behavior signs of autism emerge, life is different for people with ASD. These differences are biologically-based and result in lifelong differences in processing information and experiencing the world. In addition to these core aspects of ASD, people with ASD are likely to have co-occurring challenges in areas such as sleeping, eating, sensory processing, attention, and anxiety, among others. People with ASD may find the unpredictability of office visits to be disconcerting. The unfamiliar people with unclear intentions in the midst of strange sights, smells, and sounds may be overwhelming. Some people with ASD may react with outbursts that are frightening to those not familiar with the person, or they may just shut down and not respond. A person with ASD may not be able to tell you where it hurts, or that they even have pain in the first place. Even before the appointment it may take extra steps and preparation to get ready for an office visit. Then, supports throughout the visit may be necessary. In these busy times, many healthcare professionals may not be interested in taking the time necessary to address the special needs that someone with ASD may have. Getting routine health care can be a challenge for many reasons, but the main barrier comes from the breakdown in efficient communication between provider and patient when they are not able to understand each other. This book provides the tools and information so the healthcare professional can think differently about caring for this patient, and see through his or her eyes.

Given the current prevalence estimates and improvements in awareness of ASD, it is very likely that most healthcare offices will have patients on the spectrum at some time or another. Ideally, each person has access to a Medical Home that provides accessible and family-centered care across the lifespan. People with ASD may have unique developmental challenges, but they face a range of health issues like all people. Many of these may be compounded by an ASD. Access to quality care is a challenge and many individuals have no one to transition to when aging out of pediatric care. We know very little about the long-term health effects of activity limitations, restricted diets, or other compounding behavioral challenges. For too many, basic healthcare needs have been overshadowed by ASD with potentially treatable health issues explained away as just another part of the ASD. There is a great need to change that bias so that each person has access and is involved in what is needed to help them live healthy lives.

This volume edited by Dr. Ellen Giarelli and Dr. Kathleen Fisher is a much-needed resource with important information from the 2014 conference "Creating Integrated Healthcare Services for people with Autism Spectrum Disorder" sponsored by Drexel University College of Nursing and Health Professions and the AJ Drexel Autism Institute. The information and tools are essential to improve the care and support of people with ASD. Compilation of the information shared during the conference can help move health care forward by recognizing that people with ASD face the range of issues that all individuals may encounter in addition to more complicated and unique challenges requiring specialized strategies and attention. The presentations summarized here and the additional chapters share the importance of early, continuous, coordinated, and individualized care that is integrated into the existing health care system. Examples of models and policies that have improved the access, experience, and outcomes for patients with ASD are shared. In addition, the importance of continuous quality improvement through data collection and monitoring of outcomes is emphasized. This information is essential for addressing the capacity crisis we have in providing routine, specialized, and emergency care for individuals with ASD.

This volume brings together a wealth of expertise with information and strategies across the lifespan. As a result of these efforts, I hope that more people with ASD will feel they are part of a trusted health care team that provides meaningful information, prevention, and intervention throughout their lives.

CATHERINE E. RICE, PH.D.

PREFACE

This book is the product of an interdisciplinary conference funded in 2014 by a grant from the U.S. Department of Health and Human Services, Agency for Health Care Research and Quality (1R13HS023035-01) and matching grants from Drexel University College of Nursing and Health Professions, Drexel University Online, and the A.J. Drexel Autism Institute. The purpose of the conference was to start a conversation among experts, professionals and consumers. We presumed that if we brought together healthcare providers to learn about and discuss these conversations it would stimulate new and creative approaches to the provision and coordination of medical care for people with autism spectrum disorder (ASD) across the lifespan. The conference provided a forum for the discussion of a research agenda to evaluate the outcomes of integrated care and policy efforts.

We hope that improving such coordination of care derived from creative problem solving will reduce miscommunication among providers, family members and patients, and control the confusion that compromises patient safety or delays in the delivery of needed services. We also hope that, over time, better integration of care will reduce costs, improve treatment outcomes, and improve the quality of life for people with ASD. This book continues the conversation and proposes ways to test these presumptions and affect changes.

We conceptualized this book as a service to our colleagues and a responsibility to our patients with autism spectrum disorder and their families. It satisfies a need for a clear, comprehensive collection of interdisciplinary perspectives on how to provide quality health care when a patient is also diagnosed with autism spectrum disorder (ASD). The conference had a key address, summarized by Doctor Catherine Rice in the Foreword. The book is divided into four sections that correspond with the four sessions of the conference and reflect the overarching need to understand the scope of the problem, consider different solutions, examine different environment and contextual factors, and recognize the need for research and policy changes. The chapters offer perspectives from leaders across multiple health care services and in public policy and research. The authors include nurses (women's health, primary care, urgent care), physicians (psychiatry, pediatrics, gerontology), educators, occupational therapists, physical therapists, epidemiologists, psychologists, public health professionals, and genetic counselors.

In Section 1, the chapters examine and explore the type and scope of the factors that contribute to the problem of providing comprehensive health care to people with ASD. In Chapter 1, I outline how a fragmented healthcare system results in rising costs and diminished quality of care. In Chapter 1, I call attention to urgent need for healthcare providers to learn to manage a complex set of symptoms and anticipate the potential side effects of polypharmacy. In Chapter 2, Michael J. Brenner, Kate E. Wallis and Jennifer A. Pinto-Martin discuss the epidemiology of ASD, the evolution of diagnostic codes, global prevalence, and proposed etiological theories. They make a convincing case for continuing research. In Chapter 3, Kathleen G. Freeman and Jennifer Harrison Elder share their personal and professional experience with ASD. They assert that healthcare providers must try to comprehend the complexity of the problem faced by parents of children and adults with ASD. They advocate for trying to comprehend the patient's and parent's reality, working closely with parents, and considering ways to prepare for medical visits. Care does not just flow from the healthcare provider to the patient. It is coextensive with sensations that flow from the environment in which care is delivered. In Chapter 4, Elizabeth Pfeiffer and Leah I. Stein Duker discuss sensory processing, anxiety and related obstacles to care. They offer anticipatory strategies and recommend environmental modifications to removed barriers to optimizing therapeutics. In Chapter 5, Paul A. Kettl considers the complexity of prescribing medications to the patient with ASD. He considers the comorbidities, side effects and polypharmacy, and introduces the reader to some promising pharmacotherapeutics presently under investigation.

Section 2 includes chapters that address the solutions to some of the problems described in Section 1, beginning with a framework to guide practice and research descried presented by Joan Rosen Bloch in Chapter 6. A broad view of healthcare services is used to point out the ways equity, effectiveness, and efficiency can be improved. In Chapter 7, services settings are further examined and the pediatric Medical Home is described as the exemplar for comprehensive care. The author, Renee Turchi, illustrates further the ways to provide patient and family centered care and how to engage community partners and how partnerships are key. In Chapter 8, James E. Connell, Margaret C. Souders and Connor M. Kerns extend the idea and apply the principles of the Medical Home to the adult ASD services. They share their Case Consultation Model as a way to address the complex challenges and needs of the adult population. Selecting optimal intervention from among a host of treatment options can be daunting for patients and family members. In Chapter 9, Jennifer Harrison Elder advises on how healthcare providers can assist parents and other family caregivers to best navigate the healthcare system and make informed circles. She offers advice on how to support family members and informal caregivers and summarizes the key instructional points when discussing complementary and alternative therapies. Genetic testing is becoming the standard of care in diagnosing cases of ASD. In Chapter 10, Marian Reiff and Surabhi Mulchandani share their expertise to explain first-line genetics testing, psychosocial implications, and practice implications. They offer recommendations for pre- and post-counseling and practice and policy changes.

The knowledge base of the health provider, the immediate environment, and other contextual factors such as social variables will have an effect on how health services can be integrated. These are explored in Section 3. In Chapter 11, Marcia R. Gardner describes how professional nurses conceptualize their role in the care of patients with ASD. She uncovers faculty and curriculum obstacles and offers her advice on designing training programs that are effective and innovative. In urban centers, emergency departments may be the principal source of care for patients without health insurance. In Chapter 12, Romy Nocera describes common medical emergencies among patients with ASD, along with the process for admitting, assessing, and designing treatment plans for urgent care. A consideration of core symptoms is necessary, and environmental modifications, along with appropriate triage questions, will enhance the benefit of inter-professional communication and help to insure a therapeutic encounter. Physical therapy is often prescribed for people with ASD to promote motor function and sensory modulations. In Chapter 13, Margaret E. O'Neil and Maria Fragela-Pinkham present a case study illustrating optimum integrated care from the perspective of the physical therapist. Section 3 is completed with Chapter 14 in which the author, Carl V. Tyler, Jr., describes how to use Big Data to direct quality improvement. He illustrates an analytic platform and its key functions and makes a convincing argument that these data can facilitate the integration of healthcare services.

Section 4 contains chapters offering perspectives on research, policy development, and the process for selecting patient outcomes to monitor. Judith Miller, Meghan N. Davignon, Terisa P. Gabrielsen, and Eron Y. Friedlaender begin the section with Chapter 15 in which they describe the characteristics of a good healthcare experience for a person with ASD. They advise that measuring and evaluating are essential components of care and can be guided by the application of an ecological systems perspective. They introduce various approaches to researching treatment choices and outcomes. In Chapter 6, Lindsay Shea, David S. Mandell, and Craig Newschaffer tackle the important issue of policy develop and systematic change. They outline policy issues related to Medicaid and insurance mandates as they pertain to ASD. The authors provide a model of success and strategies for engaging policy makers. Section 4 culminates with frequently asked questions and answers from the experts on the integration of healthcare for people with ASD.

Many important people contributed to the preparation of the book and the success of the conference. I am most grateful to my co-editor Kathleen Fisher for sharing her expert knowledge of caring for people with special needs, her attention to detail, and her untiring willingness to take on more responsibility. Doctor Jennifer Plumb was co-investigator on the grant, directed marketing efforts, and orchestrated the flow of questions and answers for Chapter 17. The moderators of each of four panel discussions lent their unique expertise and skill in fielding questions and guiding discussion. They were Mrs. Jean Ruttenberg, Dr. Diana Robins, Dr. Margaret O'Neil, and Dr. Paul Shattuck.

I wish to thank the conference committee, Kathy Freeman, Kartikeya Puranik, Margaret O'Neil, and Elizabeth Nolan, for the many roles they played and the marketing/advertising/website group from Drexel University College of Nursing and Health Profession (DU-CNHP). Included in this cohort are Laura Valenti, Wayne Miller, Christine Migeot, and Craig Schlanser. Also included are Anna Auch, Joan Bloch, Andrea Bricklin, Rebecca Charuk, Nicole Davis, Rachel Ewing, Janelle Gillis, Kirsten Glaser, Christina Klassis, Christine McAuliffe, Mary Kate O'Keefe, Jessica Rast, Margaret Rowen, Mahmoud Shurbaji, Laura Valenti, and John Zabinski. A special thanks goes to Doctor Fran Cornelius for help in establishing and enrolling students in the Post-baccalaureate Certificate Program in the Nursing Care of Autism Spectrum Disorder at DU-CNHP.

Finally, I am grateful to the following individuals for their support of the conference and support and advocacy for the larger, social endeavor to improve the quality of health care and the quality of life for people with ASD and their families. These advocates are: Mr. John A. Fry, President of Drexel University (DU); Dr. Gloria Ferraro Donnelly, Dean of the DU College of Nursing and Health Professions; Dr. Albert Rundio, Associate Dean for Post Licensure Nursing Programs at DU College of Nursing and Health Professions; Dr. Elizabeth Gonzalez, Doctoral Nursing Chair; and Dr. Craig Newschaffer, Director of the AJ Drexel Autism Institute.

E.G.

CONTENTS

Section 1
THE PROBLEM: SCOPE/BREADTH OF THE PROBLEM OF PROVIDING COMPREHENSIVE HEALTH CARE TO PEOPLE WITH ASD

Section 2
THE SOLUTIONS: EFFECTIVE, SAFE, COORDINATED CARE

Section 3
ENVIRONMENTS, SERVICES, AND CONTEXT

Section 4
MONITORING PATIENT OUTCOMES:
RESEARCH AND POLICY DEVELOPMENT

INTEGRATED HEALTH CARE FOR PEOPLE WITH AUTISM SPECTRUM DISORDER

Section 1

THE PROBLEM: SCOPE/BREADTH OF THE PROBLEM OF PROVIDING COMPREHENSIVE HEALTH CARE TO PEOPLE WITH ASD

Chapter 1

INTEGRATING KNOWLEDGE OF AUTISM WITH COMPREHENSIVE HEALTH CARE

ELLEN GIARELLI

Health Care in a Fragmented System

The United States (US) has a fragmented healthcare system with limited primary care resources and a large uninsured population. According to the Institute of Medicine and the National Research Council (Woolf, Aron, Committee on Population of the Division of Behavioral and Social Sciences and Education, & Board on Population Health and Public Health Practice of the Institute of Medicine, 2013), the US health disadvantage is expressed as higher rates of chronic disease and mortality among adults and as higher rates of untimely death and injuries among adolescents and small children. One explanation for the health disadvantage of the US might be its deficiencies in the planning and delivery of health services. Another factor that diminishes the effectiveness of health care in the US is its disruptions in the care delivery process.

For many years, quality improvement programs and health services research have recognized that the fragmented nature of the US healthcare system, miscommunication, and incompatible information systems create lapses in care; oversights and errors; and unnecessary repetition of testing, treatment, and associated risks, because records of prior services are unavailable (Fineberg, 2012; Institute of Medicine & Committee on Public Health Strategies to Improve Health, 2012; Kohn, Corrigan, Donaldson, & Committee on Quality of Health Care in America, 2000). These problems exist for the general population and may be compounded for the patients with autism spectrum disorder (ASD).

Cost of Care

Care has monetary and human costs. Monetarily, the health expenditures in the US have grown annually from $256 billion (9.2 % of gross domestic product [GDP]) in 1980 to $2.6 trillion (17.9 percent of GDP) in 2010 (Martin et al., 2012). When compared with the average for other high-income countries, the US fares worse in nine health domains, one of which is disability, and persons within the disability domain, including those with ASD, also suffer from fragmentation in the healthcare system.

The human cost of care includes wasted provider time and the effort spent during inefficient communication with other providers. Human costs also include the emotional distress associated with frustrated efforts to provide quality care to patients and the burden to patients and families struggling to secure optimal services. When the efforts of physicians, nurses, assistive personnel, and families are consolidated, medical care for people with mental health problems will be improved.

A diagnosis of ASD is associated with a higher rate of comorbid medical and mental health conditions that increase the patient's need for treatments in acute care and other services settings. The cascading effect of multiple health conditions may lead to a higher mortality rate among people with ASD through multiple causal pathways (Thornicroft, 2011; Wahlbeck, Westman, Nordentoft, Gissler, & Laursen, 2011). At this point, there are no reports of the impact. Patient-centered care requires that treatments be tailored to the specific health needs of the individual. This chapter addresses the nexus of a consistently rising prevalence of ASD and the persistent fragmentation of acute care services.

Rising Prevalence and Narrowing Services

The rising prevalence of people with neurodevelopmental disorders, such as ASD (Centers for Disease Control and Prevention, 2014; USDHHS/ Centers for Disease Control and Prevention, 2012), translates to a rise in the use of acute and chronic care services for this population across the lifespan. Acute care is defined as the branch of secondary health care where a patient receives active but short-term treatment for a severe injury or episode of illness, an urgent medical condition, or treatment during recovery from surgery, rather than long-term residential care for chronic illness. Acute care may require a stay in a hospital emergency department, ambulatory surgery center, urgent care center or other short-term stay facility, along with the assistance of diagnostic services, surgery, or follow-up outpatient care in the community. Acute care settings include but are not limited to: Emergency departments, intensive care, coronary care, cardiology, neonatal intensive care, and many general areas where a patient might be admitted for acute illness, stabilization, and transfer to another higher dependency unit for further treatment (American Psychiatric Association, 2013). In acute care settings, services are often coordinated by a nurse and delivered by a multidisciplinary team composed of both generalists and specialists. The coordinator sets the tone and possibly the pace of care. Safe and effective health care for the patient with ASD requires an understanding of the complex nature of the diagnosis and treatment of co-occurring conditions.

Health Care Needs of People with ASD

The most recent statistics from the Centers for Disease Control and Prevention (CDC) identified that one in 68 children aged eight years old in 2010 are on the autism spectrum (Centers for Disease Control and Prevention, 2014). This prevalence rate has increased by 30% from the last report in 2012. ASD continues to increase and continues to be an important public health concern in the United States (US) (US; CDC, 2014; (USD-HHS/Centers for Disease Control and Prevention, 2012). Patients with ASD may require healthcare services at a higher rate than the general population.

The years of life affected by developmental disabilities can be substantial, because these disorders often first appear in early childhood and persist throughout life (Kessler, 2007). Each individual with an ASD will also have multiple needs for healthcare services over a lifetime, in addition to those associated with ASD. According to Palloni and Yonker (Palloni & Yonker, 2012), neuropsychiatric disorders claimed approximately 75 percent of days lost to disability at ages 15 to 29 years and approximately 50% of days lost at ages 30 to 44 years. Neurodevelopmental disorders may act as both a cause and a manifestation of the US health disadvantage. A person's emotional and neuropsychiatric health can affect disease, and ASD is itself a significant health problem (US Department of Health and Human Services, 2001).

Comorbidities

According to Levy, Giarelli, Lee et al. (Levy et al., 2010), 82% of individuals diagnosed with ASD also exhibit medical, psychiatric, neurological, and/or behavior co-morbidities–any one of which might require medical intervention. People with ASD have a high risk for developing and receiving treatment for comorbid neuropsychiatric disorders such as depression, obsessive compulsive disorders, and anxiety (Levy et al., 2010). Individuals with depression face a higher risk of physical illnesses such as diabetes, hypertension and heart disease, pulmonary, and infectious diseases (Newcomer, 2007) and, in the US at least, may die years earlier than the general population (Felker, Yazel, & Short, 1996; Parks, Svedsen, Singer, & Foti, 2006). Furthermore, McEwen's and Gianaros' (B.S. McEwen, 2000; B.S. McEwen & Gianaros, 2010) theory of allostasis purported that stress and anxiety may affect the brain and the endocrine system, alter the behavior of the immune system, and damage end organs. People with ASD suffer from high levels of anxiety and they experience a high rate of sensory processing dysfunctions that may significantly interfere with the delivery of care in certain environments (Lane, Young, Baker, & Angley, 2010).

Pharmacotherapeutics

In addition, management of many comorbid disorders relies heavily on the use of pharmacotherapeutics. In 2003, Aman and colleagues (Aman, Lam, & Collier-Crespin, 2003) reported that between 45% and 55% of children diagnosed with ASD were treated with one or more psychopharmacologic agents. When considering the use of any biomedical treatment, these rates appeared to be as high as 65% (Martin, Scahill, Klin, & Volkmar, 1999).

Considering the high rate and complexity of comorbidity, the rate of polypharmacy, and the use of complementary and alternative medications, at this time, we must take a cautious, informed, and anticipatory approach to assessing the interaction of these factors when planning and delivering care.

Assuring Quality Health Care

The Agency for Healthcare Research and Quality (AHRQ) recognizes that the best new science occurs when someone combines the knowledge gained by other scientists in nonobvious ways to create a new understanding of how the world works (Geonnotti et al. 2015)). There is a lack of scientific literature on the effect of integrated care on patient outcomes thus highlighting the need to promote high-level (among experts) discourse on the practice and delivery of health care for a population of US citizens who are at high risk for health disparities by virtue of this developmental disability. One place to start is at primary prevention and those services, such as screening, that have well-established guidelines.

Risk Management and Disease Prevention

Preventing disease helps keep healthcare costs down and is critical to helping people live longer, healthier lives. Patients' poor diets, physical inactivity, tobacco use, and alcohol misuse are just some of the challenges faced by health care providers. People with ASD, across the lifespan, are at higher risk for poor diets and physical inactivity due to higher incidence of eating abnormalities and food sensitivity, and social isolation that might limit their exercise and activity options. Nurses, physicians, and public health professionals know that many of the strongest predictors of health and well-being fall outside of the healthcare setting. Housing, transportation, education, workplaces, and environment are major elements that impact the physical and mental health of Americans. All these factors are issues for people with ASD, thus confirming the need for a comprehensive approach to case management that integrates primary, secondary, and tertiary prevention.

Integrated Preventive Health Care

Members of the National Prevention Council of the US Department of Health and Human Services (National Prevention Council, 2011) described a National Prevention Strategy to identify and meet the preventative healthcare needs of the general US population. The Council, created by the Affordable Care Act in 2010, identified priorities and recognized the need to lower healthcare costs, improve the quality of care, and provide coverage options for the uninsured. Building partnerships was a key aspect. Partnership among healthcare providers, ASD case managers, patients with ASD, and family members can adapt scientifically evaluated and proven programs and policies. There are various resources available to assist public health and medical professionals to be prepared for improving evidence-based practice. Box 1.1 contains a list of resources for program planning and evaluation.

Box 1.1. Resources for Training Professionals and Creating Planning Tools for Evidence-Based (EB) Integrated Health Care for Patients with ASD.

The tools can be adapted and used to plan evidence-based health care for a patient with autism spectrum disorder.

Training Tool

Evidence-based Behavioral Project Training Portal

http://www.ebbp.org

The site contains nine modules illustrating evidence-based practice for both individuals and populations with special needs and offers continuing education for social workers, nurses, psychologists, and physicians.

---

continued

Box 1.1–*Continued*

Training Tool

Evidence-based Public Health (EBPH) Online Course

http://ebph.ihrp.uic.edu/

This online course provides an overview of the EBPH process and includes additional resources.

Planning Tool

Cancer Control P.L.A.N.E.T.

http://cancercontrolplanet.cancer.gov

This portal walks practitioners through an EB process for cancer control including easy access to data and resources.

Planning Tool

Community Health Assessment and Group Evaluation Tool and Action Guide (CHANGE)

www.cdc.gov/healthycommunitiesprogram/tools/change.htm

This tool focuses on assessment and planning and establishing tracking procedures.

Planning Tool

Mobilizing for Action through Planning and Partnerships (MAPP)

www.naccho.org/topics/infrastructure/mapp/index.cfm

The site guides practitioners through organizational steps from assessment through planning. Includes a comprehensive user handbook and clearinghouse of resources.

Planning Tool

CDC Program Evaluation

www.cdc.gov/eval/index.htm

continued

Box 1.1–*Continued*

The site contains step-by-step manuals and other evaluation resources including the CDC framework for program evaluation.

Economic Evaluation

Cost-effectiveness Analysis Registry

https://research.tufts-nemc.org/cear4/home.aspX

The registry offers detailed information on approximately 3,000 cost-effectiveness analyses covering a range of diseases and interventions.

Preventing Disease in People with ASD

Preventing disease in people on the autism spectrum requires more than simply providing individuals with tailored instructions for making decisions that promote health. All sectors of the community contribute in some way to the prevention of illness and the promotion of health and well-being. The sectors include housing, transportation, labor, and education, and they all can be modified to promote health through prevention-oriented environments and policies, tailored to people with developmental disabilities. The communities in which these people reside should reinforce and support these efforts. People with ASD will ultimately benefit from any community-based efforts to improve air quality and reduce exposure to carcinogens and other toxic substances in the environment; however, they have unique needs with respect to safe and affordable housing, and access to safe and affordable public transportation. Obtaining healthy foods and engaging in healthy physical activities may be blocked when transportation and community infrastructure do not provide options that take into account these special needs.

Physical inactivity is a primary contributor to one-third of the adult population being overweight or obese; contributing to diabetes, and heart disease. With one in six children and adolescents being obese and activity levels declining with age (Sallis, Prochaska, & Taylor, 2000; Trost, Owen, Bauman, Sallis, & Brown, 2002), work environments must be designed to support emotional and physical health.

Five causes account for the majority (66%) of deaths among the general population: Heart disease (17%), cancer (23%), chronic lower respiratory disease (5%), stroke (5%), and unintentional injuries (5%) (Adams, Barnes, &

Vickerie, 2008). Each has been targeted for a modest reduction 1-2% by 2020. For each, there are evidence-based recommendations for improving health and wellness, but none has included advice on how to tailor the recommendations for the patient with ASD. Such tailoring will be accomplished in the future by knowledgeable and motivated health care providers who desire to put evidence to work (Jacobs, Jones, Gabella, Spring, & Brownson, 2012).

Less than half of older adults are up to date on a core set of clinical preventive services (e.g., cancer screening and immunizations) (Bolen, Seeff, & Blackman, 2005; Howerton et al., 2007; Shenson, Bolen, & Adams, 2007; Shenson, Bolen, Adams, Seeff, & Blackman, 2005).

CANCER RISK ASSESSMENT. Cancer risk assessment and reduction can have a significant impact on population health. We know very little about cancer care among people with ASD. However, we know some risks among patient populations with related disorders. Approximately 30% have an intellectual disability and people with intellectual disability (ID) have an increased risk of cancer in the gallbladder, thyroid, and brain (Patja et al., 2001).

In 2008, Liu and Clark reported that women with disabilities faced significant barriers accessing health care and routine preventive services, and were less likely to report having screening tests (Liu & Clark, 2008). In general, the incidence of lung cancer among people with ASD is comparable to the general population, despite low prevalence of smoking and low prevalence of diagnostic screening activity. Less is known about cancer prevalence of testicular and prostate cancer, or breast cancer among patients who are diagnosed with ASD (Mehta, Fung, Kistler, Chang, & Walter, 2010). There are no statistics on cancer risk management for adults with ASD. In addition, physical inactivity is a primary contributor to one-third of the adult population being overweight or obese; contributing to diabetes and heart disease.

The following example is offered to illustrate how risk management through routine screening can be adapted to the special needs of the patient with ASD. The basic principles are relevant for any type of cancer screening and in general for any effort to establish a primary prevention program.

EXAMPLE: COLORECTAL CANCER. Colorectal cancer (CRC) is the leading cause of cancer-related death in the US (U.S. Cancer Statistics Working Group, 2010). It is one of the most preventable cancers and for decades, health care providers have known that regular screening colonoscopy could prevent most of these deaths by early detection and removal of both cancer and precancerous polyps (Winawer et al., 1993). A national study of colonoscopies performed on 1,418 patients with polyps suggested that periodic colonoscopy could prevent 76% to 90% of colon cancers (Winawer et al., 1993). Despite this evidence, screening rates remain low–especially among African

Americans (the group most likely to die of the disease) and Hispanics. Screening rates among patients with ASD is unknown.

Most neurotypical patients tolerate colonoscopy well with conscious sedation. However, there are no descriptions or statistics on how patients with ASD tolerate the procedure. Currently, the standard calls for conscious sedation using benzodiazepine plus a narcotic. This regimen is low-cost, safe, and effective, in general, but may not be optimal for the patient with ASD. Patient comfort and satisfaction are key indicators of intention to return for follow-up procedures. Therefore, the patient care team may determine that a sedative-hypnotic agent from a class of intravenous anesthetics called alkylphenols (e.g., Propofol or Diprivan®) is more appropriate. Currently, the use of propofol is not standard in most GI practices for first colonoscopies, but some experts recommend using the drug selectively in patients who have had prior difficulty with operative or invasive procedures (Nelson, Barkun, Block, & Technology Committee of the American Society for Gastrointestinal Endoscopy, 2001). An advantage is that recovery time is generally not problematic and besides increased tiredness and decreased concentration for approximately 12 hours, there are no side effects (Levin et al., 2006).

Some have suggested that if screenings were implemented at recommended levels, more than 18,000 lives could be saved each year (Joseph, Rim, & Seef, 2008; Maciosek, Solberg, Coffield, Edwards, & Goodman, 2006). Risk assessment for CRC includes self-assessment and invasive clinical diagnostic tests; two interventions that may be especially difficulty for the person with ASD. Table 1.1 provides a list of best practices for CRC screening and corresponding strategies for patients with ASD.

An exemplar. The Department of Health and Mental Hygiene (DoHMH) in New York City has developed a Colonoscopy Navigator Program designed to eliminate barriers to care, improve patient understanding of colonoscopy, reduce patient "no-show" rates, and improve colonoscopy screening rates. In the program, the navigators explain to patients the importance of the procedures, and how to prepare and alleviate fears. In a 12-month period, the DoHMH reported a 61% increase in colonoscopy volume in hospitals and a 25% increase in the number of patients completing the procedure. The program website includes instructional materials, links to additional information, and tools for patient self-management and clinician tracking (New York City Department of Health and Mental Hygiene, 2015). The complete program is available at http://www.nyc.gov/html/doh/html/living/cancer-colon .shtml.

This model can easily be adapted for the patient population with ASD by modifying the content and process of instruction to consider the patient's limitations in expressive and receptive communication, and include family

Table 1.1
BEST PRACTICES FOR INCREASING COLORECTAL SCREENING
AMONG PATIENTS WITH AUTISM SPECTRUM DISORDER (ASD)

BEST PRACTICE OVERALL	*STRATEGIES TO ACCOMPLISH*
Identify eligible patients	• Identify primary care providers via insurance provider databases (i.e., Independence Blue Cross) serving ASD patients • Query electronic medical record or billing systems monthly: For patients turning 50 and to identify patients aged 50 to 80 w/o documented CRC screening • Identify residential facilities with adult populations
Promote routine colonoscopy referral for outpatients 50 and older. • Community outreach	• Distribute information to primary care providers • Internal medicine • Family medicine • Geriatric medicine • Distribute services information to residential facilities • Distribute materials to ambulatory clinics including • Mammography • Diabetes • Distribute materials to • Places of worship • Community-based • Nonprofit organizations • Community health clinics • Senior centers • Libraries
Referral Indicators	• Colorectal cancer screen in patients aged 50 to 75 years • Positive fecal occult blood test (FOBT) or rectal bleed in a patient < 75 years of age with no prior GI endoscopic workup • Iron deficiency anemia in patients < 75 years of age with NO prior GI endoscopic workup

Table 1.1–*Continued*

	• Family history of colorectal cancer (provided patient is at least 5 yrs younger than the age at which relative was diagnosed) • Personal history of adenomatous colon polyps in a patient aged 50 to 75 years whose last colonoscopy was at least 5 years prior to referral • Colonic mass lesion seen on barium enema or CT scan
Identify patients likely to slow "throughput"	Accommodations for the individual with ASD: • Schedule each patient individually • Consult with caregivers on optimal time of day • Include family caregiver in scheduled visit • Allocate quiet, environmentally modified procedure rooms • Keep pre-procedure time less than 30 hours • Include ancillary personnel who have specialized knowledge of ASD • Avoid handling paperwork/electronic data management during visit • Have patients send in their paperwork in advance • Call, text, otherwise confirm appointment and answer last-minute questions • Schedule practice session and pre-visits to familiarize • Start IVs in the holding area, after sedated if possible • Have anti-anxiety medications prescribed and ready • Aim to keep median colonoscopy procedure time less than 30 minutes • Use personnel trained in care of patients with ASD to handle recovery room issues • Expand GI suite hours to evenings and weekends
Establish Follow-up protocol	• Annual outreach • Tracking those screened • Tracking outcomes of care

caregivers in every phase of instruction and preparation. Box 1.2 contains a list or the roles of the CRC Navigator with expertise in the care of patients with ASD (Bassett et al., 2005).

Box 1.2. Roles of the Navigator for a Patient with Autism Spectrum Disorder Undergoing Colorectal Cancer Screening

- Coordinate the daily scheduled appointments for the GI clinic, the colorectal surgery clinic, and the endoscopy suite with the schedules activities and/or routines of the patient
- Communicate with the family or professional caregiver specific barriers to care
    - financial
    - logistical, or
    - psychosocial
- Ascertain from family or professional caregiver the patients behavioral triggers, sensory processing problems
- Ascertain from family or professional caregiver the patient's self-regulatory behaviors and any devices or activities that are calming
- Provide each patient with the navigator's name and phone number
- Schedule the preadmission testing appointment
- Assist eligible patients with preadmission testing and paperwork
- Accompany patients to the preadmission testing office for financial and medical clearance, if necessary
- Check to see if each patient is medically and financially cleared and then booked for colonoscopy
- Call each patient the day before the scheduled colonoscopy
- Secure safe and reliable transportation
- Review bowel prep procedure with each patient, repeat as needed
- Make sure each patient, and/or the family or professional caregiver knows the name and location of the clinic
- Give each patient clear directions to the facility and instructions on precisely where to go on arrival
- Greet patients on arrival to clinic
- Answer questions and explain delays, repeat as needed
- Record patient data:
    - colonoscopy results,
    - disposition

Box 1.2–*Continued*

- • behavorial triggers
- • effective communication aids
- • waiting time for colonoscopy to be performed
- • follow-up recommendations
- • Monitor monthly for ASD patient population
  - • Total number contacted through in-reach/outreach, by facility
  - • Total number referred for screening
  - • Total number that declined screening
  - • Total number screened by type of screening
  - • Total number with pathologic findings
  - • Total number referred for case management
  - • Average waiting time for colonoscopy to be performed
  - • Total number of screening vs. diagnostic colonoscopies
- • Demographics of patients

ASD and Health Disparities

Reports on the health disparities for individuals on the autism spectrum are not yet available; however, key facts on disparities for other subgroups of the population are transferrable to individuals with ASD. Like other vulnerable subgroups, people with ASD systematically experience greater obstacles to health on the basis of their mental health, and cognitive, sensory, or physical disability. Adults with disabilities are more likely to report their health to be fair or poor (Wolf, Armour, & Campbell, 2008) and experience unmet health care needs due to cost (Anonymous, 2009). On average, adults with serious mental illness die 25 years earlier than their peers, largely due to preventable health conditions (Manderscheid, Druss, & Freeman, 2008). This particular health statistic may be most applicable to the individual who lives outside of a residential facility. In addition, residents in rural areas are more likely to have a number of chronic conditions (e.g., diabetes, heart disease) and are less likely to receive the recommended preventative services in part due to reduced access to trained mental health professionals and physicians (Larson & Fleishman, 2003).

Conclusion

Integration of healthcare services has been recommended to improve overall care but is generally untested among people with ASD. Prevention of disease and risk management for patients with ASD is best delivered during primary care visits. In an effort to improve healthcare delivery systems, many payers, providers, and other organizations are supporting the use of quality improvement (QI) initiatives (Geonnotti et al., 2015). These may be designed to improve the performance of primary care practices and can be tailored to the ASD population. They require that practices continually assess performance, plan changes in areas where improvement is needed, and track the outcomes of the changes (Wagner, Austin, & Von Korff, 1996). Figure 1.1 illustrates the basic relationship between willingness to change one's practice and the resources needed to do so.

Engaging primary care practices in these activities, with respect to the ASD patient, is an important component of any efforts to improve the health of this group; enhance the quality of the patient, caregiver, and provider

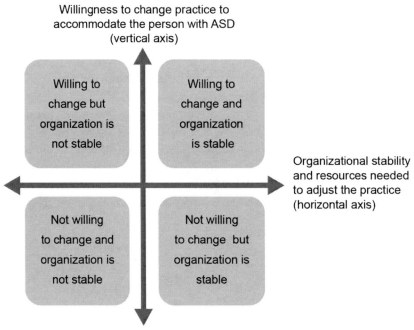

Figure 1.1. Readiness of practice to modify care delivery to accommodate the needs of people on the autism spectrum. Adapted from: Geonnotti, K., Taylor, E. F., Peikes, D., Schottenfeld, L., Burak, H., McNeillis, R., & Genevro, J. (2015). *Engaging primary care practices in quality improvement: Strategies for practice facilitators* (p. 13). AHRQ Publication No. 15-0015-EF. Rockville, MD: Agency for Healthcare Research and Quality.

experience; and possibly reduce cost. Health care is trending toward precision medicine and tailored therapies. Health care for patients with ASD should do no less. Organizations that pay for health care are searching increasingly for value in the care they purchase. They look for high-quality care at reasonable cost, with an eye toward continually improving care over time for their patients. A number of federal programs and private payer initiatives encourage primary care practices to engage in improvement efforts by offering financial support (in the form of incentive payments, grants, and other funding) and providing other resources and supports.

References

Adams, P. F., Barnes, P. M., & Vickerie, J. L. (2008). National Center for Health Statistics. *Vital Health Statistics, 10*(238), http://www.cdc.gov/nchs/data/series/sr_10/sr10_238.pdf

Aman, M. G., Lam, K. S., & Collier-Crespin, A. (2003). Prevalence and patterns of use of psychoactive medicines among individuals with autism in the Autism Society of Ohio. *Journal of Autism and Developmental Disorders, 33,* 527–534.

American Psychiatric Association. (2013). *Diagnostic and Statistical Manual of Mental Disorders (DSM-V)* (5th ed.). Washington, DC: American Psychiatric Association.

Anonymous. (2009). QuickStats: Delayed or forgone medical care because of cost concerns among adults aged 18–64 years, by disability and health insurance coverage status–National Health Interview Survey, United States, 2009. *MMWR, 59*(44), 1456.

Bassett, M., Bogler, B., Feldman, G., Rosenberg, R., Silver, L., Winawer, S., & New York Citywide Colon Cancer Control Coalition. (2005). *A practical guide to increasing screening.* New York: New York City Department of Health and Mental Hygiene. Available at http://www.nyc.gov/html/doh/html/living/cancer-colon.shtml

Centers for Disease Control and Prevention. (2014). Prevalence of autism spectrum disorder among children age 8 years–Autism and Developmental Disabilities Monitoring Network, 11 sites, United States, 2010. *Morbidity and Mortality Weekly Report, Surveillance Summaries, 63*(2), 1–21.

Felker, B., Yazel, J. J., & Short, D. (1996). Mortality and medical comorbidity among psychiatric patients: A review. *Psychiatric Service, 47*(1), 1,356–351, 363.

Fineberg, H. V. (2012). A successful and sustainable health system–How to get there from here. *New England Journal of Medicine, 366*(11), 1020–1027.

Geonnotti, K., Taylor, E. F., Peikes, D., Schottenfeld, L., Burak, H., McNellis, R., & Genevro, J. (2015). *Engaging primary care practices in quality improvement: Strategies for practice facilitators.* Rockville, MD: Agency for Healthcare Research and Quality.

Howerton, M. W., Gibbons, M. C., Baffi, C. R., Gary, T. L., Lai, G. Y., Bolen, S. S., . . . Ford, J. (2007). Provider roles in the recruitment of underrepresented populations to cancer clinical trials. *Cancer, 109*(3), 465–476.

Institute of Medicine, & Committee on Public Health Strategies to Improve Health. (2012). For the public's health: Investing in a healthier future. Washington, DC: The National Academies Press.

Jacobs, J. A., Jones, E., Gabella, B. A., Spring, B., & Brownson, R. C. (2012). Tools for implementing an evidence-based approach in public health practice. *Preventing Chronic Disease, 9,* 1–9, http://dx.doi.org/10.5888/pcd5889.110324

Joseph, D. A., Rim, S. H., & Seef, L. C. (2008). Use of colorectal cancer tests–United States, 2002, 2004, and 2006. *MMWR, 57,* 253–258.

Kessler, R. C. (2007). The global burden of anxiety and mood disorders: Putting the European Study of the Epidemiology of Mental (ESEMeD) findings into per-spective. *Journal of Clinical Psychiatry, 68*(Suppl. 2), 10–19.

Kohn, L. T., Corrigan, J. M., Donaldson, M. S., & Committee on Quality of Health Care in America (Eds.). (2000). *To err is human: Building a safer health system.* Washington, DC: National Academy Press.

Lane, A. E., Young, R. L., Baker, A. E. Z., & Angley, M. T. (2010). Sensory process-ing subtypes in autism: Association with adaptive behavior. *Journal of Autism & Developmental Disorders, 40,* 112–122.

Larson, S. L., & Fleishman, J. A. (2003). Rural urban differences in usual source of care and ambulatory service use: Analyses of national data using Urban Influence Codes. *Medical Care, 31*(7 Suppl), III-65–III-75.

Levin, T. R., Zhao, W., Conell, C., Seeff, L. C., DManniner, L., M., Shapiro, J. A., & Schulman, J. (2006). Complications of colonoscopy in an integrated health care delivery system.[Summary for patients in Ann Intern Med. 2006 Dec 19;145(12):I39; PMID: 17179055]. *Annals of Internal Medicine, 145*(12), 880–886.

Levy, S. E., Giarelli, E., Lee, L., Scheve, L. A., Kirby, R. S., Cuniff, C., & Rice, C. (2010). Autism spectrum disorder and concurrent developmental, psychiatric, and medical conditions among children in multiple populations in the United States. *Journal of Developmental and Behavioral Pediatrics, 31*(4), 267–275.

Liu, S. Y., & Clark, M. A. (2008). Breast and cervical cancer screening practices among disabled women aged 40–75: Does quality of the experience matter? *Journal of Women's Health, 17*(8), 1321–1329.

Maciosek, M. V., Solberg, L. I., Coffield, A. B., Edwards, N. M., & Goodman, M. J. (2006). The health impact and cost effectiveness of colorectal cancer screening. *American Journal of Preventative Medicine, 31,* 80–89.

Manderscheid, R., Druss, B., & Freeman, E. (2008). Data to manage the mortality crisis: Recommendations to the Substance Abuse and Mental Health Services Administration. *International Journal of Mental Health, 37*(2), 49–68.

Martin, A., Lassman, D., Washington, B., Catlin, A., & The National Health Expenditure Accounts Team. (2012). Growth in U.S. health spending remained slow in 2010; health share of gross domestic product was unchanged from 2009. *Health Affairs* (31), 1, 208–219. http://content.healthaffairs.org/content/31/1/208 .full.html

Martin, A., Scahill, L., Klin, A., & Volkmar, F. R. (1999). Higher-functioning perva-sive developmental disorders: Rates and patterns of psychotropic drug use. *Journal of the American Academy of Child and Adolescent Psychiatry, 38,* 923–931.

McEwen, B. S. (2000). The neurobiology of stress: From serendipity to clinical relevance. *Brain Research in Developmental Disabilities, 886*(1–2), 172–189.

McEwen, B. S., & Gianaros, P. J. (2010). Central role of the brain in stress and adaptation: Links to socioeconomic status, health, and disease. *Annals of the New York Academy of Sciences, 186*(1), 190–222.

Mehta, K. M., Fung, K. Z., Kistler, C. E., Chang, A., & Walter, L. C. (2010). Impact of cognitive impairment on screening mammography. *American Journal of Public Health, 100*(10), 1917–1923.

National Prevention Council. (2011). National prevention strategy. Washington, DC: U.S. Department of Health and Human Services, Office of the Surgeon General.

Nelson, D. B., Barkun, A., Block, K. P., & Technology Committee of the American Society for Gastrointestinal Endoscopy. (2001). Technology status evaluation report: Colonoscopy preparations. *Gastrointestinal Endoscopy, 54*(6), 829–832.

New York City Department of Health and Mental Hygiene. (2015). Colon cancer. Retrieved April 5, 2015 from http://www.nyc.gov/html/doh/html/living/cancer-colon.shtml

Newcomer, J. W. (2007). Metabolic syndrome and mental illness. *American Journal of Managed Care, 13*(7 Suppl.), S170–S177. Erratum in *American Journal of Managed Care,* 2008 Feb; *14*(2), 76.

Palloni, A., & Yonker, J. (2012). Health in the U.S. at young ages: Preliminary findings (CDE Working Paper 2012-04). Madison, WI: Center for Demography and Ecology, University of Wisconsin.

Parks, D., Svedsen, J., Singer, P., & Foti, M. E. (2006). Morbidity and mortality in people with serious mental illness. http://www.nasmhpd.org/general_files/publications/med_directors_pubs/Technical%20Report%

Sallis, J. F., Prochaska, J., & Taylor, W. C. (2000). A review of correlates of physical activity of children and adolescents. *Medical Science and Sports Exercise, 32,* 963–975.

Shenson, D., Bolen, J., & Adams, M. (2007). Receipt of preventive services by elders based on composite measures, 1997–2004. *American Journal of Preventative Medicine, 32,* 11–18.

Shenson, D., Bolen, J., Adams, M., Seeff, L., & Blackman, D. (2005). Are older adults up-to-date with cancer screening and vaccinations? *Preventing Chronic Disease, 2*(3), A04.

Thornicroft, G. (2011). Physical health disparities and mental illness: The scandal of premature mortality. *British Journal of Psychiatry, 199,* 441–442.

Trost, S. G., Owen, N., Bauman, A. E., Sallis, J. F., & Brown, W. (2002). Correlates of adults' participation in physical activity: Review and update, 1996–2001. *Medical Science and Sports Exercise, 34*(12), 1996–2001.

U. S. Cancer Statistics Working Group. (2010). United States cancer statistics: 1999–2006 incidence and mortality web-based report. (Vol. http://www.cdc.gov/uscs). Atlanta, GA: Department of Health and Human Services, CDC, and National Cancer Institute.

U. S. Department of Health and Human Services. (2001, February 2013). Mental health: Culture, race, and ethnicity–A supplement to mental health: A report of the Surgeon General. from http://137.187.25.243/library/mentalhealth/cre/execsummary-1.html

USDHHS/Centers for Disease Control and Prevention. (2012). Prevalence of autism spectrum disorders–Autism and Developmental Disabilities Monitoring Network, 14 sites, United States, 2008. *Morbidity & Mortality Weekly Report, Surveillance Summaries, 61*(3), 1–25.

Wagner, E. H., Austin, B. T., & Von Korff, M. (1996). Organizing care for patients with chronic illness. *Milbank Quarterly, 74*(4), 511–544.

Wahlbeck, K., Westman, J., Nordentoft, M., Gissler, M., & Laursen, T. M. (2011). Outcomes of Nordic mental health systems: Life expectancy of patients with mental disorders. *British Journal of Psychiatry, 199*(6), 453–458.

Winawer, S. J., Zauber, A. G., Ho, M. N., O'Brien, M. J., Gottlieb, L. S., Sternberg, S. S., . . . Stewart, E. T. (1993). Prevention of colorectal cancer by colonoscopic polypectomy. The National Polyp Study Workgroup. *New England Journal of Medicine, 329*(27), 1977–1981.

Wolf, L. A., Armour, B. A., & Campbell, V. A. (2008). Racial/Ethnic disparities in self-rated health status among adults with and without disabilities–United States, 2004–2006. *MMWR 57*(39), 1069–1073.

Woolf, S. H., Aron, L., & Committee on Population of the Division of Behavioral and Social Sciences and Education, & Board on Population Health and Public Health Practice of the Institute of Medicine. (2013). *US health in international perspective: Shorter lives, poorer health* (pp. 405). Washington, DC: National Research Council and the Institute of Medicine.

Chapter 2

THE EPIDEMIOLOGY OF AUTISM SPECTRUM DISORDER: PREVALENCE AND RISK FACTORS

Michael J. Brennan, Kate E. Wallis, and Jennifer A. Pinto-Martin

Introduction

Autism spectrum disorder, or ASD, represents a heterogeneous group of disorders, which may or may not share common etiology. In clinical practice, the term ASD is operationalized to include many disorders with separate etiologies. Each etiology may represent a distinct disorder that shares the phenotypic characteristics used to define ASD. While there is no biomarker for autism, elucidating the etiology of ASD may facilitate improved detection through establishing objective laboratory values, radiological studies, dysmorphology measurements, and/or genetic testing.

The focus of this chapter is the epidemiology of autism spectrum disorders, including: A review of the changing diagnostic criteria and how this has contributed to the increase in reported prevalence; a summary and discussion of the Center for Disease Control (CDC) prevalence data and additional data from other sites in the world; a discussion of the underlying etiology including genetic factors, immune dysfunction, and brain development and dysmorphology; and finally, a review of the epidemiologic data on preterm delivery/low birthweight, one of the factors with a significant and growing body of evidence linking it to ASD. The relevance of these topics to the delivery of health care services, in general, will be introduced. Understanding the etiology of ASD will help clinicians to improve diagnosis and will help to guide and refine the treatments prescribed to ensure the delivery of better services to children with ASD and their families.

Evolution of the Autism Diagnosis:
From Kanner to The DSM-V

In 1943, Leo Kanner published a report in which he used the term "autism" to describe children who were born with a condition characterized by social isolation, insistence on sameness, and speech disorders. Over the last 70 years, the definition and diagnostic criteria for autism have evolved, contributing to complex methodological challenges surrounding the estimation of the prevalence of the disorder. However, the gold standard of autism diagnosis continues to be based on clinical observation. In Leo Kanner's 1943 landmark paper, five-year-old Donald T. was distinguished from other boys his age by his obsession with spinning toys, preference for social isolation, and abnormal speech (Kanner, 1943). Kanner's highly detailed accounts of Donald T. and ten other children with similar presentation provided the framework for the newly described autism diagnosis.

In 1978, Michael Rutter (Rutter, 1978) called on the psychiatric community to return to Kanner's observations by putting forth diagnostic criteria in his *Diagnosis and Definition of Childhood Autism.* Closely resembling Kanner's criteria, Rutter's definition of autism required deficits in three domains: Social development, language development, and insistence on sameness. By emphasizing these domains as requisites for an autism diagnosis, Rutter clearly differentiated autism from childhood schizophrenia.

With the 1980 publication of the *Diagnostic and Statistical Manual of Mental Disorders III (DSM-III),* autistic disorders were incorporated into the heading of pervasive developmental disorders (PDDs) (American Psychiatric Association, 1980). This group of disorders included infantile autism, atypical PDDs, and childhood-onset PDDs. By grouping these disorders into one umbrella term, *PDD,* the DSM-III served as a precursor to the concept of the autism spectrum. In order to include children who did not meet all of the criteria for infantile autism or childhood PDD, atypical PDD served as a catch-all diagnosis (American Psychiatric Association, 1980).

The 1994 publication of the DSM-IV and the Text Revision in 2000 further refined the PDD checklist. Collapsing the 16 criteria outlined in the DSM-III-R to 12, the DSM-IV introduced Asperger syndrome, Rett syndrome, and childhood disintegrative disorder to the list of PDDs. According to the DSM-IV criteria, autistic disorder required the presence of at least six of the 12 symptoms from the appropriate domains (APA, 2000).

Concerned that the DSM criteria were introducing unwarranted heterogeneity, the APA formed a workgroup tasked with redefining PDDs for the recent DSM-5. After five years of deliberation, the group recommended subsuming PDD-NOS, childhood disintegrative disorder, and Asperger syndrome into the overarching category of ASD (APA, 2013; Swedo, Baird, Cook Jr, Happé, Harris, Kaufmann et al., 2012; Tsai & Ghaziuddin, 2014).

The implications of grouping the ASD subtypes into one overarching disorder and how this will affect patients, families, and clinicians remain unclear. A recent review of 12 empirical papers investigating the effect of the DSM-5's stricter criteria for ASDs has shown a 33% median reduction in diagnosis (Sturmey & Dalfern, 2014). This effect was more pronounced in milder phenotypes with reductions of up to two-thirds, as compared to those captured by DSM-IV-TR criteria. Concerns about how the new diagnostic criteria will affect a child's access to services are particularly troublesome to the families of individuals with ASD, and could potentially disrupt the delivery of integrated care services to affected individuals (Coury, 2013). The DSM-5 workgroup has stressed that changes to the diagnostic criteria will not affect those currently diagnosed with an Asperger syndrome or PDD (Coury, 2013; Swedo et al., 2012), and a "grandfather clause" is included to ensure that patients who previously met diagnostic criteria will continue to be included.

The evolution of the criteria required for ASD diagnosis is outlined in Table 2.1. Clinicians will determine how to integrate the diagnostic changes to ensure that qualifying patients can continue to access integrated health care services and receive optimal care that is appropriately reimbursed by insurance companies and accepted by school districts. Clinicians will need to remain up-to-date to ensure they are making appropriate diagnoses based on the accepted diagnostic criteria.

Table 2.1
CHANGING CRITERIA FOR DIAGNOSING AUTISM SPECTRUM DISORDER

Source/Date	*Criteria for a Diagnosis*
Kanner (1943)	*Autism: Two Essential Criteria* 1. A profound lack of affective contact 2. Repetitive, ritualistic behavior
Rutter et al. (1978)	*Autism: Four Essential Criteria* 1. Onset before the age of 30 months 2. Impaired social development which has a number of special characteristics and is out of keeping with the child's intellectual development 3. Delayed and deviant language development which also has certain defined features and which is out of keeping with the child's intellectual level 4. Insistence on sameness, as shown by stereotyped play patterns, abnormal preoccupations or resistance to change

continued

Table 2.1—*Continued*

DSM-III (1980)	*Subgroup: Infantile Autism* 1. Lack of responsiveness to others 2. Language absence or abnormalities 3. Resistance to change or attachment to objects 4. The absence of schizophrenic features 5. Onset before 30 months * *Also with provisions for childhood onset (>30months and <12years) and atypical PDDs
DSM-III-R (1987)	Checklist of symptoms requiring at least 8 of 16 symptoms for diagnosis. At least two must be from the Item A, one from the Item B, and one from Item C. (A) impairment in reciprocal social interaction (5 items) (B) impairment in verbal and nonverbal communication (6 items) (C) markedly restricted repertoire of activities and interests (5 items) (D) onset in infancy or early childhood
DSM-IV (1994, 2000 text revision)	*Autistic Disorder* 1. A total of six (or more) items from (A), (B), and (C), with at least two from (A), and one each from (B) and (C) 　(A) qualitative impairment in social interaction 　(B) qualitative impairments in communication as 　(C) restricted repetitive and stereotyped patterns of behavior, interests and activities 2. Delays or abnormal functioning in at least one of the following areas, with onset prior to age 3 years: 　(A) social interaction 　(B) language as used in social communication 　(C) symbolic or imaginative play 3. The disturbance is not better accounted for by Rett syndrome or childhood disintegrative disorder
DSM-5 (2013)	*Autism Spectrum Disorder* 1. Persistent deficits in social communication and social interaction across multiple contexts 2. Restricted, repetitive patterns of behavior, interests, or activities (2 items) 3. Symptoms must be present in the early developmental period (but may not become fully manifest until social demands exceed limited capacities, or may be masked by learned strategies in later life) 4. Symptoms cause clinically significant impairment in social, occupational, or other important areas of current functioning 5. These disturbances are not better explained by intellectual disability (intellectual developmental disorder) or global developmental delay. Intellectual disability and autism spectrum disorder frequently co occur; to make comorbid diagnoses of autism spectrum disorder and intellectual disability, social communication should be below that expected for general developmental level

*Specify severity of symptoms

Prevalence of Autism Spectrum Disorder

Due to constantly evolving diagnostic criteria, subtyping, variable screening protocols, and a wide range of external factors, measuring the prevalence of autism has been a notoriously difficult task for public health professionals. During the era of Kanner and Rutter, autistic disorder was considered a rare condition. One of the first estimates in a 1966 report found a prevalence of only 4.5/10,000 eight to ten-year-olds in a United Kingdom (UK) sample (Lotter, 1966). As diagnostic criteria were refined and surveillance systems were established, an upward trend was recognized and persists into the twenty-first century. In spite of the challenges of accurate measurement of ASD prevalence, studies on autism continue to shape policy discussions, service provision, and research funding.

Historically, prevalence studies examining ASD have been hindered by several methodological limitations, and therefore must be interpreted with care. With no established biomarkers, the gold standard for autism diagnosis is the combination of the clinical exam and expert opinion. Even with the challenges related to diagnostic criteria aside, many children living with what would qualify as an ASD may remain undiagnosed. Social, socioeconomic, and geopolitical factors, such as differing public health policies, community awareness, education services, and variable access to care may in fact account for the discrepancies observed across geographic areas in various studies. After finding poor interrater reliability among the diagnostic outcomes at clinics screening for autism, Lord suggested the most important predictor of an autism diagnosis is the clinic to which the individual presents (Lord, Petkova, Hus, Gan, Lu, Martin et al., 2012). Mandell and Lecavalier (2014) contended that reported prevalence estimates more closely approximate variation in access to clinicians who diagnose autism than any true regional differences in prevalence.

Tracking Autism through the US Department of Education (USDE)

Under the 1990 revision to the Individuals with Disabilities Education Act (IDEA), autism became one of the 13 disability categories monitored by the United States Department of Education (USDE), with all 50 states reporting the number of special education students in this category by 1994 (Individuals with Disabilities Education Act, Pub L. 101-476, 20 USC § 1400, 1990). USDE data provided the first national surveillance system for ASDs, producing some of the early prevalence studies reporting 31 cases per 10,000 children in 2003, up from 6 per 10,000 in 1994 (Shattuck, 2006). This prevalence was lower than that reported by other studies conducted during the same decade, as other studies began using population-based samples with medical record abstraction components, while the USDE data used case enumeration from education data alone (Yeargin-Allsopp, Rice, Karapurkar, Doernberg, Boyle, & Murphy, 2003).

Although USDE data provided the first glimpse into the extent of the national burden of ASD, it was limited by several important methodological challenges. Shattuck's 2006 report on the prevalence of autism in the USDE sample based its diagnoses on USDE criteria instead of on those established in the DSM-IV (Shattuck, 2006). With researchers unable to validate diagnoses coupled with variation in reporting between states, the USDE system likely underreported the national ASD burden.

Centers for Disease Control and Prevention ADDM Network

In 1991, the Centers for Disease Control and Prevention (CDC) established the *Metropolitan Atlanta Developmental Disabilities Surveillance Program* (MADDSP) with the aim of determining the prevalence of intellectual disability, cerebral palsy, hearing loss, and vision impairment in five counties in the state of Georgia in the United States (US) (CDC, 2014). Trained abstractors obtained medical records of eight-year-olds through a process known as *active record review,* identifying the specific developmental disorders tracked by MADDSP. In 1996, ASDs were added to this list of target conditions to be tracked (CDC, 2014). Based on this methodology, the CDC established and funded the *Autism and Developmental Disabilities Monitoring Network* (ADDM), consisting of surveillance centers in 12 US states as of 2014 (CDC, 2015). Since 2000, ADDM has provided information on the prevalence of and sociodemographic factors related to autism in the US.

In 2014, the CDC ADDM network reported a prevalence 147.1/10,000 (or 1 in 68) eight-year-olds, up from the 2011 estimate of 113.6/10,000 (Developmental Disabilities Monitoring Network Surveillance Year Principal Investigators, Centers for Disease Control and Prevention, 2014). Boys were almost five times more likely than girls to be diagnosed with ASD. These data reveal a pronounced geographic variation between study centers, with estimates ranging from 1 in 175 in Alabama, to 1 in 45 in New Jersey. These findings, subject to several important limitations, have often been the subject of intense debate.

Global Prevalence of ASD

Studies from other countries report a range of prevalence estimates. Figure 2.1 illustrates some of these estimates and compares them to studies conducted in the US. In general, international prevalence figures tend to support the notion that the prevalence of autism is increasing globally. However, recent studies conducted in developing countries have shown estimates that

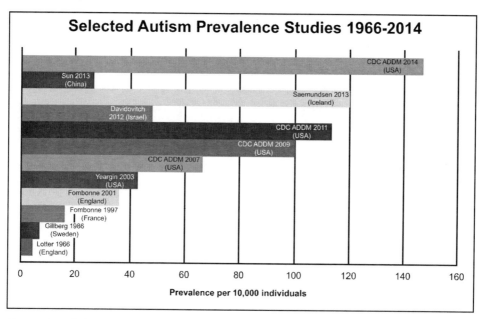

Figure 2.1. Selected autism prevalence studies, 1966 to 2014, showing variable rates across different countries.

are lower than those in the US and other developed nations (Davidovitch, Hemo, Manning-Courtney, & Fombonne, 2013; Saemundsen, Magnússon, Georgsdóttir, Egilsson, & Rafnsson, 2013; Sun, Allison, Matthews, Sharp, Auyeung, Baron-Cohen et al., 2013). This observation is often ascribed to underascertainment in areas with poor access to specialized child psychiatric care.

Clinicians will ultimately determine how to integrate the new diagnostic criteria to ensure steady access to integrated healthcare services for qualifying patients. Insurance plans, school districts, and other governmental and healthcare agencies will have to determine appropriate reimbursement for these services and thresholds for qualification. In order to maintain a high standard of care for this vulnerable population, clinicians will need access to the most current information regarding any changes in diagnostic criteria and incorporate them into their practice. Using standardized diagnostic definitions will allow us to more accurately estimate ASD prevalence, which will consequently determine funding for integrated healthcare services and research. Unveiling risk factors for the disease is vital for targeting public health programming. Until the causes of ASD can be determined, healthcare providers will continue to work toward a balance between research-oriented and practical diagnostic definitions for this complex condition.

Etiology of ASD

Researchers continue to seek etiologic factors that will help us to understand the causes of autism. Consequently, this will help us to focus our diagnostic techniques and guide the therapies if we can identify specific etiologies implicated in producing autism in particular patients. The sections that follow will introduce the research supporting the predominant etiological mechanisms that are currently being considered.

Genetics

Since the earliest studies of autism when heritability was questioned (Hanson & Gottesman, 1976), our understanding of the genetics of ASD has become much more nuanced; we now appreciate the complexity of the genetic mechanisms involved. Identifying the genes responsible for autism heritability has been a decades-long endeavor that seems more complicated each year, as more distinct genes thought to contribute to autism symptomatology are identified. For example, one paper published in May 2014 listed at least 124 candidates for autism genes (Pinto, Delaby, Merico, Barbosa, Merikangas, Klei et al., 2014), reflecting a locus on almost every chromosome (C. P. Johnson & Myers, 2007). Case ascertainment and changing diagnostic criteria have made genetic studies challenging, as the heterogeneity of the disorder makes it particularly difficult to find common genes.

Researchers originally became interested in the genetics of autism when twin concordance was first recognized. Estimates for ASD concordance in monozygotic twins range from 60% (Bailey, Le Couteur, Gottesman, Bolton, Simonoff, Yuzda et al., 1995) to 91% (Steffenburg, Gillberg, Hellgren, Andersson, Gillberg, Jakobsson et al., 1989), while for dizygotic twins, concordance is estimated at 31% (Hallmayer, Cleveland, Torres, Phillips, Cohen, Torigoe et al., 2011). In nontwin siblings, concordance ranged from 3.94% in a survey study (Chakrabarti & Fombonne, 2001), 10.9% in a national registry (Constantino, Zhang, Frazier, Abbacchi, & Law, 2010), to 18.7% in an autism database (Ozonoff, Young, Carter, Messinger, Yirmiya, Zwaigenbaum et al., 2011).

The broader autism phenotype (BAP) represents a constellation of traits that are consistent with, but below threshold for an autism diagnosis. When the BAP is included in the evaluation of phenotype, 92% of monozygotic and 10% of dizygotic twin pairs are concordant (Bailey et al., 1995) and 20–22% of nontwin siblings qualify for the BAP (Constantino et al., 2010; Lauritsen, Pedersen, & Mortensen, 2005).

Recent data show that autism affects between two and three times as many males than females (Lai, Lombardo, & Baron-Cohen, 2014). Interestingly, this male predominance translates into a higher recurrence risk in male siblings than in female siblings (25.9% versus 9.6%, respectively) (Ozonoff et al., 2011). Families with more than one child already diagnosed with autism have a significantly increased risk, for example, 32.2% in multiplex families compared to 13.5% of simplex families (Ozonoff et al., 2011).

While ongoing research continues to discover new chromosomal regions of interest, testing for genetic abnormalities in children diagnosed with autism has left the experimental laboratory and become standard clinical practice. Routinely, children diagnosed with ASD are referred to a geneticist as part of the initial work-up, and genetic counseling is recommended for all families that are open to it (Simonoff, 1998). In fact, the American College of Medical Genetics and Genomics (ACMG) has issued guidelines recommending routine tiered testing for children diagnosed with ASD (Schaefer & Mendelsohn, 2013). Testing requires obtaining a three-generation family history, performing a full physical exam, and offering families a chromosomal microarray analysis (CMA) and targeted genetic testing. Specifically, the physical exam should identify dysmorphic features, as well as other "phenotypic variables," such as seizure disorder, macrocephaly or microcephaly, regressive characteristics, and IQ. Results may help identify specific genotypic correlates (Miles, 2011).

Genetic mechanisms known to account for subsets of the ASD phenotype include large copy number variants (CNVs, 10–20% of autism cases), chromosomal abnormalities (5%), and single-gene disorders (5%) (Miles, 2011). Mitochondrial diseases are thought to affect as many as 7.2% of children with autism (Oliveira, Diogo, Grazina, Garcia, Ataide, Marques et al., 2005), and may comprise the largest individual etiological subgroup found to date (Miles, 2011).

In particular, CNVs, or alterations in the genes that result in a duplication or a deletion, have received much attention. These mutations can be either be inherited from the parent, or occur *de novo* and arise endogenously in the germline. Each individual CNV is thought to account for no more than 1% of cases (Heil & Schaaf, 2013), although, in their entirety, CNVs are thought to account for a large proportion of cases of ASD (Pinto et al., 2014). It is theorized that autism follows a "multiple hit model," requiring multiple CNVs to result in disease. Loci of particular interest for CNVs associated with the phenotype include chromosome 15q11 (duplications), 16p (duplications and deletions), and 7q (duplications) (Miles, 2011).

ASD is known to co-occur with several recognized single-gene disorders, such that a better name for these conditions may be "autism of known etiology" (Miles, 2011). These disorders include tuberous sclerosis, neurofibromatosis, Angelman's syndrome, Rett disorder, and fragile-X syndrome, as well as many more rare syndromes. Despite high rates of comorbidity, these disorders are still thought to contribute to a small proportion of total cases of ASD (C. P. Johnson et al., 2007; Miles, 2011).

It has been estimated that the yield for performing testing is quite high, with 20–25% of children with autism having a detectable genetic abnormality (Miles, 2011). These estimates imply that a particular genetic cause can be identified in many patients. For this reason, genetic testing is encouraged, including a chromosomal microarray. However, the ethical implications of performing such expensive tests are concerning, given that there are no targeted therapies for most genetic abnormalities and that testing can be hard to interpret. Not all genetic variations that are detected will have clinical relevance. Additionally, as with all genetic testing, results invoked important privacy concerns. The ACMG provided a clinical rationale for justifying these evaluations by arguing that assisting families in establishing a definitive etiology and diagnosis, helping clinicians to be aware of related medical comorbidities that will require management, allowing clinicians to offer genetic counseling about risk in future pregnancies, and targeting future therapies supersedes the potential risks.

Ongoing analyses of large genetic databases will undoubtedly lead to the discovery of additional candidate genes (Buxbaum, Daly, Devlin, Lehner, Roeder, & State, 2012). Ideally, these studies will also lead to the refined understanding of current mechanisms through which genetic abnormalities are thought to produce the neurological and social impairments that define autism. This will ultimately aid in the identification of biomarkers to enhance detection and diagnosis of autism, in providing more focused genetic counseling for families, and in the development of therapies targeted to specific genetic abnormalities. The implications for the use of genomic testing for individuals with ASD and detailed descriptions of CMA are discussed in Chapter 10.

Inflammation

As early as 1971, researchers began to recognize an association between familial autoimmune diseases and autism (Money, Bobrow, & Clarke, 1971), a relationship that continues to be demonstrated in subsequent large-population samples. One descriptive survey-based study, vulnerable to significant selection and recall biases, found that among families with an autistic child, the number of family members with autoimmune disease was significantly higher than among controls, such that more children with ASD had two or more family members with an autoimmune disease compared to those without autism (Comi, Zimmerman, Frye, Law, & Peeden, 1999). A case-control study including families with a child with PDD, families with autoimmune disease, and healthy families found that families with an autistic child had a significantly higher frequency of autoimmune disorders than both the auto-immune and the healthy control families (Sweeten, Bowyer, Posey, Halber-stadt, & McDougle, 2003). An association between autism and mothers with psoriasis (Croen, Grether, Yoshida, Odouli, & Van de Water, 2005), rheuma-toid arthritis, and celiac disease have also been demonstrated (Atladottir, Ped-ersen, Thorsen, Mortensen, Deleuran, Eaton et al., 2009).

Given this relationship between familial autoimmune disease and autism, researchers have implicated autoimmune processes, inflammation, and im-mune dysfunction in the etiology of autism, with ongoing research continu-ally refining each of these conceptual models (Ashwood & Van de Water, 2004). The proposed mechanism through which aberrant immune system functioning produces autism may occur through two pathways: Autoim-munity, with antibodies reacting to CNS proteins and causing destruction of neurons; or through a dysfunctional immune system, with the body not re-sponding appropriately to pathogens (Ashwood et al., 2004).

Some researchers have theorized the presence of autoantibodies in the CNS of children with autism. However, results have been conflicting when specific antibodies are sought (Ashwood et al., 2004). Nonetheless, antibod-ies may have an effect during the early developmental period even though they may be undetectable later.

Other studies propose that maternal antibodies may have a role in autism pathogenesis. One group of researchers designed an experiment in which serum from a mother who had two children with developmental de-lays (one child with autism and the other with severe speech delay) was in-jected into pregnant mice. The mouse offspring were found to have alter-ations in their exploration behavior and motor coordination. Researchers attributed these deficits to the transfer of maternal antibodies as producing autistic-like behaviors in the mouse models (Dalton, Deacon, Blamire, Pike, McKinlay, Stein et al., 2003). Similarly, another group injected purified IgG antibodies from mothers with multiple children affected by autism into Rhesus monkeys and found autistic-like behaviors in offspring (Martin, Ashwood, Braunschweig, Cabanlit, Van de Water, & Amaral, 2008). This suggests that gestational exposure to specific maternal antibodies may produce autism. These findings need to be reproduced, but ethical concerns make replicating this study in humans impossible.

Increased gastrointestinal abnormalities were long considered a feature of autism, with some studies demonstrating higher prevalence of GI inflammato-ry conditions in autistic patients than in controls. These data, however, have been inconsistent and a consensus statement from the American Academy of Pediatrics questions the evidence supporting an autism-specific GI disturbance and inflammation (Buie, Campbell, Fuchs, Furuta, Levy, Vandewater et al., 2010). Additional study is recommended to further elucidate these processes.

An additional proposed site of inflammation is the brain. A study of postmortem brain tissue from patients with autism found increased levels of pro-inflammatory cytokines, as well as increased microglial and astroglial activation (Vargas, Nascimbene, Krishnan, Zimmerman, & Pardo, 2005). Microglia are small nonneural cells forming part of the supporting structure of the central nervous system. They are migratory and act as phagocytes to waste products of nerve tissue responsible for brain modeling and cortical organization during brain development, and their dysfunction may be related to observed differences in the autistic brain.

At the molecular level, many studies have showed altered levels of immunological markers in children with autism, including aberrant T-cells, cytokines (including interleukins and chemokines), complement proteins, adhesion molecules, and growth factors (for a review, see Ashwood et al., 2004). Differential human leukocyte antigen (HLA) expression in autistic subjects has received significant attention, given the crucial role of HLA molecules in brain development and synaptic plasticity (Boulanger & Shatz, 2004; Torres, Sweeten, Cutler, Bedke, Fillmore, Stubbs et al., 2006). While many of the studies are compelling, contradicting results and small sample sizes have made interpretation difficult. Large, systematic studies are needed to establish the pathogenesis of any of these differences.

One of the most important weaknesses in the inflammatory model of autism has been unsuccessful treatment of autism with immune suppression. Studies that have implemented intravenous immunoglobulins (IVIG) or steroid therapies have not been effective (Gesundheit, Rosenzweig, Naor, Lerer, Zachor, Prochazka et al., 2013). To date, there is no prospective model that explains how immune system dysfunction affects the developing brain. Such a neurodevelopmental model will be crucial in understanding how each of these mechanisms can produce altered brain development and neurological functioning. An enhanced understanding of the role of inflammatory processes as a cause of autism would serve to enhance clinicians' ability to target therapies more directly to the underlying etiological process. Employing anti-immunologic therapies will likely require careful care coordination between multiple practitioners, including immunologists and primary care practitioners.

Prenatal and Perinatal Risk Factors

Emerging data from brain imaging studies on the structural differences in brain development and function among those with ASD has led naturally to a focus on risk factors during the prenatal and perinatal period when fetal and early neonatal brain development is ongoing. Numerous risk factors have been examined, and data of varying quality and quantity exist to suggest an increase in the risk of ASD for the following: Advanced maternal and paternal age, meconium staining of amniotic fluid, breech presentation, uterine bleeding, hyperbilirubinemia, preterm birth (PTB), low birthweight (LBW), C-section delivery, and neonatal brain hemorrhage, among others (Gardener, Spiegelman, & Buka, 2011). Many of these studies combine all events into an index of "perinatal sub-optimality," rendering the delineation of a causal pathway difficult, if not impossible.

Other researchers have attempted to estimate the attributable risk of perinatal factors for ASD and report that perinatal risk factors may account for 11–13% (population attributable fraction) of ASD etiology (Schieve, Tian, Baio, Rankin, Rosenberg, Wiggins et al., 2014). While preventing these risk factors may reduce the incidence of autism, further studies are needed to characterize the remaining approximate 87% of risk.

The challenge inherent in identifying the other factors for this complex disorder is made apparent when one focuses on the numbers from a recent large case-control study in Finland that included 4,713 cases of ASD with four controls per case. When one examines the prevalence of any given risk factor, it is often in the single digits (Polo-Kantola, Lampi, Hinkka-Yli-Salomaki, Gissler, Brown, & Sourander, 2014). When one considers the potential for multiple etiologies for the various phenotypes that fall under the umbrella of ASD, one can appreciate the challenges faced by epidemiologists and other researchers who are attempting to elucidate a unifying cause.

ASD AND PRETERM BIRTH/LOW BIRTHWEIGHT. There is a growing body of literature that supports an association between preterm birth/low birthweight and ASD. Screening studies in early childhood reveal that features of ASD are more common in the preterm population compared to the general population (Kuban, O'Shea, Allred, Tager-Flusberg, Goldstein, & Leviton, 2009; Limperopoulos, Bassan, Sullivan, Soul, Robertson, Moore et al., 2008; Moore, Johnson, Hennessy, & Marlow, 2012; Wong, Huertas-Ceballos, Cowan, & Modi, 2014). For example, studies using the M-CHAT, a commonly used ASD-screening tool (Robins & Dumont-Mathieu, 2006; Robins, Fein, Barton, & Green, 2001), found that among preterm infants, 21% to 41% screened positive, while in the general population, a positive screen rate of 5.7% was found (Kleinman, Robins, Ventola, Pandey, Boorstein, Esser et al., 2008). Two studies using multiple screening instruments found comparable rates across the various tools (Dudova, Kasparova, Markova, Zemankova, Beranova, Urbanek et al., 2014; Stephens, Bann, Watson, Sheinkopf, Peralta-Carcelen, Bodnar et al., 2012). In addition, two recent studies reported a gestational age gradient, with shorter gestational ages leading to an increased risk of ASD (Kuzniewicz, Wi, Qian, Walsh, Armstrong, & Croen, 2014; Leavey, Zwaigenbaum, Heavner, & Burstyn, 2013).

Screening for ASD in late childhood and early adolescence revealed similar results. Hack et al. (2009) examined a group of eight-year-old, extremely low-birthweight children (birth weight < 1000 g) and found higher rates of ASD traits in these children compared with term peers. In addition, scores on the *Autism Spectrum Screening Questionnaire* were higher for a group of adolescents who were preterm (gestational age < 32 weeks) (Indredavik, Vik, Evensen, Skranes, Taraldsen, & Brubakk, 2010).

While the screening data are intriguing, it is important to remember that indicators of ASD risk in toddlers include problems with communication, social reciprocity, sensory hypersensitivity, and repetitive movements. The presence of these behaviors at ages 12–36 months among children who were born preterm may represent a "preterm phenotype" and may be due to general cognitive deficits, or other neurocognitive deficits rather than a direct indication of the risk of ASD. These behaviors that reflect comorbid language, cognitive, motor, neurosensory, and behavioral deficits pose a major methodological challenge for ASD-specific screening in very preterm infants (S. Johnson & Marlow, 2009).

Concern that the high frequency of neurological, cognitive, and sensory difficulties in the functioning of preterm children may give rise to false-positive screening classifications for ASD has led to the design of studies which include a diagnostic evaluation to confirm true rates of ASD. One study reported on the 15.8% children in the EPIcure cohort (S. Johnson, Hollis, Kochhar, Hennessy, Wolke, & Marlow, 2010b) with a positive screen on the *Social Communication Questionnaire* (SCQ) who underwent psychiatric evaluation at 11 years; only 8% were diagnosed with ASD (S. Johnson, Hollis, Kochhar, Hennessy, Wolke, & Marlow, 2010a). A second study evaluated a cohort with birthweight of less than 2000 grams screened with the SCQ in later adolescence (16–21 years) and reported an estimated prevalence rate of ASD of 5% (Pinto-Martin, Levy, Feldman, Lorenz, Paneth, & Whitaker, 2011). At least two recent studies are in the process of publishing data on the diagnostic prevalence in preterm or low birthweight cohorts and new data will emerge over time.

It is well established that LBW/PTB is a risk factor for white matter injury (Grunewaldt, Fjortoft, Bjuland, Brubakk, Eikenes, Haberg et al., 2014). White matter injury, in turn, is a risk factor for a number of neurodevelopmental conditions, including ASD. One study reported an almost seven-fold increased risk of ASD associated with ventricular enlargement on cranial ultrasound compared to those with no abnormality (Movsas, Pinto-Martin, Whitaker, Feldman, Lorenz, Korzeniewski et al., 2013). Another study showed that children who developed autism showed significant differences in white matter development compared to those who did not. This suggests problems in the development of brain wiring during early infancy in advance of core clinical symptoms (Wolff, Gu, Gerig, Elison, Styner, Gouttard et al., 2012).

Other studies have suggested that autism involves abnormal connectivity between different brain regions (Belmonte, Allen, Beckel-Mitchener, Boulanger, Carper, & Webb, 2004). In theory, this could explain the impaired communication and social behaviors that are hallmarks of ASD. For example, a typical infant trying to communicate something of shared interest uses a combination of gestures, babbling, and eye contact. This requires several brain regions to communicate with each other simultaneously, which may be a difficult or impossible task for an autistic brain.

In summary, while there is a growing body of evidence in support of an increased risk for ASD among those born LBW/ preterm, the mechanism remains to be elucidated. Is it a common factor that causes LBW/PTB and ASD or is ASD a consequence of early birth, and the subsequent health challenges and neonatal intensive care interventions? Of course, what we are all searching for is a presymptomatic marker for ASD. It is too early to tell whether some form of brain imaging could be used to identify children at risk for ASD in early infancy, but the discovery of an early biomarker would offer the possibility of intervention before behavioral symptoms become obvious and harder to reverse.

Interesting models are being developed that link many of the etiological considerations described above. For example, the laboratory of David Geschwind at University of California at Los Angeles (Geschwind, 2014) looks at gene expression, brain anatomy, and immunologic phenomena (Parikshak, Luo, Zhang, Won, Lowe, Chandran et al., 2013; Scudellari, 2011; Voineagu, Wang, Johnston, Lowe, Tian, Horvath et al., 2011). It is likely that multiple early insults–whether genetic, inflammatory, or related to preterm birth/low birthweight–may result in changes to the "vulnerable embryonic and infantile brain," thus producing autism (Gesundheit et al., 2013).

Summary and Conclusions

Given the compelling but incomplete evidence for genetic, autoimmune, and perinatal risk factors as possible etiologies, we speculate that etiological heterogeneity may go along with the phenotypic heterogeneity observed in children with autism. Even the most promising etiological mechanisms have not been consistently found in 100% of autistic children sampled. Perhaps as evidence mounts to support specific etiological models, we will be able to further distinguish autism subtypes that go along with each etiology and determine specific treatments to address distinct etiologies.

To better enumerate ASD incidence and prevalence and to explain the perceived increasing prevalence of the condition, we hope that further research helps to identify early markers to aid in more objective autism diagnosis. Until etiological mechanisms are better elucidated—which may perhaps result in the recognition that what we recognize as ASD today may in fact be a group of related but distinct conditions—our best estimates at prevalence will continue to be limited by variable data quality related to case ascertainment and identification.

Understanding the etiological mechanisms will affect our ability to accurately diagnose ASD, help us to refine our diagnostic criteria, and consequently improve our ability to estimate the prevalence of the disorder. Armed with knowledge about what causes ASD in their patients, clinicians can better prescribe treatments more targeted to the affected causal pathways producing autism, enhancing our ability to act early to improve the sociability and independence of affected individuals throughout the lifespan. For all of these reasons, the importance of understanding the etiologies of ASD cannot be overstated, and we encourage research funding to be targeted to further refine the mechanisms presented here to ensure improved care of individuals with ASD.

References

American Psychiatric Association. (1980). *Diagnostic and statistical manual of mental disorders: DSM-III*. Washington, DC: American Psychiatric Association American Psychiatric Association.

American Psychiatric Association. (2000). *DSM-IV-TR: Diagnostic and statistical manual of mental disorders, text revision*. Washington, DC: American Psychiatric Association.

American Psychiatric Association. (2013). *Diagnostic and statistical manual of mental disorders: DSM-5*. Washington, DC: American Psychiatric Association.

Ashwood, P., & Van de Water, J. (2004). A review of autism and the immune response. *Clinical Developmental Immunology, 11*(2), 165-174.

Atladottir, H. O., Pedersen, M. G., Scient, C., Thorsen, P., Mortensen, P. B., Deleuran, . . . Parner, E. T. (2009). Association of family history of autoimmune diseases and autism spectrum disorders. *Pediatrics, 124*(2), 687–694. http: //pediatrics.aappublications.org/content/124/2/687.short

Bailey, A., Le Couteur, A., Gottesman, I., Bolton, P., Simonoff, E., Yuzda, E, & Rutter, M. (1995). Autism as a strongly genetic disorder: Evidence from a British twin study. *Psychological Medicine, 25*(1), 63–77.

Belmonte, M. K., Allen, G., Beckel-Mitchener, A., Boulanger, L. M., Carper, R. A., & Webb, S. J. (2004). Autism and abnormal development of brain connectivity. *Journal of Neuroscience, 24*(42), 9228–9231.

Boulanger, L. M., & Shatz, C. J. (2004). Immune signalling in neural development, synaptic plasticity and disease. *Nature Reviews in Neuroscience, 5*(7), 521–531.

Buie, T., Campbell, D. B., Fuchs, G. J., 3rd, Furuta, G. T., Levy, J., Vandewater, J., . . . Winter. H. (2010). Evaluation, diagnosis, and treatment of gastrointestinal disorders in individuals with ASDs: A consensus report. *Pediatrics, 125*(Suppl 1), S1–S18. http://pediatrics.aappublications.org/content/125/Supplement_1/S1.short

Buxbaum, J. D., Daly, M. J., Devlin, B., Lehner, T., Roeder, K., & State, M. W. (2012). The autism sequencing consortium: Large-scale, high-throughput sequencing in autism spectrum disorders. *Neuron, 76*(6), 1052–1056.

CDC. (2015). Autism and Developmental Disabilities Monitoring (ADDM) Network. Retrieved Jan 6, 2015, from http://www.cdc.gov/ncbddd/autism/addm.html

Centers for Disease Control and Prevention (CDC). (2014). Metropolitan Atlanta Developmental Disabilities Surveillance Program (MADDSP). Retrieved 22 Dec, 2014, from http://www.cdc.gov/ncbddd/developmentaldisabilities/MADDSP.html

Chakrabarti, S., & Fombonne, E. (2001). Pervasive developmental disorders in preschool children. *JAMA, 285*(24), 3093–3099.

Comi, A. M., Zimmerman, A. W., Frye, V. H., Law, P. A., & Peeden, J. N. (1999). Familial clustering of autoimmune disorders and evaluation of medical risk factors in autism. *Journal of Child Neurology, 14*(6), 388–394.

Constantino, J. N., Zhang, Y., Frazier, T., Abbacchi, A. M., & Law, P. (2010). Sibling recurrence and the genetic epidemiology of autism. *American Journal of Psychiatry, 167*(11), 1349–1356.

Coury, D. L. (2013). DSM-5 and autism spectrum disorders: Implications for families and clinicians. *Journal of Developmental and Behavioral Pediatrics, 34*(7), 494–496.

Croen, L. A., Grether, J. K., Yoshida, C. K., Odouli, R., & Van de Water, J. (2005). Maternal autoimmune diseases, asthma and allergies, and childhood autism spectrum disorders: A case-control study. *Archives of Pediatric & Adolescent Medicine, 159*(2), 151–157.

Dalton, P., Deacon, R., Blamire, A., Pike, M., McKinlay, I., Stein, J., . . . Vincent, A. (2003). Maternal neuronal antibodies associated with autism and a language disorder. *Annals of Neurology, 53*(4), 533–537.

Davidovitch, M., Hemo, B., Manning-Courtney, P., & Fombonne, E. (2013). Prevalence and incidence of autism spectrum disorder in an Israeli population. *Journal of Autism & Developmental Disorders, 43*(4), 785–793.

Developmental Disabilities Monitoring Network Surveillance Year Principal Investigators, Centers for Disease, Control, & Prevention. (2014). Prevalence of autism spectrum disorder among children aged 8 years–autism and developmental disabilities monitoring network, 11 sites, United States, 2010. *Morbidity and Mortality Weekly Report Surveillance Summaries* (Washington, D.C.: 2002), 63(2), 1–21.

Dudova, I., Kasparova, M., Markova, D., Zemankova, J., Beranova, S., Urbanek, T., . . . Hrdlicka, M. (2014). Screening for autism in preterm children with extremely low and very low birth weight. *Neuropsychiatric Disease & Treatment, 10,* 277–282. http://www.ncbi.nlm.nih.gov/pmc/articles/PMC3931701/

Eisenberg, L., & Kanner, L. (1956). Childhood schizophrenia: Symposium, 1955: 6. Early infantile autism, 1943–55. *American Journal of Orthopsychiatry, 26*(3), 556.

Gardener, H., Spiegelman, D., & Buka, S. L. (2011). Perinatal and neonatal risk factors for autism: A comprehensive meta-analysis. *Pediatrics, 128*(2), 344–355.

Geschwind, D. H. (2014). Geschwind Lab. Retrieved 28 Dec 2014, from http://geschwindlab.neurology.ucla.edu/

Gesundheit, B., Rosenzweig, J. P., Naor, D., Lerer, B., Zachor, D. A., Prochazka, V., . . . Ashwood, P. (2013). Immunological and autoimmune considerations of autism spectrum disorders. *Journal of Autoimmunology, 44,* 1–7. http://www.sciencedirect.com/science/article/pii/S0896841113000735

Grunewaldt, K. H., Fjortoft, T., Bjuland, K. J., Brubakk, A. M., Eikenes, L., Haberg, A. K., . . . Skranes, J. (2014). Follow-up at age 10 years in ELBW children–Functional outcome, brain morphology and results from motor assessments in infancy. *Early Human Development, 90*(10), 571–578.

Hack, M., Taylor, H. G., Schluchter, M., Andreias, L., Drotar, D., & Klein, N. (2009). Behavioral outcomes of extremely low birth weight children at age 8 years. *Journal of Developmental & Behavioral Pediatrics, 30*(2), 122–130.

Hallmayer, J., Cleveland, S., Torres, A., Phillips, J., Cohen, B., Torigoe, T., . . . Risch, N. (2011). Genetic heritability and shared environmental factors among twin pairs with autism. *Archives of General Psychiatry, 68*(11), 1095–1102. http: //archpsyc.jamanetwork.com/article.aspx?articleid=1107328&maxtoshow=&hits=10&resultformat=&fulltext=hallmayer%20j&searchid=1&firstindex=0&resourcetype=hwcit

Hanson, D. R., & Gottesman, I. (1976). The genetics, if any, of infantile autism and childhood schizophrenia. *Journal of Autism Childhood Schizophrenia, 6*(3), 209–234.

Heil, K. M., & Schaaf, C. P. (2013). The genetics of autism spectrum disorders–a guide for clinicians. *Current Psychiatry Reports, 15*(1), 334.

Individuals with Disabilities Education Act, Pub L. 101-476, 20 USC § 1400, (1990).

Indredavik, M. S., Vik, T., Evensen, K. A., Skranes, J., Taraldsen, G., & Brubakk, A. M. (2010). Perinatal risk and psychiatric outcome in adolescents born preterm with very low birth weight or term small for gestational age. *Journal of Developmental & Behavioral Pediatrics, 31*(4), 286–294.

Johnson, C. P., & Myers, S. M. (2007). Identification and evaluation of children with autism spectrum disorders. *Pediatrics, 120*(5), 1183–1215.

Johnson, S., Hollis, C., Kochhar, P., Hennessy, E., Wolke, D., & Marlow, N. (2010a). Autism spectrum disorders in extremely preterm children. *Journal of Pediatrics, 156*(4), 525–531.

Johnson, S., Hollis, C., Kochhar, P., Hennessy, E., Wolke, D., & Marlow, N. (2010b). Psychiatric disorders in extremely preterm children: Longitudinal finding at age 11 years in the EPICure study. *Journal of the American Academy of Child & Adolescent Psychiatry, 49*(5), 453–463.

Johnson, S., & Marlow, N. (2009). Positive screening results on the Modified Checklist for Autism in Toddlers: Implications for very preterm populations. *Journal of Pediatrics, 154*(4), 478–480.

Kanner, L. (1943). Autistic disturbances of affective contact. *Nervous Child, 2*(3), 217–250.

Kleinman, J. M., Robins, D. L., Ventola, P. E., Pandey, J., Boorstein, H. C., Esser, E. L., . . . Fein, D. (2008). The Modified Checklist for Autism in Toddlers: A follow-up study investigating the early detection of autism spectrum disorders. *Journal of Autism & Developmental Disorders, 38*(5), 827–839.

Kuban, K. C., O'Shea, T. M., Allred, E. N., Tager-Flusberg, H., Goldstein, D. J., & Leviton, A. (2009). Positive screening on the Modified Checklist for Autism in Toddlers (M-CHAT) in extremely low gestational age newborns. *Journal of Pediatrics, 154*(4), 535–540.

Kuzniewicz, M. W., Wi, S., Qian, Y., Walsh, E. M., Armstrong, M. A., & Croen, L. A. (2014). Prevalence and neonatal factors associated with autism spectrum disorders in preterm infants. *Journal of Pediatrics, 164*(1), 20–25.

Lai, M. C., Lombardo, M. V., & Baron-Cohen, S. (2014). Autism. *Lancet, 383*(9920), 896–910.

Lauritsen, M. B., Pedersen, C. B., & Mortensen, P. B. (2005). Effects of familial risk factors and place of birth on the risk of autism: A nationwide register-based study. *Journal of Child Psychology & Psychiatry, 46*(9), 963–971.

Leavey, A., Zwaigenbaum, L., Heavner, K., & Burstyn, I. (2013). Gestational age at birth and risk of autism spectrum disorders in Alberta, Canada. *Journal of Pediatrics, 162*(2), 361–368.

Limperopoulos, C., Bassan, H., Sullivan, N. R., Soul, J. S., Robertson, R. L., Jr., Moore, M., . . . du Plessis, A.J. (2008). Positive screening for autism in ex-preterm infants: Prevalence and risk factors. *Pediatrics, 121*(4), 758–765. http://pediatrics.aappublications.org/content/121/4/758.short

Lord, C., Petkova, E., Hus, V., Gan, W., Lu, F., Martin, D.M., . . . Risi, S. (2012). A multisite study of the clinical diagnosis of different autism spectrum disorders. *Archives of General Psychiatry, 69*(3), 306–313.

Lotter, V. (1966). Epidemiology of autistic conditions in young children. *Social Psychiatry, 1*(3), 124–135.

Mandell, D., & Lecavalier, L. (2014). Should we believe the Centers for Disease Control and Prevention's autism spectrum disorder prevalence estimates? *Autism, 18*(5), 482–484.

Martin, L. A., Ashwood, P., Braunschweig, D., Cabanlit, M., Van de Water, J., & Amaral, D. G. (2008). Stereotypies and hyperactivity in rhesus monkeys exposed to IgG from mothers of children with autism. *Brain Behavavior and Immunology, 22*(6), 806–816.

Miles, J. H. (2011). Autism spectrum disorders–a genetics review. *Genetics in Medicine, 13*(4), 278–294.

Money, J., Bobrow, N. A., & Clarke, F. C. (1971). Autism and autoimmune disease: A family study. *Journal of Autism & Childhood Schizophrenia, 1*(2), 146–160.

Moore, T., Johnson, S., Hennessy, E., & Marlow, N. (2012). Screening for autism in extremely preterm infants: Problems in interpretation. *Developmental Medicine & Child Neurology, 54*(6), 514–520.

Movsas, T. Z., Pinto-Martin, J. A., Whitaker, A. H., Feldman, J. F., Lorenz, J. M., Korzeniewski, S. J., . . . Paneth, N. (2013). Autism spectrum disorder is associated with ventricular enlargement in a low birth weight population. *Journal of Pediatrics, 163*(1), 73–78.

Oliveira, G., Diogo, L., Grazina, M., Garcia, P., Ataide, A., Marques, C., . . . Olivieri, C. R. (2005). Mitochondrial dysfunction in autism spectrum disorders: A population-based study. *Developmental Medicine & Child Neurology, 47*(3), 185–189. http://onlinelibrary.wiley.com/doi/10.1111/j.1469-8749.2005.tb01113.x/full\

Ozonoff, S., Young, G. S., Carter, A., Messinger, D., Yirmiya, N., Zwaigenbaum, L., . . . Stone, W.L. (2011). Recurrence risk for autism spectrum disorders: A Baby Siblings Research Consortium study. *Pediatrics, 128*(3), e488–e495.

Parikshak, N. N., Luo, R., Zhang, A., Won, H., Lowe, J. K., Chandran, V., . . . Geschwind, D. H. (2013). Integrative functional genomic analyses implicate specific molecular pathways and circuits in autism. *Cell, 155*(5), 1008–1021.

Pinto, D., Delaby, E., Merico, D., Barbosa, M., Merikangas, A., Klei, L., . . . De Jonge, M. V. (2014). Convergence of genes and cellular pathways dysregulated in autism spectrum disorders. *American Journal of Human Genetics, 94*(5), 677–694.

Pinto-Martin, J. A., Levy, S. E., Feldman, J. F., Lorenz, J. M., Paneth, N., & Whitaker, A. H. (2011). Prevalence of autism spectrum disorder in adolescents born weighing <2000 grams. *Pediatrics, 128*(5), 883–891.

Polo-Kantola, P., Lampi, K. M., Hinkka-Yli-Salomaki, S., Gissler, M., Brown, A. S., & Sourander, A. (2014). Obstetric risk factors and autism spectrum disorders in Finland. *Journal of Pediatrics, 164*(2), 358–365.

Robins, D. L., & Dumont-Mathieu, T. M. (2006). Early screening for autism spectrum disorders: Update on the modified checklist for autism in toddlers and other measures. *Journal of Developmental & Behavioral Pediatrics, 27*(2 Suppl), S111–S119.

Robins, D. L., Fein, D., Barton, M. L., & Green, J. A. (2001). The Modified Checklist for Autism in Toddlers: An initial study investigating the early detection of autism and pervasive developmental disorders. *Journal of Autism & Developmental Disorders, 31*(2), 131–144.

Rutter, M. (1978). Diagnosis and definition of childhood autism. *Journal of Autism & Childhood Schizophrenia, 8*(2), 139–161.

Saemundsen, E., Magnússon, P., Georgsdóttir, I., Egilsson, E., & Rafnsson, V. (2013). Prevalence of autism spectrum disorders in an Icelandic birth cohort. *BMJ Open, 3*(6). http://bmjopen.bmj.com/content/3/6/e002748.short

Schaefer, G. B., & Mendelsohn, N. J. (2013). Clinical genetics evaluation in identifying the etiology of autism spectrum disorders: 2013 guideline revisions. *Genetics in Medicine, 15*(5), 399–407. doi: 310.1038/gim.2013.1032. Epub 2013 Mar 1021.

Schieve, L. A., Tian, L. H., Baio, J., Rankin, K., Rosenberg, D., Wiggins, L., . . . Devine, O. (2014). Population attributable fractions for three perinatal risk factors for autism spectrum disorders, 2002 and 2008 autism and developmental disabilities monitoring network. *Annals of Epidemiology, 24*(4), 260–266. http://www.sciencedirect.com/science/article/pii/S104727971400009X

Scudellari, M. (2011, May 25). An autism brain signature? *The Scientist.* Retrieved 18 August 2014, from http://www.the-scientist.com/?articles.view/articleNo/29713/title/An-autism-brain-signature-/

Shattuck, P. T. (2006). The contribution of diagnostic substitution to the growing administrative prevalence of autism in US special education. *Pediatrics, 117*(4), 1028–1037.

Simonoff, E. (1998). Genetic counseling in autism and pervasive developmental disorders. *Journal of Autism & Developmental Disorders, 28*(5), 447–456.

Steffenburg, S., Gillberg, C., Hellgren, L., Andersson, L., Gillberg, I. C., Jakobsson, G., & Bohman, M. (1989). A twin study of autism in Denmark, Finland, Iceland, Norway and Sweden. *Journal of Child Psychology & Psychiatry, 30*(3), 405–416.

Stephens, B. E., Bann, C. M., Watson, V. E., Sheinkopf, S. J., Peralta-Carcelen, M., Bodnar, A., . . . Vohr, V. R. (2012). Screening for autism spectrum disorders in extremely preterm infants. *Journal Developmental & Behavioral Pediatrics, 33*(7), 535–541.

Sturmey, P., & Dalfern, S. (2014). The effects of DSM-5 autism diagnostic criteria on number of individuals diagnosed with autism spectrum disorders: A systematic review. *Review Journal of Autism & Developmental Disorders, 1,* 249–252.

Sun, X., Allison, C., Matthews, F. E., Sharp, S. J., Auyeung, B., Baron-Cohen, S., . . . Brayne, C. (2013). Prevalence of autism in mainland China, Hong Kong and Taiwan: A systematic review and meta-analysis. *Molecular Autism, 4*(1), 7. http://www.molecularautism.com/content/4/1/7

Swedo, S. E., Baird, G., Cook Jr., E. H., Happé, F. G., Harris, J. C., Kaufmann, W. E., . . . Wright, H. H. (2012). Commentary from the DSM-5 Workgroup on Neurodevelopmental Disorders. *Journal of the American Academy of Child & Adolescent Psychiatry, 51*(4), 347–349.

Sweeten, T. L., Bowyer, S. L., Posey, D. J., Halberstadt, G. M., & McDougle, C. J. (2003). Increased prevalence of familial autoimmunity in probands with pervasive developmental disorders. *Pediatrics, 112*(5), e420.

Torres, A. R., Sweeten, T. L., Cutler, A., Bedke, B. J., Fillmore, M., Stubbs, E. G., . . . Odell, D. (2006). The association and linkage of the HLA-A2 class I allele with autism. *Human Immunology, 67*(4–5), 346–351. http://www.sciencedirect.com/science/article/pii/S0198885906000425

Tsai, L. Y., & Ghaziuddin, M. (2014). DSM-5. ASD moves forward into the past. *Journal of Autism & Developmental Disorders, 44*(2), 321–330.

Vargas, D. L., Nascimbene, C., Krishnan, C., Zimmerman, A. W., & Pardo, C. A. (2005). Neuroglial activation and neuroinflammation in the brain of patients with autism. *Annals of Neurology, 57*(1), 67–81.

Voineagu, I., Wang, X., Johnston, P., Lowe, J. K., Tian, Y., Horvath, S., . . . Geschwind, D. H. (2011). Transcriptomic analysis of autistic brain reveals convergent molecular pathology. *Nature, 474*(7351), 380–384.

Wolff, J. J., Gu, H., Gerig, G., Elison, J. T., Styner, M., Gouttard, S., . . . Piven, J. (2012). Differences in white matter fiber tract development present from 6 to 24 months in infants with autism. *American Journal of Psychiatry, 169*(6), 589–600.

Wong, H. S., Huertas-Ceballos, A., Cowan, F. M., & Modi, N. (2014). Evaluation of early childhood social-communication difficulties in children born preterm using the Quantitative Checklist for Autism in Toddlers. *Journal of Pediatrics, 164*(1), 26–33.e21.

World Health Organization (WHO). (2014). ICD-11 beta draft. Retrieved 1 Oct 2014, from http://apps.who.int/classifications/icd11/browse/f/en

Yeargin-Allsopp, M., Rice, C., Karapurkar, T., Doernberg, N., Boyle, C., & Murphy, C. (2003). Prevalence of autism in a US metropolitan area. *JAMA, 289*(1), 49–55.

Chapter 3

FACILITATING THE ROLE OF
PARENTS IN HEALTHCARE
MANAGEMENT AND ADVOCACY

KATHLEEN G. FREEMAN AND JENNIFER HARRISON ELDER

Historically, parents have been at the vanguard as experts in understanding autism. They persevered when their concerns were dismissed, "Don't worry, he's a boy. He'll talk when he's ready." They have had to do research, find funding sources, implement treatments, and survive the impact of raising a child with autism. Adding to these challenges, are parents' low confidence and dissatisfaction with healthcare practitioners (HCPs) (Harrington, Patrick, Edwards, & Brand, 2006; Liptak, Orlando, Yingling, Therurer-Kaufman, Malay, Thompkins, & Flynn, 2006). Parental dissatisfaction is unfortunate as strong parent-HCP teams can be highly effective in facilitating timely diagnosis and treatment over a lifetime. The purpose of this chapter is to assist HCPs to understand how parents perceive the health care system and suggest ways for improving access to early diagnosis. The first author, a mother of a son with autism spectrum disorder (ASD) and faculty at a school of nursing, introduces this discussion by sharing her unique insights from her journey in the following vignette.

A Parent's Journey to the Diagnosis

When my son was born, I was already a mother of a three-year-old daughter and employed full-time. The only pregnancy complication was severe hyperemesis gravidarum beginning at six weeks gestation. My obstetrician prescribed hydroxyzine to alleviate the nausea and vomiting in lieu of admission for intravenous therapy. I was concerned about taking medications during pregnancy, and fortunately the nausea and vomiting stopped at

13 weeks. The remainder of the pregnancy was unremarkable. During labor, my son's heart rate dipped briefly corresponding with the epidural administration. Once fully dilated, he was delivered after two pushes.

My son was born full-term but small for gestational age (SGA) at 6 pounds 2 ounces. APGARs were 8, at one minute; and 9, at five minutes. His bilirubin climbed due to ABO incompatibility, but phototherapy was not required. He was an efficient breast-feeder and extremely healthy, rarely needing episodic visits to the pediatrician. At his 18 month check-up, the pediatrician asked if I had any concerns. I reported, "He isn't talking" and the pediatrician asked, "Do you think he can hear?" I responded, "I know he can." Although, I recall that my mother-in-law had commented that she was afraid my son could not hear because he was not turning to his name, and there was a history of hearing loss in her family. The assessment ended, and I left with only a vague sense of concern. His two-year check-up was much the same, and he was considered to be "developing normally."

Within a week of that visit, I was in the company of two other toddlers. My niece had asked me for "more milk." My neighbor's son pointed to a plane in the sky. I thought to myself, my son never asked me for anything or tried to get my attention. My experience as a HCP led me to administer the Denver Developmental Screening Tool, and his results were lower than peers in social interaction and language. I contacted his pediatrician and requested an evaluation for possible "developmental delay." Within two weeks of his two-year well check-up, I returned, fearing my son was autistic.

The pediatrician was surprised to see me and seemed reluctant to use the term "autistic" and suggested we first rule out hearing loss followed by a neurological evaluation. Getting an appointment for a hearing test took a month. The hearing test was normal. Getting an appointment for a neurologist took two months. That visit was long and stressful. He conducted a Bayley Developmental test, evaluated for nystagmus, by spinning him in a chair. He commented to his medical student, "See how he goes back to touch his mother's leg (periodically) for reassurance, he definitely is not autistic. An autistic child would not do that." The neurologist recommended early intervention services, although I was not told for what specific developmental delay. I was relieved for the moment. The neurologist's report described a communication language disorder and a pervasive developmental disorder–not otherwise specified (PPD-NOS).

Immediately after the visit, I contacted several early intervention programs which were closed for the month of August. Over the next two months, my relief of hearing that he was not autistic was fading. He was not speaking, pointing, or making eye contact. He developed an interest in lining up his trains, lying on the floor to visually inspect them, and sitting in the mulch at the playground dropping mulch in front of his eyes. In September, he started early intervention with two 45-minute sessions per week. He never missed an appointment.

The uncertainty of a clear diagnosis continued to gnaw at me. My neighbor, a neonatologist, suggested that I get an appointment with a developmental pediatrician who was a friend. Months passed, and I was ready to hear the autism diagnosis. I made sure my husband was there with me. When we were told that our son had PDD-NOS, I asked, "Is the treatment any different than for autism?" The pediatrician said, "It is the same." I said, "Are we just talking about a continuum here, with PDD-NOS on one end?" She said, "Yes," and used the word "spectrum." My worst fears were confirmed. My son was finally diagnosed at age 30 months.

Partnering with Parents: What Parents Know and HCPs Need to Know

Parents are often the best resource to identify young children whose behavior and development does not appear to be typical (Glascoe, 2003). Frequently it is the parents' concerns brought to the HCP that are the primary trigger of medical and behavioral conditions diagnosed at health care visits. Eliciting key information from parents may facilitate earlier diagnosis. As daily observers of their children, parents have contributed to the expert understanding of ASD because they see nuances of behavior and treatment responses that may be invisible to the HCP (Silverman & Brosco, 2007). Parents are skilled observers. As far back as 1999, Howlin and Asgharia found that 49 percent of parents (n=770) indicated that they were either "not very" or "not at all satisfied" with the diagnostic process. This finding was supported more recently by Crais and colleagues (2006) who reported that parents were frustrated when their "initial instincts" were not acknowledged. Similarly, Harrington et al. (2006) noted that 75% of parents (n=62) expressed little to no confidence in their HCP's ability to recognize ASD and that a perceived delay in the diagnosis might have contributed to their reported low confidence level (p=0.20).

Concerns Related to Diagnosis and Referrals

Studies regarding the timing of the diagnosis have demonstrated that a significant lag exists between the critical time points of: When parents first become concerned, seek treatment, and obtain an ASD diagnosis (Wiggins, Baio, & Rice, 2006; Rosenberg, Landa, Law, Stuart, & Law, 2011). Wiggins and colleagues (2006) reviewed 115 records of eight-year-olds with ASD identified by the Centers for Disease Control and Prevention (CDC) population-based surveillance program to assess the diagnostic timeline. The delay between mean age at first documented evaluation (mean 48 months, range 16–103 months) and mean age at first ASD diagnosis (mean 61 months, range 17–105) was 13 months. Likewise, Rosenberg et al. (2011) reviewed records from a national online registry of 6,214 children aged 0–21 years diagnosed with ASD between 1994 and 2010 in the US. They reported a mean age of documented parental concern of 19.6 months (SD 15.0) and a mean age of diagnosis of 47.9 months (SD 30.8). Explicitly probing for parental concerns about development is useful for identifying those needing closer monitoring, surveillance, and possible testing (Ozonoff et al., 2011).

NEED FOR TRAINING. The delay from symptom recognition to diagnosis could be due to insufficient training, a lack of understanding of diagnostic criteria, inconsistent use of screening and assessment tools, or time constraints limiting behavioral observations (Golnik, Ireland, & Borowsky, 2009; Gabrielsen, Farley, Speer, Villalobos, Baker, & Miller, 2015). Daniels and Mandell (2014) suggested that providers may benefit from greater training on how to respond to parental concerns and encourage parents to contact early intervention programs as soon as concerns arise. Supporting the need for additional training, Shah (2001) found that fourth-year medical students averaged fewer than five correct responses on a 10-item questionnaire about ASD and in a qualitative study by Fisher, Frazer, Hasson, and Orkin (2007); emergency room nurses reported their educational preparation to care for those with developmental disabilities, such as ASD, was inadequate. HCP's with limited experience or training may have difficulty distinguishing among subtle cognitive or language delays and social communication delays associated with ASD (Caronna, Augustyn, & Zuckerman, 2007).

In addition, HCPs might be reticent to diagnose a child since behavior problems and speech delays are common developmental concerns in children between the ages of one and three years (Filipek et al., 2000). Also interesting are findings by Gabrielsen, Farley, Speer, Villalobos, Baker, and Miller (2015) who reported that children with ASD showed more typical behavior (89% of the time) than atypical (11%). In their study, even clinicians who had experience and expertise in ASD could not detect atypical: Typical behavior ratios in a 10–20 minute observation. The HCP's limited opportunities for observing key developmental delays suggestive of ASD combined with reluctance in identifying ASD makes the HCP-parent interactions paramount for identifying children who need greater surveillance, screening, or possible referral.

SCREENING AND DIAGNOSTIC PROCESSES. Another concern is that HCPs may not consistently use developmental screening tools even though the American Academy of Pediatrics recommended routine developmental surveillance and targeted screenings with standardized developmental screening tools at well child visits (Sand et al., 2005). The inconsistent use of screening tools has been attributed to time constraints or lack of insurance reimbursement (Filipek et al., 2000; Sand, Silverstein, Glascoe, Gupta, Tonniges, & O'Connor, 2005; Sices, Feudtner, McLaughlin, Drotar, & Williams, 2003).

The delay from the time of expressed concern until eventual diagnosis contributes to low satisfaction and frustration for parents. These reports substantiate the need for effective early screening, careful listening to parents and inviting their input, and timely referrals to appropriate resources. Attention to these could bolster parental confidence and enhance the HCP-parent partnership that is essential not only in the early stages but throughout the lifetime of the individual with ASD (Bultas, 2012; Harrington et al., 2006). Also promising is the parent completed 20-item Modified Checklist for Autism in Toddlers, Revised with Follow-up (M-CHAT-R/F) that has resulted in 95% of those identified at risk to be later diagnosed with a developmental disability; and 47% of the 95%, were later diagnosed with ASD (Robins, Casagrande, Barton, Chen, & Dumont-Mathieu, 2014). The children in this study received a diagnosis two years earlier than the national median age of diagnosis.

REFERRALS. HCPs may be hesitant to raise the suspicion of ASD, especially if the child is young, and/or the HCP feels the diagnosis is outside of his or her expertise. Therefore, referral, not diagnosis, is the appropriate step (Caronna, Augustyn, & Zuckerman, 2007). Parents often view the HCP as the authority on the child's health and development. Thus, if concerns are dismissed or signs of ASD missed, parental confidence in, and respect for, the HCP diminishes. Delayed referral could adversely affect future parent-HCP collaboration and partnership. Additionally, a HCP can encourage parents who suspect a developmental delay to initiate an evaluation to obtain services provided under the Individuals with Disabilities Education Act (IDEA). IDEA is a federally mandated service for children with disabilities.

Developing the Partnership with Parents

Providing the required comprehensive assessment and treatment planning for a patient with ASD requires time, patience, and skill. Fathers are involved in childcare, but mothers more often fulfill a greater role related to childrearing in the typical American family (Tehee, Honan, & Hevey, 2009), and make the first contact with the HCP (Bultas, 2012).

Experiences of Mothers

In a study by Bultas (2012), mothers felt stress and anxiety over their need to continually "drive" the health care visit by repeating patient-specific instructions and information on every visit. To ameliorate this, mothers suggested creating a child profile, rather than medical history and the parent serves as the consultant. The profile included important information about routines and behaviors that could negatively impact their child's visit (Marshall, Sheller, Mancl, & Williams, 2008). It also incorporated suggestions from the parents and thus fostered a true-family-centered approach that reflected the mutual goal of achieving the best outcome for the child (Inglese, 2009). The HCP should recognize that mothers can also be stressed during a healthcare visit, and their attention will be divided between listening to the HCP and monitoring their child. Keeping this in mind, the HCP's understanding and empathy will lead to a collaborative and satisfying long-term parent-HCP relationship.

The Environment and Physical Barriers

Giarelli and colleagues (2014) described the intensity and variety of stimuli in the environment of the hospital emergency department as posing significant obstacles to the delivery of medical care to a patient with ASD. This is especially true for the patient who has co-occurring sensory processing dysfunction. A patient profile may describe the patient's specific sensory dysfunction (e.g., hypersensitivity to sounds, smells, touch, and textures), past reactions to sensory stimuli, and interventions that have been successfully used to mitigate the effects. For example, a crowded and noisy waiting room is particularly challenging. Ear muffs and devices with headphones can help reduce noises that can elicit aberrant behavior. Find a quiet area in the waiting room and use tech devices. Figure 3.1 illustrates the use of diversions.

Waiting can be challenging for the parent in constant anticipation of a stimulus that will trigger an unwanted behavior. Fortunately, there are several strategies that can help. For example, reducing the actual time patients with ASD are exposed to environmental stressors can be beneficial. Scheduling the appointment for the first appointment of the day or immediately after lunch can greatly diminish wait times. Allowing a parent to "call ahead" to determine if the HCP is behind schedule and being given a new time to arrive is helpful. Similarly, entering by a rear entrance, having a quiet area to wait, or going directly to an exam room can eliminate the risk of encountering a sensory obstacle, and greatly lessen a parent's stress level. Another strategy is allowing the parent and patient to remain in the "safe haven" of their car until staff and the exam room are ready. Using this approach, the parent can call the office when they arrive, provide any necessary information and ask the desk to text them when it is time for the exam.

Core Behavioral Characteristics as Barriers

Patients with ASD exhibit impaired functioning in two critical domains: Age-appropriate social skills and communication, and the abnormal devel-

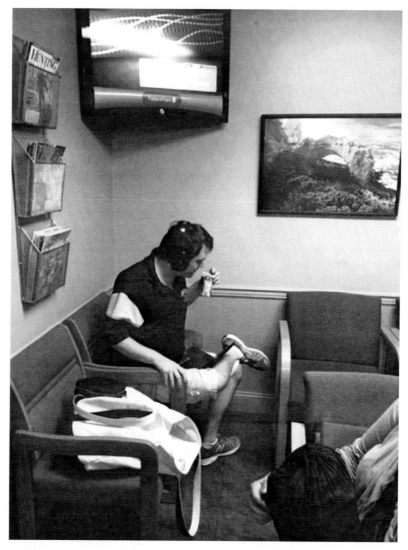

Figure 3.1. This young adult with autism is made more comfortable in the waiting room when he has some devices to distract him. This picture is printed with permission from the legal guardian. K. Freeman.

opment of restricted interests or stereotyped behaviors (American Psychological Association, 2013). Each behavioral characteristic may interfere with treatments. A HCP should seek the advice of a parent on which core features are most prominent, disruptive, and easily triggered in the child.

Stereotypical behaviors such as repetitive motor movements or object use may be difficult to interrupt. Restricted interests may take the form of preoccupation with a toy or hobby, or a topic so intense that they have difficulty transitioning to another topic or activity. Patients may also have emotional and sensory issues such as low frustration tolerance, moods swings, and overreactivity, which could lead to tantrums, aggression, and/or self-injurious behavior (Ming, Brimacombe, Chaaban, Zimmerman-Bier, & Wagner, 2008; Souders, Freeman, DePaul, & Levy, 2002).

The Medical Visit

Ideally, a nontreatment visit to the office environment prior to an actual visit to the HCP should occur. During this visit, the patient becomes acquainted with staff and oriented to the waiting area and exam room. This "trial visit" can also help identify potential environmental obstacles and establish a positive association to the health office experience. New patient paperwork including insurance information can be given to the parent in advance to complete and return on the next visit. For the patient who may benefit from a social story, pictures taken by the caregiver on a smart phone can be used to create the story in anticipation of the return visit. At this visit, the patient profile may be further developed.

Patient-Specific Profile

Many of the child's interests and preoccupations, such as preferred toys, books, videos, or objects already present in the HCP's office, can be identified and noted on a profile form (see Box 3.1). The HCP can then ensure that the preferred objects are available during the actual visit. Knowledge of a child's preferences is instrumental for engaging conversation and/or gaining attention, building trust and rapport, and identifying reinforcers as well as potential distractors. These preferences can also be a window through which the HCP can ascertain the patient's developmental age.

A simple scale, such as the one developed by Hudson (2006), groups patient abilities and needs better than chronological age and parent descriptors such as "mild" and "severe." On the scale, Level 1 corresponds with a child who responds to his or her name and is aware of another's presence or attends to a person speaking. Level 2 corresponds with a child who interacts functionally with toys, has developed beginning language, is curious about his or her environment, and demonstrates repetition in play and tasks. At Level 3, a child interacts with others, recognizes order and sequence, and is able to control his or her own behavior. Level 4, the highest level of function, corresponds with a child who is curious to learn with detailed description, maintains control when provoked, verbalizes feelings, and understands rules and regulations. These levels may guide the interactions.

Box 3.1. Sample Profile Form		
Autism level:		
Chronological age:		
Developmental age:		
Preferred wait area: Car (text cell phone #) Waiting room Empty exam room		
What should be placed in exam room: (specific toys from office, books, white board, iPad, computer)?		
Mode of communication: Parent/caregiver:		
Device:	Patient:	
Reciprocal Conversation:	Yes	No
Able to read:	Yes	No
Verbalizes:		
Pain	Yes	No
Feelings	Yes	No
Likes	Yes	No
Desires/Wants	Yes	No
Favorite characters, interests:		
Reinforcers		
Distractors		

continued

Box 3.1–*Continued*
Known antecedents to behavior:
Behaviors:
Appropriate HCP response:
Will extra time be needed with this visit?   Yes   No
What we have learned from previous visits:
Strategies that work:
Strategies that don't:
Anticipated procedures for next visit:
Prescriptions needed/referrals requested:
Instructions/literature needed:

If a nontreatment visit is not possible, a phone interview to obtain the information for the profile should be done. Requests for a list of anticipated procedures, immunization history, and all health history information should be sent to the parents prior to the visit.

Preparing for the Medical Visit

In addition to preparing the individual profile and conducting a preliminary nontreatment visit, there are other methods to help reduce fear and anxiety for both parents and their child. For young children, there are numerous children's books which tell the story of a popular character going to see the doctor. Characters range from Elmo® to SpongeBob®. In 2012, Doc McStuffins®, a popular television animated series (http://disneyjunior.com /doc-mcstuffins) was created and familiarized children with health care visits.

SOCIAL STORIES AND VIDEO MODELING. For children with a more advanced developmental and/or functional level, social stories may be used

(Gray, 1994). Social stories are individualized and help familiarize the patient with what is going to happen. Words, illustrations, and photographs are used to tell the story. Such social stories allow the patient to anticipate each step of the visit, and mitigate anticipatory fear or anxiety. Pictures might include: The exterior of the building, waiting room, exam room, and office and medical personnel on the HCP's office website. A parent can download the pictures to place them in a social story "book."

Video modeling uses recordings and display equipment to provide a visual model of the targeted behavior or skill. Providing a video of a patient calmly visiting the health care office, effectively engaging in different aspects of a physical exam, and receiving procedures peacefully. This video can be viewed by the patient prior to the visit. Collaborate with the parents to develop social stories designed specifically for their child.

ANTICIPATING INTRUSIVE PROCEDURES. Painful procedures are particularly challenging for all patients especially those with ASD. Medications such as lidocaine-prilocaine (EMLA) cream and lidocaine-epinephrine-tetracaine (LET) gel, both applied topically, can eliminate pain caused by venipuncture, injections, or administration of a local anesthetic. Typically, the cream or gel is applied to the antecubital, deltoid, or *vastas lateralis* areas and covered with plastic wrap at home prior to coming to the office. Its use requires planning because, generally, it must be applied to the skin 45 minutes prior to a procedure for EMLA and 20–30 minutes prior for LET. Having the patient wear long sleeve or long pant clothing over the site prevents the patient from removing it prematurely. A prescription for the topical anesthetic with preprinted administration instructions could be given in advance to the parent.

Since painful procedures are typically performed last, there usually is a sufficient amount of time that has lapsed during a typical office visit that the anesthetic has had time to take effect. Therefore, for the HCP, there is time efficiency despite the extra time needed for the anesthetic to numb the skin. For the patient with ASD, it allows for a potentially painless visit, which may eliminate fear, anxiety, and phobic avoidance behaviors commonly associated with previous negative experiences which have induced pain and distress.

Although obtaining blood samples in the HCP's office is not typical, it is appreciated by parents because it eliminates another potential traumatizing visit to a lab. Using proactive strategies, sometimes even chemical restraint, is preferable over aggressive physical restraint. However, parents may vary in how they view pharmacological and/or physical restraint and thus, they should be active partners with the HCP in deciding the best approach for their child.

The Day of the Medical Visit

A successful visit is one that accomplishes the purpose, is not stressful for the parent, and does not result in aberrant child behaviors. Negative experiences can have long-lasting effects, making every subsequent visit a difficult one for everyone (Souders et al., 2002). Further, they can result in phobic avoidance behaviors often characterized as fear or anxiety (Jennett & Hagopian, 2008). The objective is to reduce the antecedents that trigger unwanted behaviors before the HCP walks in the exam room.

For the parent of the child with ASD and HCP, the best case scenario is that the patient is cooperative; exhibits no aberrant behaviors; the goal of the visit is met; and the stress level for parent, patient, and HCP is kept to a minimum. It is possible that the visit may go smoothly, but anticipating some of the challenges that have been mentioned is important. See Table 3.1 for potential problems related to the medical visit and recommendations.

Table 3.1
SUMMARY OF POTENTIAL PROBLEMS RELATED
TO THE HCP VISIT AND RECOMMENDATIONS

Potential Problem	*Recommendation*
Before the Visit	
Patient may fear associated new experiences	Advise caregiver to visit the site prior to the scheduled visit • show the treatment rooms, provide pictures • introduce to the staff • allow exploration • allow rehearsal by staff • provide prescriptions in advance, i.e., antianxiety
Environmental factors may pose barriers to receiving care	Establish an individual patient profile • request from parent or caregiver prior to visit • review prior to the encounter • revise after the encounter
Wait time prior to encounter	Anticipate and mitigate problems • schedule first appointment of the day • complete paperwork ahead of visit • ask for payment /insurance information in advance

Table 3.1–*Continued*

	• advise to call ahead to determine wait time • enter by the rear entrance • designate a quiet waiting place • provide beeper or other notification devices so patient and caregiver may wait in car until called

During the Visit

Compliance	Facilitate rapport • allow parent to maintain close proximity to child • allow use of technology such as iPAD®, DVD, etc. • use support personnel • ensure equipment is ready and out of sight.
Disruptive behaviors caused by common negative triggers such as hunger, boredom, overstimulation	Advise to bring distractors or provide • snacks • technology devices or toys • ear muffs or headsets with music • personal security items • reduce wait time
Unexpected mishaps	Be prepared • have available diapers, wipe-ups • advise parent to bring a change of clothing
Caregiver stress related to HCP visit	Recognize and acknowledge • caregiver stress • need for extra time and special accommodations • need for skilled listening

After the Visit

Lack of consistency and follow-up	Consider the next encounter • encourage parent follow-through on promised rewards/consequences • instruct on timing of follow-up and referrals • chart the effectiveness of recommendations: those were or were not successful

HCP PREPARATION. A quick review before walking in the door, the HCP should remind themselves that individuals with ASD are often concrete thinkers, rigid, like repetition and predictability, may engage in stereotypy, like choices, and need more time to process, especially auditory stimuli (American Psychological Association, 2013; Autism Speaks, 2013; Giarelli et al., 2014; Lytle & Todd, 2009; Souders et al., 2002). The visit will take more time to complete due to the occurrence of behaviors or other factors that could reduce efficiency (Bultas, 2012). Therefore, it is helpful to build in additional time to discuss health concerns and comprehensive, interdisciplinary, integrated care-planning.

ANTECEDENT-BASED INTERVENTION. Referring to the patient-specific profile, the white coat, the necktie, or anything that has been identified as an antecedent resulting in disruptive behavior should be out of sight. Environmental stimuli should be reduced. The door should be closed, and a "do not disturb" sign used if necessary (Scarpinato, Bradley, Kurbjun, Bateman, Holtzer, & Ely, 2010). The parent should be in close proximity to the patient and be consulted on the best mode of communication. The HCP should attempt to make eye contact and connect with the patient before speaking, but not insist. Speech should be clear without abstract terms. The HCP should also wait patiently for responses and not repeat a question, statement, or request multiple times. When possible, the HCP should pair himself/herself with the identified highly preferred items and "share." It is best if initial interactions are playful, nonthreatening, and without demands.

The HCP should state what is going to happen next or use picture schedules (Chebuhar, McCarthy, Bosch, & Baker, 2013). Visual cues alert the patient to a change in activity or a transition coming. Visual schedules can be made from icons or actual pictures from the medical office taken by a smart phone, laminated, and placed on a board with Velcro®. Other resources for creating schedules include Chebuhar and colleagues (2013) literature search on use and benefits, websites: Do 2 Learn, Boardmaker, Google Images, and Autism Speaks Tool Kits that contain helpful tips and icons for blood draws, and dental and vision exams. See Box 3.2 for links to sites with information on using visual supports.

For the patient who can read, a simple white board could list activities of the visit, the steps of a procedure, or for writing questions. Providing a multiple choice of possible answers facilitates a quick response and giving the patient some sense of control by offering choices or allowing them to choose the order of events is beneficial. Devices, such as a charged iPad with WiFi access, are effective tools that many patients with ASD are familiar with or able to quickly adapt to their use. The iPad (with a protective case) could be used for typing a schedule or questions, accessing a popular communication

---

Box 3.2. Links for Visual Supports

Autism Speaks Tool Kits

    http://www.autismspeaks.org/family-services/tool-kits

    Autism Speaks (2013). About Autism: What you need to know.

    http://www.autismspeaks.org/sites/default/files/afyo_about_autism.pdf

Do 2 Learn

    http://www.dotolearn.com/picturecards/howtouse/schedule.htm)

Boardmaker™

    http://www.mayer-johnson.com/products/boardmaker/

Google Images

    https://images.google.com/

---

application, such as Proloquo2Go™, or viewing YouTube videos, can be used to improve compliance or to distract.

Behaviors, whether desirable or maladaptive, are followed by a consequence. A consequence may be positive, negative, or neutral. Combined with an antecedent condition, consequences determine what is learned and affect future behavior. Therefore, the frequency of compliance is determined by the history of consequences (Cooper et al., 2007). A healthcare visit for a patient with ASD is full of demands (antecedents). If the patient responds to a demand appropriately, the behavior is reinforced (consequence). This consequence (reinforcer) increases the frequency of compliance.

REINFORCEMENT FOR SUCCESSFUL ENCOUNTERS. The patient-specific profile has identified the patient's preferences. These preferences should be available to use as rewards or reinforcers. These rewards may have been previewed in the social story and/or a visual schedule. Prior to placing any demands on the patient, the HCP has already established that he/she is the source of their preferred objects by interacting with the patient without placing demands. The HCP can deliver the reinforcers or work in tandem with the parent to establish when the patient complies with a demand, and thus receives the reinforcer. This is also called contingent reinforcement. For some patients, the reinforcer can simply be descriptive praise ("Great job!" or "Way to go!"). For others, it may have to be more tangible, like receiving a preferred item or something edible. Mentioned above, hand-held digital device can be used as a reinforcer, or creatively to assist in the evaluation. For example, by just moving the video screen, an eye gaze can be diverted for a neurological exam, to accomplish a position change, or move the patient to a different location. If distraction is all that is needed, the HCP can use a smart TV or computer capable of accessing websites and videos from YouTube. If ready to play, a remote control can turn the distraction to a reinforcer very quickly. See Figure 3.2 for an illustration.

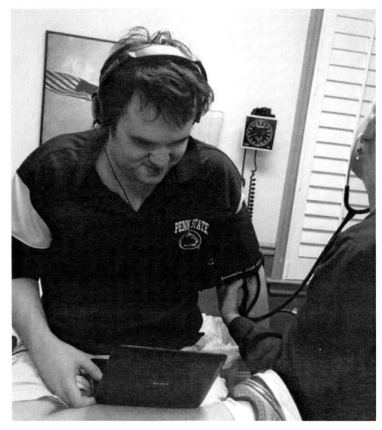

Figure 3.2. Young adult usig a DVD player as a distraction. This picture is printed with permission from the legal guardian. K. Freeman.

MANAGING UNSUCCESSFUL ENCOUNTERS. According to Johnson and Rodriguez's (2013) systematic review, four categories of challenging behaviors emerged for children with ASD in the healthcare setting. These categories were: (1) Noncompliance, (2) hyperactivity, (3) sensory defensiveness/self-stimulatory, and (4) self-injury. The HCP needs to be prepared for behaviors which interfere with completion of the health care visit.

NON-COMPLIANCE. Patients with ASD were reported to have difficulty with cooperation (noncompliance) in healthcare settings, although often not intentional (Johnson & Rodriguez, 2013). Noncompliance can be defined as poor adherence to requests by HCPs or a way for the patient to escape a demand. It can extend to emotional outbursts (Bellando & Lopez 2009) and temper tantrums or behavioral outbursts when patients are asked to comply with instructions related to their health care (Browne, 2006; Lowe, Allen, Jones, Brophy, Moore, & James, 2007; Searcy, 2001; Thorne, 2007). Patients can also exhibit aggression (Golnik & Maccabee-Ryaboy, 2010; Lowe et al., 2007; Skinner, Ng, McDonald, & Walters, 2005); destroy property (such as small items, furniture, fittings, fixtures) (Lowe et al., 2007); and scratch, head butt, bite, punch, and slap others (Souders et al., 2002). Patients with ASD are prone to agitation (Scarpinato et al., 2010) with kicking/yelling and rolling to/on the floor (Gardner, 2011).

Allowing the patient to escape when exhibiting these behaviors reinforces the behaviors and makes it more likely that the patient will try the strategy again when the demands or requests are repeated. Extinction/blocking is a strategy during which the participant is not permitted to escape the current demand. This is typically done through physically guiding the patient to engage in the desired behavior or blocking the patient from escaping (Jennett & Hagopian, 2008). Most parents would prefer that the situation not escalate to the level of requiring a restraint; therefore, it is important to establish a health care visit routine that is positive in which any difficult behavior for the patient has not been rewarded in previous encounters.

HYPERACTIVITY. Hyperactivity and impulsivity are common among people with ASD (Aman, 2004). Young children with ASD may bolt from the exam room, find stray accessible objects without a sense of selection or purpose, and appear to be in constant motion. Those with ASD with verbal skills may display their hyperactivity by pestering (Lowe et al., 2007). The primary concern for the parent with a child who is hyperactive is safety. The environment must be childproof regardless of the patient's age. For the hyperactive patient, a quiet safe area where he/she can pace or even run in an enclosed space is good for the patient and those waiting.

MEDICATIONS. The use of medications are an antecedent-based strategy. When hyperactivity is the target symptom, psychostimulants are considered, but they may not be effective and often produce side effects (Golnik & Maccabee-Ryaboy, 2010). The newer antipsychotics (especially risperidone) seem to be effective for hyperactivity, but their use may be difficult to justify if hyperactivity is the sole target symptom (Aman, 2004).

SENSORY DEFENSIVENESS/SELF-STIMULATORY. Patients with ASD with sensory dysfunction who are overstimulated or understimulated may find solace with self-stimulatory behaviors (Beard-Pfeuffer, 2008). Self-stimulatory behaviors are referred to as automatic reinforcement such that the reinforcement occurs independent of social mediation by others (Cooper, Heron, & Heward, 2007); much like scratching relieves an itch. HCPs should not interrupt self-stimulatory behaviors. Many authors report it to be a way that anxiety is reduced (Browne, 2006; Scarpinato et al., 2010). Parents can readily note the self-stimulatory behavior and advise the HCP on when to initiate a procedure.

SELF-INJURIOUS BEHAVIOR. Self-injurious behavior (SIB) is a bizarre and often chronic form of aberrant behavior. The etiology of which is at best poorly understood (Iwata, Dorsey, Slifer, Bauman, & Richman, 1982). It is a repetitive act directed toward oneself that often results in physical harm. The topography manifests as, but is not limited to, eye-poking/gouging, face slapping, head banging, hand mouthing, hair pulling, self-biting, pinching, scratching, and rubbing (Iwata et al., 1982; Lowe et al., 2007). It may be the result of frustration at being unable to communicate, or attempts to express physical pain, and manifested by slapping or biting a limb that hurts (Inglese, 2009). Improved communication may reduce the likelihood of a SIB. Unfortunately, SIBs, like all undesirable behaviors, can also result from overstimulation, loud noises, smells; or demands placed on a patient who is already experiencing anxiety, has had to wait, and/or does not know what to expect.

All common antecedents, as well as, unknown antecedents can bring a range of behaviors from simple agitation to a complete meltdown. There are times when even the parent does not know why their child exhibits a behavior. The HCP should ask the parent about the history of self-stimulatory and/or SIBs before the visit.

From Pursuing a Cure to Improving the Quality of Life

The lack of simple medical interventions contributes to the frantic search for miracle cures for desperate parents (Silverman & Brosco, 2007). Resolving the myriad issues of comorbidities along with the core symptoms of ASD has prompted parents to seek answers. Ideally this help should come from reputable sources as parents continue to endeavor to relieve the distress they see in their children and reduce the turmoil in the family life. See Table 3.1 for some recommendation on how to deal with problems during the medical visit.

Parents as Advocates

ASD would not be the household word it is today without the efforts of parents. The movement from obscurity to a national health priority has largely been the result of the love, dedication, and commitment parents have for their children with ASD. Silverman and Brosco (2007) investigated the role of parents and advocates in ASD research and treatment over a 50-year span. By reviewing scientific publications and archival sources, they found parents and advocacy groups had (1) organized research funding, (2) assembled clinical research networks, (3) suggested new avenues for research, (4) popularized empirically based therapies, and (5) anticipated the need for paradigmatic shifts necessary in the understanding of ASD. The advocacy will continue to spur efforts to uncover a cause and improve treatments.

In 1965, Bernard Rimland, a father with a son with autism, was at the forefront starting the Autism Society of America. Parents, Eric and Karen London, established the National Alliance for Autism Research (NAAR) in 1994 followed by the start of Cure Autism Now (CAN) in 1995 by Jon Shestak and Portia Iverson, also parents. These organizations were responsible for amassing data and genetic samples from families which eventually led to the Autism Genome Project. Since its creation in 2005 by Bob and Suzanne Wright, grandparents of a child with autism, Autism Speaks has grown into the world's leading ASD science and advocacy organization. The combined efforts of parents over the last 50 years have been instrumental in advancing the science and increasing the funding for ASD research.

Parents have also been the proponents of, and popularized, empirically based therapies. One of the first groundbreaking studies was done by Lovaas in 1987 using applied behavioral analysis (ABA), widely recognized as safe and effective behavioral intervention in ASD. Widespread adoption of ABA techniques came in part from the activism of parents who sought the best treatments for their children, despite the opposition of those who argued their children were untreatable. ABA remains the theory behind many models of intervention used today such as verbal behavior (VB), pivotal response training (PRT), and Early Start Denver Model (ESDM). A 2014 update to the US Agency for Healthcare Research and Quality Report reinforced the overwhelming record of evidence supporting the efficacy of ABA as a beneficial intervention in treating children with ASD (Weitlauf et al., 2014). Parents have been and are already partners in the process.

Conclusion

The supportive HCP is one who acknowledges parents as experts, partners, and advocates. The caring HCP inquires about the requirements of their patients with ASD, and proactively plans and implements strategies that accommodate the unique clinical presentation. The HCP must understand the complex healthcare needs and recognize the impact of ASD on the entire family—emotionally, financially, and physically. As a parent, there is one final word of advice when providing medical care—PEARL. This acronym is easy to remember (see Box 3.3.).

Parents need your patience and time. They have already spent much time preparing for the visit and have been challenged just getting to the exam room. Families face numerous multifaceted challenges every day and may easily collaborate with an empathetic HCP who anticipates the individual needs of the patient being seen and accommodates his or her special needs. Anticipation of these needs increases the likelihood of a positive and efficacious visit. Referring the patient to services provided by Part B or C under IDEA or another specialist is essential when there is a suspicion of a delay or a parent expresses concern. Last, HCPs should listen carefully to parents' concerns and opinions regarding their child.

Box 3.3. A Parent's PEARL

PEARL

P   *Patience* and adequate time allocated

E   *Empathy* for patient and parents

A   *Anticipate* the individualized needs of the patient with accommodations

R   *Refer* early to facilitate conclusive diagnoses and expeditious treatment

L   *Listen* carefully to parent and caregivers who live with the patient

References

Aman, M. G. (2004). Management of hyperactivity and other acting-out problems in patients with autism spectrum disorder. *Seminars in Pediatric Neurology, 11,* 225–228.

American Psychological Association. (2013). *Diagnostic and statistical manual of mental disorders* (5th ed.). Washington, DC: American Psychiatric Association.

Beard-Pfeuffer, M. (2008). Understanding the world of children with autism. *RN, 71*(2), 40–45.

Bellando, J., & Lopez, M. (2009). The school nurse's role in treatment of the student with autism spectrum disorders. *Journal for Specialists in Pediatric Nursing, 14*(3), 173–182.

Browne, M. E. (2006). Communicating with the child who has autistic spectrum disorder: A practical introduction. *Pediatric Nursing, 18*(1), 14–17.

Bultas, M. (2012). The health care experiences of preschool children with autism. *Journal of Pediatric Nursing, 27*(5), 460–470.

Caronna, E. B., Augustyn, M., & Zuckerman, B. (2007). Revisiting parental concerns in the age of autism spectrum disorders. *Archives of Pediatric Medicine, 161*(4), 406–408.

Chebuhar, A., McCarthy, A. M., Bosch, J., & Baker, S. (2013). Using picture schedules in medical settings for patients with an autism spectrum disorder. *Journal of Pediatric Nursing, 28,* 125–134.

Cooper, J. O., Heron, T. E., & Heward, W. L. (2007). *Applied behavior analysis* (2nd ed.). Columbus, OH: Merrill.

Crais, E. R., Watson, L. R., Baranek, G. T., & Resnick, J. S. (2006). Early identification of autism: How early can we go? *Seminars in Speech and Language, 27,* 143–160.

Daniels, A. M., & Mandell, D. S. (2014). Explaining differences in age at autism spectrum diagnosis: A critical review. *Autism, 18*(5), 583–597.

Filipek, P. A., Accardo, P. J., Ashwal, S., Baranek, G. T., Cook, E. H., Dawson, G., ... Volkmar, F. R. (2000). Practice parameter: Screening and diagnosis of autism: Report of the quality standards subcommittee of the American Academy of Neurology and the Child Neurology Society. *Neurology, 55,* 468–79.

Fisher, K., Frazer, C., Hasson, C., & Orkin, F. (2007). A qualitative study of emergency room nurses' perceptions and experiences of caring for individuals with intellectual disabilities in the United States. *International Journal of Nursing in Intellectual and Developmental Disabilities, 3*(1), 1. Available at http://ddna.org/publications/journal/vol-3-issue-1-article-1/

Gabrielsen, T. P., Farley, M., Speer, L., Villalobos, M., Baker, C. N., & Miller, J. (2015). Identifying autism in a brief observation. *Pediatrics, 135*(2), e330–e338.

Gardner, M. R. (2011). Preparing nurses to care for people with developmental disabilities. *Nursing Clinics of North America, 47,* 517–527.

Giarelli, E., Nocera, R., Turchi, R., Hardie, T. L., Pagano, R., & Yuan, C. (2014). Sensory stimuli as to emergency care for children with autism spectrum disorder. *Advanced Emergency Nursing Journal, 36*(2), 145–163.

Glascoe, F. P. (2003). Parents' evaluation of developmental status: How well do parents' concerns identify children with behavioral and emotional problems? *Clinical Pediatrics, 42,* 133–138.

Golnik, A., Ireland, M., & Borowsky, I. W., (2009). Medical homes for children with autism: A physician survey. *Pediatrics, 123*(3), 966–971.

Golnik, A., & Maccabee-Ryaboy, N. (2010). Autism: Clinical pearls for primary care. *Contemporary Pediatrics,* (November) 42–45. Retrieved from http://contemporary pediatrics.modernmedicine.com/contemporarypediatrics/news/modern medicine/modern-medicine-feature-articles/autism-clinical-pearls-

Gray, C. (1994). *The new social story book.* Arlington, TX: Future Horizons.

Harrington, J. W., Patrick, P. A., Edwards, K. S., & Brand, D. A. (2006). Parental beliefs about autism: Implications for the treating physician. *Autism, 10*(5), 452–462.

Howlin, P., & Asgharian, A. (1999). The diagnosis of autism and Asperger syndrome: Findings from a systematic survey. *Developmental Medicine and Child Neurology, 41,* 834–839.

Hudson, J. (2006). *Prescription for success: Supporting children with autism spectrum disorders in the medical environment.* Shawnee Mission, KS: Autism Asperger Publishing.

Hyman, S., & Levy, S. E., (2005). Introduction: Novel therapies in developmental disabilities–Hope, and evidence. *Mental Retardation and Developmental Disabilities Research Reviews, 11*(2), 107–109.

Inglese, M. D. (2009). Caring for children with autism spectrum disorder, part II: Screening, diagnosis, and management. *Journal of Pediatric Nursing, 24*(1), 49–59.

Iwata, B. A., Dorsey, M. F., Slifer, K. J., Bauman, K. E., & Richman, G. S. (1982). Toward a functional analysis of self-injury. *Analysis and Intervention in Developmental Disabilities, 2*(1), 3–20.

Jennett, H. K., & Hagopian, L. P. (2008). Identifying empirically supported treatments for phobic avoidance in individuals with intellectual disabilities. *Behavior Therapy, 39,* 151–161.

Johnson, C. P., Meyers, S. M., & The Council on Children with Disabilities. (2007). Identification and evaluation of children with autism spectrum disorders. *Pediatrics, 120*(5), 1183–1215.

Johnson, N. L., & Rodriguez D. (2013). Children with autism spectrum disorder at a pediatric hospital: A systematic review of literature. *Pediatric Nursing, 39,* 131–141.

Kanner, L. (1949). Problems of nosology and psychodynamics in early infantile autism. *American Journal of Orthopsychiatry, 19*(3), 416–426.

Levy S. E., Mandell, D. S., Merhar, S., Ittenbach, R. F., & Pinto-Martin, J. A. (2003). Use of complementary and alternative medicine among children recently diagnosed with autistic spectrum disorder. *Developmental and Behavioral Pediatrics, 24*(6), 418–423.

Liptak, G. S., Orlando, M., Yingling, J. T., Theurer-Kaufman, K. L., Malay, D. P., Tompkins, L. A., & Flynn, J. R. (2006). Satisfaction with primary health care received by families of children with developmental disabilities. *Journal of Pediatric Health Care, 20*(4), 245–252.

Lovaas, O. I. (1987). Behavioral treatment and normal educational and intellectual functioning in young autistic children. *Journal of Consulting and Clinical Psychology, 55,* 3–9.

Lowe, K., Allen, D., Jones, E., Brophy, S., Moore, K., & James, W. (2007). Challenging behaviours: Prevalence and topographies. *Journal of Intellectual Disability Research, 51*(8), 625–636.

Lytle, R., & Todd, T. (2009). Stress and the student with autism spectrum disorders: Strategies for stress reduction and enhanced learning. *Teaching Exceptional Children, 41*(4), 36–42.

Marshall, J., Sheller, B., Mancl, L., & Williams, B. (2008). Parental attitudes regarding behavior guidance of dental patients with autism. *Pediatric Dentistry, 30,* 400–407.

Ming, X., Brimacombe, M., Chaaban, J., Zimmerman-Bier, B., & Wagner, G. C. (2008). Autism spectrum disorders: Concurrent clinical disorders. *Journal of Child Neurology, 23*(1), 6–13.

Ozonoff, S., Young, G. S., Carter, A., Messinger, D., Yirmiya, N., Zwaigenbaum, L., . . . Stone, W. L. (2011). Recurrence risk for autism spectrum disorders: A Baby Siblings Research Consortium Study. *Pediatrics, 128,* e488–e495.

Robins, D. L., Casagrande, K., Barton, M., Chen, C. M., Dumont-Mathieu, T., & Fein, D. (2014). Validation of the Modified Checklist for Autism in Toddlers, Revised with follow-up (M-CHAT-R/F). *Pediatrics, 133*(1), 37–45.

Rosenberg, R. R., Landa, R. J., Law, J. K., Stuart, E. A., & Law, P. A. (2011). Factors affecting age at initial autism spectrum disorder diagnosis in a national survey. *Autism Research and Treatment, 2011,* 1–11. Article ID 874619.

Sand, N., Silverstein, M., Glascoe, F. P., Gupta, V. B., Tonniges, T. P., & O'Connor, K. G. (2005). Pediatricians' reported practices regarding developmental screening: Do guidelines work? Do they help? *Pediatrics, 116,* 174–179.

Scarpinato, N., Bradley, J., Kurbjun, K., Bateman, X., Holtzer, B., & Ely, B. (2010). Caring for the child with an autism spectrum disorder in the acute care setting. *Journal for Specialists in Pediatric Nursing, 15*(3), 244–254.

Searcy, E. (2001). Helping the patient who has pervasive development disorder. *Journal of the American Academy of Physician Assistants, 14*(10), 44–45.

Shah, K. (2001). What do medical students know about autism? *Autism, 5*(2), 127–133.

Sices, L., Feudtner, C., McLaughlin, J., Drotar, D., & Williams, M. (2003). How do primary care physicians identify young children with developmental delays? A national survey. *Journal of Developmental and Behavioral Pediatrics, 24,* 409–417.

Silverman, C., & Brosco, J. P. (2007). Understanding Autism: Parents and pediatricians in historical perspective. *Archives of Pediatric and Adolescent Medicine, 161*(4), 392–398.

Skinner, S., Ng, C., McDonald, A., & Walters, T. (2005). A patient with autism and severe depression: Medical and ethical challenges for an adolescent medical unit. *Medical Journal of Australia, 183*(8), 422–424.

Souders, M. C., Freeman, K. G., DePaul, D., & Levy, S. E. (2002). Caring for children and adolescents with autism who require challenging procedures. *Pediatric Nursing, 28*(6), 555–562.

Tehee, E., Honan, R., & Hevey, D. (2009). Factors contributing to stress in parents of individuals with autistic spectrum disorders. *Journal of Applied Research in Intellectual Disabilities, 22,* 34–42.

Thorne, A. (2007). Are you ready to give care to a child with autism? *Nursing, 37,* 59–61.

Weitlauf, A. S., McPheeters M. L., Peters, B., Sathe, N., Travis, R., Aiello, R., . . . Warren, Z. (2014). *Therapies for children with autism spectrum disorder: Behavioral interventions update, comparative effectiveness review no. 137.* (Prepared by the Vanderbilt Evidence-based Practice Center under Contract No. 290-2012-00009-I.) AHRQ Publication No. 14-EHC036-EF. Rockville, MD: Agency for Healthcare Research and Quality. www.effectivehealthcare.ahrq.gov/reports/final.cfm.

Wiggins, L. D., Baio, J., & Rice, C. (2006). Examination of the time between first evaluation and first autism spectrum diagnosis in a population-based sample. *Journal of Developmental and Behavioral Pediatrics, 27*(2 Suppl), S79–S87.

Chapter 4

THE IMPACT OF THE SENSORY ENVIRONMENT ON CARE

ELIZABETH PFEIFFER AND LEAH I. STEIN DUKER

Introduction

There are multiple barriers that have the potential to impact the provision of effective health care for individuals with autism spectrum disorders (ASD). Frequently consideration is often given to behavioral characteristics that may impede optimal interactions and the implementation of care, with interventions commonly targeting individual person factors. However, consideration of the potential impact of the sensory environment on patient care should also be taken into account. Best practices in healthcare settings may require interventions aimed at modifying the sensory factors in the physical and social environments.

Individuals with ASD have a significantly higher risk for sensory processing differences across the lifespan (Ben-Sasson et al., 2009; Crane, Goddard, & Pring, 2009; Leekam, Nieto, Libby, Wing, & Gould, 2007; Tavassoli, Miller, Schoen, Nielson, & Baron-Cohen, 2014). These differences can impact behaviors and participation in the health care process. There are a number of interventions that target changing an individual's sensory responses to environmental stimuli, although these often require longer term interventions that are not appropriate or feasible in primary healthcare settings. Therefore, strategies to adapt the sensory features inherent to the health care environment are essential.

Parents of children with ASD have reported dissatisfaction with the primary care their children receive and elevated levels of stress related to obtaining and coordinating health care for their child (Carbone, Behl, Azor, &

Murphy, 2010; Liptak et al., 2006). Interestingly, one study found significantly greater satisfaction when medical care was provided in the home environment, suggesting that environmental factors may contribute to satisfaction with care (Golnik, Scal, Wey, & Gaillard, 2012).

Stimulating environments, such as those found in healthcare settings, can increase anxiety and maladaptive behavioral responses, impacting the ability of healthcare professionals to provide effective care for both children and adults with ASD. Therefore, families and caregivers for individuals with ASD, as well as those with ASD, may avoid or minimize access to health care due to the intense behavioral and emotional responses related to the sensory environment and the elevated anxiety that occurs in these settings. Primary care providers should consider an approach that modifies the environment in order to provide more integrated opportunities and successful health care experiences for individuals with ASD of all ages.

Sensory Processing and Autism Spectrum Disorders

It is well documented that individuals with ASD process sensory stimuli in the environment differently (Baranek, 2002; Ben-Sasson et al., 2009; Crane et al., 2009; Davidson, 2010; Leekam et al., 2007; Perry, Minassian, Lopez, Maron, & Lincoln, 2007; Tomchek & Dunn, 2007), resulting in an impact on behavior and inclusion in a variety of settings, including the health care environment. Prevalence rates of sensory processing differences have varied from 42% to 100% across studies inclusive of individuals across the lifespan with ASD (Baranek, 2002; Talay-Ongan & Wood, 2000; Tomchek & Dunn, 2007), which is significantly greater than their neurotypical peers (Ben-Sasson et al., 2009). A meta-analysis examining sensory processing differences of mostly children and adolescents with ASD, indicated an increase in prevalence in sensory processing differences in individuals with more severe ASD symptomatology (Ben-Sasson et al., 2009).

Sensory processing difficulties can lead to a wide array of responses, including sensory seeking, overresponsivity, and underresponsivity to sensory stimuli, or a combination of these (Ben-Sasson et al., 2009), and can occur across all sensory domains (e.g., visual, auditory, tactile, olfactory, gustatory, vestibular (movement), and proprioception). For example, individuals with overresponsivity may notice stimuli present in daily life more than others, leading to exaggerated and/or aversive responses, that others would consider nonnoxious. Individuals with underresponsivity may not notice or respond to sensory events around them, leading to decreased responses during interactions in their environment, and at times show sensory-seeking behaviors such as self-stimulation. Ultimately, sensory processing differences have the potential to negatively impact daily functioning, social interactions, and participation in the health care process in a variety of ways.

Sensory Processing and Core Symptoms

Physiological research with both children and adults further supports the presence of sensory differences and suggests that sensory abnormalities contribute to some of the core symptoms of ASD. In a review of the literature, such physiological differences were identified in auditory, tactile, visual, and multisensory integration (Marco, Hinkley, Hill, & Nagarajan, 2011). This research suggested that deficits in auditory processing might cause or contribute to the language delays common in ASD, and deficits in visual processing may contribute to challenges in reading faces and emotions. Another study found a positive correlation between level of sensory overresponsivity and activity in areas of the brain responsible for sensory processing, as well as those important for emotion processing and regulation in children/ adolescents with ASD (Green et al., 2013). This may help to explain some of the behavioral responses to sensory stimuli.

Not only does the social-behavioral and physiological research support the presence of significant sensory processing differences in ASD, but there is similar evidence documented in personal accounts in the literature from individuals with ASD. Davidson (2010) compiled information from 45 autobiographical texts written by adults with ASD to identify the barriers to sociospatial inclusion. In their autobiographies, authors wrote at length about how external sensory stimuli was perceived very differently from that of neurotypical (NT) individuals, resulting in a sense of exclusion related to being "out of place in mainstream space" (p. 306). These atypical sensory responses vary from overresponsivity, during which a person is overwhelmed and overloaded by the sensory stimuli in the environment, to underresponsivity, during which a person does not perceive relevant stimuli for the task. Others described difficulty using their senses simultaneously, resulting in sensory confusion as a consequence of exposure to multisensory stimuli that was too intense or too complex to process. Specifically, adults with ASD described the profound impact of certain types of sensory stimuli on their daily lives. For example, one adult identified that fluorescent lights made it difficult to concentrate and think clearly, resulting in mental exhaustion. Another described hearing distracting noises, which were not perceived by others. This same individual reported that certain noises that were not averse to others were painful to his ears.

Problems across the Lifespan

Although the majority of research focusing on sensory processing difficulties has been conducted with pediatric populations, studies support that these issues continue to be problematic in adults with ASD as well. For example, 92% of adults with ASD presented with sensory symptoms in one or more sensory domains on the Diagnostic Interview for Social Communication Disorders, regardless of level of functioning (94% low functioning versus 89% high functioning) (Leekam et al., 2007). Utilizing the Adult/Adolescent Sensory Profile, Crane and colleagues (2009) found that sensory abnormalities were apparent in 94% of adults with ASD. Additionally, this over-responsivity has been reported to be present across all sensory domains (e.g., visual, auditory, tactile, olfactory, gustatory, and proprioceptive) (Tavassoli et al., 2014). Clearly, sensory processing difficulties persist throughout the lifespan in many individuals with ASD. The sensory environment has the potential to serve as a barrier for individuals across the lifespan with ASD in many health care settings. Therefore, as healthcare professionals, we must consider the impact of the sensory environment as a factor in promoting inclusive practices when providing care for individuals on the autisum spectrum.

Sensory Processing and Anxiety in the Health Care Environment

Literature contains reports of an elevated rate of anxiety among individuals with ASD (Gillott & Standen, 2007; Szatmari & McConnell, 2011; White, Oswald, Ollendick, & Scahill, 2009). In a systematic review of 40 articles published between 1990 and 2008, the authors examined the relationship between ASD and anxiety. The results clearly identified an increased prevalence rate for anxiety in children and adolescents with ASD, ranging from 11%–84%; much greater than the prevalence in typically developing individuals (White et al., 2009). Likewise, adults with ASD also experience significantly higher overall anxiety, even as compared to adults with intellectual disabilities not including ASD (Gillott & Standen, 2007). Additionally, literature contains evidence that identifies relationships between types of sensory processing difficulties and increased anxiety, with anxiety in individuals with ASD found to be strongly associated with overresponsivity to sensory stimuli in the environment (Pfeiffer, Kinnealy, Read, & Hertzberg, 2005). Also, a high rate of sensory overresponsivity has been reported in children and adults without ASD who were seeking treatment for anxiety (Conelea, Carter, & Freeman, 2014; Pfeiffer & Kinnealey, 2003).

Although general levels of anxiety are reported to be higher in individuals with ASD, medical visits are a specific event that can result in additional increases in anxiety for this group of patients. For instance, children with

ASD are reported to experience greater fear of medical procedures as compared to typically developing children matched for mental age and chronological age (Evans, Canavera, Kleinpeter, Maccubin, & Taga, 2005). In another study, 18–45% of parents reported that their child with ASD was upset or moderately upset by routine medical procedures such as examining breathing, temperature, ears, and throat (Gillis, Natof, Lockshin, & Romanczyk, 2009). These procedures all have a sensory aspect; breathing is examined with a stethoscope, temperature is assessed with a thermometer, ears with an otoscope, and the throat is examined with a tongue depressor. Interestingly, assessments that involved an intra-oral sensory component (i.e., evaluation of temperature and throat) upset the greatest number of participants (32% and 45%, respectively) and resulted in the greatest prevalence of uncooperative behavior (43% and 45%, respectively) as per parent report (Gillis et al., 2009). Likewise, state-dependent dental anxiety is correlated with parent-report of sensory processing difficulties in children with ASD. These sensory processing difficulties were also associated with uncooperative behavior during routine dental cleanings (Stein, Lane, Williams, Dawson, Polido, & Cermak, 2014).

Sensory Factors in the Health Care Environment

Sensory factors in the environment can act as barriers or facilitators to the access of health care in individuals with ASD. These barriers may include sensory factors in both physical and social environments. Research with individuals with ASD suggests that difficulties with the physical and social environments are associated with maladaptive behaviors (Baker et al., 2008; Lane, Young, Baker, & Angley, 2010), overall levels of anxiety (Gillott & Standen, 2007), and physiological stress and anxiety (Chang et al., 2012; Corbett, Mendoza, Abdullah, Wegelin, & Levine, 2006; Jansen, Gispen-de Wied, van der Gaag, & van Engeland, 2003). An analysis of 45 autobiographical texts by authors with ASD indicates that these "toxic" sensory factors can be overwhelming and impede functioning (Davidson, 2010). These stories offered examples to illustrate the ASD experience and how one may alter the environment to make it more accessible for those with ASD.

White and colleagues (2009) recommended modification of the classroom and social environments for children or adolescents with ASD to decrease stress and anxiety. However, surprisingly little research has been conducted examining the impact of the sensory environment on the function, behavioral distress, and physiological anxiety of people with ASD in a healthcare setting. In the dental office, parent-report of sensory difficulties in children with ASD was found to be associated with greater difficulty providing care, an increase in uncooperative behaviors, and an increase in physiological distress during routine care (Stein, Polido, & Cermak, 2013; Stein et al., 2014). In a subsequent pilot study comparing a sensory-adapted dental environment to a regular dental environment, results indicated that the adapted environment had moderate to large effects of decreasing: Physiological anxiety, self-report of pain, and increasing the number of people required to restrain children with ASD during care (Cermak et al., 2015). Although the aforementioned study has been conducted investigating the impact of adapting the sensory environment for dental care, no additional research currently exists in other healthcare environments.

Sensory Factors in the Physical Environment

Sensory stimuli abound in the physical environment of health care facilities in a variety of modalities (e.g., visual, auditory, tactile, olfactory, gustatory, and vestibular). In fact, healthcare environments are often designed to utilize sensory stimuli (e.g., lighting, acoustics, music, colors, and artwork) to support stress reduction and improve physiological and psychological outcomes for patients, as well as to improve satisfaction for patients, family, and staff (Sherman-Bien, Malcarne, Roesdh, Varni, & Katz, 2011; Ulrich et al., 2008).

For the patient with ASD, stimuli that may be helpful for typically developing individuals may be experienced as overwhelming and produce emotional lability and/or maladaptive behaviors, and thereby impede the patient's ability to interact with the environment in an adaptive and appropriate way (Tomchek, 2010). For example, visual stimuli such as decorations, artwork, and posters promoting proper healthcare procedures provide both education as well as a comfortable and aesthetically pleasing environment, with the intent to increase environmental satisfaction, provide distraction, and diminish stress, anxiety, fear, and pain (Norton-Westwood, 2012; Sherman, Shepley, & Varni, 2005; Ulrich et al., 2008). In contrast, these same posters, artwork, and decorations may create a visually overstimulating environment for the patient with ASD. Similarly, the noises and flickering of the bright fluorescent lights often found in the healthcare environment may be noxious to the patient with ASD. Auditory overresponsivity is frequently reported in people with ASD, yet healthcare environments are rife with noise that can originate from patients, staff, equipment, paging systems, telephones, and even music or TV programs; some of these are essential to care, while some are included to make the environment more comfortable and serve as distractors. Likewise, tactile overresponsivity is common in people with ASD, but multiple tactile stimuli may be encountered during healthcare visits, including touch and texture sensations from material covering chairs and examination tables, latex gloves, hospital gowns, bed sheets, as well as medical staff touching the patient. Distinct olfactory stimuli, which may be perceived as noxious, are frequently found in healthcare settings, often described as "sterile" from the disinfectant and cleaning supplies used. Additionally, body odor, perfume and cologne, smoke, or even smells of food may be irritants to people with ASD.

People with ASD may also be exposed to gustatory stimuli in the healthcare environment. For example, patients may be asked to drink a liquid medication or contrast agent prior to a procedure, which may be unpleasant to neurotypical patients and intolerable to patients with ASD. Lastly, a patient may be exposed to vestibular (movement/head position) stimuli in the medical or dental office as he/she may be placed in a chair that reclines, or is asked to lie down on an examination table. Some individuals with ASD can be sensitive to this type of stimuli, while others may be underresponsive. For those who are overly sensitive, changes in head movement may cause fear, anxiety, distress, or even nausea. These movements are especially threatening when someone else tries to control his/her movement or body position (e.g., when a dentist reclines the dental chair in a healthcare setting) or when asked to assume an unfamiliar position (e.g., climbing up to the examination table and then lying back) (Ayres, 2005).

Sensory Factors in the Social Environment

The social environment in a healthcare setting is complex, with a number of social rules, norms, and expectations. Social aspects of the environment may cause anxiety and distress. Individuals with ASD are reported to experience greater levels of social anxiety than their typically developing peers, but similar to people without ASD diagnosed with social phobia or social anxiety disorder (Cath, Ran, Smit, van Balkom, & Comijs, 2007; White et al., 2009). Sensitivity to sensory stimuli has been linked to anxiety as well as difficulty with social skills in individuals with ASD (Baker et al., 2008; Hilton et al., 2010; Pfeiffer et al., 2005; Pfeiffer & Kinnealey, 2003), which can further exacerbate the challenges in functioning in these complex environments.

SOCIAL DEMANDS. During encounters with healthcare professions across healthcare environments, multiple social demands are placed on individuals with ASD. These social demands may take place in a physical environment where individuals' sensory systems are already stressed or overtaxed, making social interactions even more difficult. In fact, Gillott and Standen (2007) reported a significant correlation between overall level of anxiety and the stress dimension of social and environmental interactions. Research has indicated that the more anxious an individual with autism, the more difficulty he or she will have coping with external demands or stressors, such as those found in a healthcare visit (Gillot & Standen, 2007). Joseph and colleagues (2008) identified that making and maintaining eye contact, a common social requirement in healthcare settings, can activate a sympathetic "fight or flight" nervous system response.

Sensory factors in the physical and social environments can be cumulative, impacting the experience of individuals with ASD. For instance, an individual with auditory processing difficulties may have problems filtering out familiar auditory stimuli, thereby overattending to noises and being distracted by them. For example, such a patient may be unable to draw his or her attention away from the humming of lights, the sound of footsteps in the hallway, or the beeping of a cardiac monitor. Difficulty with sensory aspects of the physical environment may then impact his or her ability to engage in needed *social* interactions with healthcare professionals in order to participate in the therapeutic encounter.

Healthcare visits include time spent in the waiting room, transition to a private room, sitting in a prescribed place for an unidentified amount of time, allowing medical staff to touch you, and following directions upon command. The waiting room may be crowded, with multiple people within it. This waiting period may set the tone for the rest of the visit if the physical and/or social environment is overwhelming. Once in the private office, an individual with ASD is expected to follow directions at the pace of a medical professional (e.g., get on the examination table, open mouth). These directions often require joint attention and multiple steps, which can be difficult for a person with ASD. Additionally, the healthcare setting and staff may be unfamiliar to the person. People with ASD, despite age, commonly experience difficulty coping with change (American Psychiatric Association, 2013). Additionally, children with ASD have also been reported to be less accepting of close proximity to unfamiliar adults (Gessaroli et al., 2014) as well as greater impairments in interactions with (Hauck, Fein, Waterhouse, & Feinstein,1995) and physiological fight or flight responses to unfamiliar adults (Van Hecke et al., 2009). These factors may also play a role in the difficulties experienced during health care visits.

Strategies for People with ASD and Sensory Processing Differences

In order to provide integrated and effective health care to individuals with ASD, it is important to implement strategies that align the unique characteristics of the person with the inherent environmental factors. When designing the person–environment fit, one must consider how a person processes sensory information in the environment and the impact that this has on behavior, interactions, and overall ability to participate in the healthcare process. Although there are interventions that target changes in the way a person processes sensory stimuli, these often require long-term therapies that are not specific to the vastly different but stimulating environments common in healthcare settings. Therefore, strategies to align the needs of the individual and the environment are needed. Three specific types include: Anticipatory, physical, and social strategies to promote inclusive healthcare services for individuals with ASD.

Anticipatory Strategies

The general definition of a strategy is the skill of making or carrying out a plan to achieve a goal. Anticipatory strategies require planning and preparation prior to going into the healthcare environment. Bedell, Cohn, and Dumas (2005) studied participation among children with disabilities. They described anticipatory planning as the "previewing of upcoming events and activities" to develop strategies promoting "positive or negative experiences" (p. 273). The intent of anticipatory strategies is to develop a plan in order to prepare the individual with ASD for the sensory environment including the physical characteristics, expected interactions, and common procedures or assessments, all of which have inherent sensory components. Additionally, anticipatory strategies are considered important in decreasing the anxiety associated with these sensory environments and the overall healthcare environment. These are strategies intended for use prior to the provision of care.

PREDICTABILITY. The perception of control and predictability are identified as two of the most prominent factors linked to anxiety symptoms in individuals with ASD. These factors can protect an individual at risk for anxiety. In contrast, the lack of predictability and perceived control can increase anxiety (Pereira, Barros, & Mendonca, 2012; Zvolensky, Eifert, Lejuez, Hopko, & Forsyth, 2000). This suggests that interventions to reduce anxious responses related to the healthcare setting may require anticipatory strategies that focus on increasing the perceived control and predictability of the typical physical and social sensory environments for individuals with ASD.

Anticipatory strategies prepare the individual, family, and caregivers for the sensory environment where care is provided. These strategies are individualized to the unique characteristics of the setting. A simple but easy to implement strategy to help a person prepare for the healthcare environment is social stories. Social stories allow a person with ASD to predict and anticipate specific situations. A social story can assist the individual with ASD to anticipate common sensory experiences in various healthcare environments, thereby diminishing anxiety.

Research suggests that when properly constructed and visually represented, social stories can create a social understanding and increase adaptive behaviors in challenging situations (Ozdemir, 2010). A caregiver or therapist of the person often develops the social story, although for the purpose of patient care environments, it is suggested that a healthcare professional or staff member provide information about what a patient would typically experience in order for the social story to accurately reflect the unique experiences in that environment. This is necessary as the healthcare professionals and staff best knows the environment, procedures, and interventions within their unique settings and specialties.

ADVANCE PREPARATION. It is highly suggested that the healthcare professional provide informational materials regarding the setting, what to expect, and common practices within their setting specific to the needs to an individual with ASD, not just to help in the development of social stories, but also as a preparatory strategy. This type of preparatory strategy has been reported by both parents and physicians as helpful to improving healthcare procedure success (Davignon, Friedlaender, Cronholm, Paciotti, & Levy, 2014) and may include a simple sheet of frequently asked questions or more extensive materials that provide specific details on the procedures or interventions to be provided. This allows families and caregivers an opportunity to practice and role-play responses that help prepare the individual for the experience. For example, injections are often a necessary procedure implemented in primary care settings. Although many perceive some mild discomfort and anxiety during this common procedure, due to the unique sensory processing responses of an individual with ASD, an injection may be perceived as painful and cause anxiety and, at times, lead to unmanageable behaviors. The ability to role-play the anticipated scenario could desensitize the individual and significantly reduce the likelihood of intense reactions. The person with ASD, who is exposed to social stories and other anticipatory strategies in early childhood and desensitized in childhood, may derive benefits with every healthcare encounter across the lifespan.

VISUAL AIDS. Visual aides are also a commonly used and successful strategy for individuals with ASD to help the person anticipate and prepare. This could include simple pictures or the use of a communication system such as the Picture Exchange Communication System (PECS) (Hart & Banda, 2010) that visually describe the expected procedures and interventions. For example, nurses and physicians completing a physical exam will assess temperature, pulse, and blood pressure. Simple pictures of the sequence of these procedures, illustrating devices to be used could reduce anxiety and maladaptive behaviors that often impact the care provided. Allowing the patient, of any age, to hold and manipulate these devices may also reduce anxiety. A visual communication system such as the PECS not only provides the individual with a method of communication that increases control and reduces anxiety, but allows the person to better communicate and participate in the care process. In fact, in a recent qualitative study, parents strongly endorsed the use of visual communication tools (Davignon et al., 2014).

Physical Strategies: Adaptations and Modifications of the Physical Environment

For individuals with ASD, especially those who exhibit overresponsiveness to sensory stimuli (hypersensitive and/or sensory avoiding), exposure to the built environment of the healthcare setting may itself increase stress and anxiety. As such, altering the physical environment may prevent or diminish this stress and anxiety.

The multisensory environment (MSE) is a built environment designed to create feelings of safety, comfort, relaxation, enjoyment, and social interaction (Fava & Strauss, 2010; Hogg, Cavet, & Smeddle, 2001; Sachs & Nasser, 2009). The MSE aims to achieve these goals by manipulating the "nature, quantity, arrangement, and intensity of sensory stimuli" encountered as the user explores his or her surroundings (Shapiro, Roth, & Marcus, 2011, p. 4). These environments can vary in their appearance, but often consist of a room with equipment designed to stimulate or calm the senses using different sensory modalities, such as: visual (e.g., colored lights, moving projections walls, fiber optics), auditory (e.g., soft, repetitive music of 72 beats per minute [a calm heartbeat]) without sudden changes in tempo), tactile (e.g., weighted blankets, toys, different types of furniture such as beanbag chairs), and olfactory (e.g., aromatherapy scents) stimuli (Shapiro, 2011). See Figure 4.1 for an illustration of a sensory-rich environment.

Sensory adaptations to the physical environment such as these have been used with positive results for a variety of populations including children and adults with developmental disabilities, children and adults with traumatic brain injuries, adults with dementia, individuals in psychiatric programs, patients in a palliative care setting, as well as individuals with chronic pain (Champagne & Stromberg, 2004; Chan, Thompson, Chau, Tam , Chiu, & Lo, 2010; Hotz, Castelblanco, Larea, Weiss, Duncan, & Klutz, 2005; Poza, Gomez, Gutierrez, Mendoza, & Hernero, 2013; Schofield, 2003; Schofield, 2005; Shapiro, 2011). Similar environments have been used for individuals with ASD with positive results in dental offices (Cermak et al., 2015), school settings (Shapiro et al., 2001), residential institutions (Fava & Strauss, 2010), and

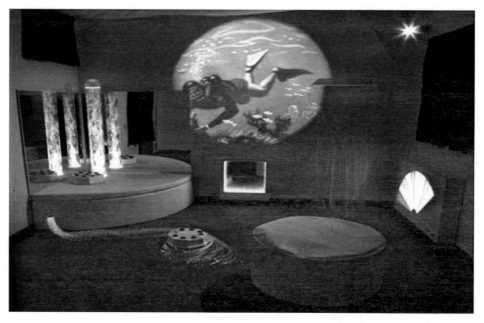

Figure 4.1. A multisensory environment. This exampe includes a darkened room equipped with bubble tubes for vibration and calming, optic fibers for visual stimulation and deep touch pressure, comfortable alternative seating, and visual projections on the wall. Picture provided by Experia USA; retrieved from http://www.experia-usa.com/c-135-sensory-room-packages.aspx.

in a day habilitation program (Kaplan, Clopton, Kaplan, Messbauer, & McPherson, 2006).

A MSE has been used in the rehabilitation units of Memorial Sloan-Kettering Cancer Center and the University of Miami/Jackson Memorial Medical Center, in the psychiatric facilities of Mercy Children's Hospital in Saint Louis and Bridgeport Hospital, part of Yale New Haven Health, as well as for women in labor in the Canadian Osborne Park Hospital. However, in many healthcare settings, private room(s) for the dedicated use of the MSE may not be feasible. Therefore, healthcare professionals, individuals with ASD, and/or their caregivers can utilize individual components of the MSE or simple sensory strategies in order to improve care. Ideally, these adaptations would be selected based on the patient's specific sensory difficulties. Parents and healthcare providers have both reported the importance and success of individualized environmental modifications for children with ASD as well as the required communication with staff to plan for the healthcare encounter (Davignon et al., 2014). See Box 4.1 for sample questions to ask a caregiver and/or individual with ASD to obtain this type of information.

Box 4.1. Questions to Ask Prior to the Visit and Strategies to Adapt Care

1. Are you the individual overresponsive or do you respond different-ly to any of the following sensory stimuli?

   Visual (sight)   Auditory (sound)   Gustatory (taste)
   Olfactory (smell)   Tactile (touch)   Vestibular (movement)

   If yes, what would help make the visit easier for you/the individual based on these responses?
   Examples: Does the individual prefer a dimly lit room? Does the individual prefer quiet or music (which kind)? Do certain tastes both-er your child (only if applicable to the current health care visit)?

2. What is the preferred method of communication for you/the indi-vidual with ASD?

   Nonverbal   Gestures   Single words/phrases
   Sentences   iPad /other Pictures

3. Does eye contact make you/the individual with ASD anxious or upset?
4. Can you/the individual with ASD follow multiple step directions?
5. Do you/the individual with ASD use visual schedules or social sto-ries to complete multiple step procedures or tasks?
6. Has the individual with ASD been to this healthcare environment before?
   a. If yes, what was his/her experience?
   b. Were there are any obvious triggers prior to distress behavior?
   c. If distress behaviors occurred, what strategies were successful to reduce or stop them?
7. Is there anything else we should know prior to the visit that may help us better prepare for a successful visit?

Anticipatory Strategies
To increase predictability of visit:
• Prepare with social story or visual schedule of pictures visually de-scribing expected procedures and/or interventions. Can the individ-ual's therapist or caregiver create this story with guidance from the healthcare professionals? Does the healthcare setting have generic social stories or visual schedules to provide to families (e.g., "Getting a check-up at the doctor," "Getting my teeth cleaned at the dentist").

continued

Box 4.1–*Continued*

- Practice visit (role play at home or, with permission, go to actual health care office). Schedule healthcare visits with the same healthcare professionals, located in the same room, and at the same time of day.

At the Healthcare Visit

Modify/adapt sensory stimuli encountered:
- Schedule appointment to be first or last of the day (quieter/less crowded)
- Minimize sensory stimuli: Sunglasses, headphones, warning before touch; speak with a clear, calm, and quiet voice, etc.
- Utilize calming sensory stimuli: Weighted blankets, calming music, etc.

To increase predictability of visit and perceived control:
- Use a visual timer
- Follow steps laid out in a visual schedule or social story
- Give choices during visit

DIMINISHING STIMULI. To diminish stimuli already present in the environment, visual adaptations would include dimming of lights or use of natural light windows instead of fluorescent lights. Additionally, if willing, individuals with ASD could wear sunglasses to decrease the brightness of the healthcare environment. Auditory adaptations would include providing a hat with ear covers, earmuffs, or noise-attenuating headphones to diminish surrounding noise. Patients and/or family caregivers should also be encouraged to bring their own devices, with which the individual with ASD is already familiar.

To diminish noxious tactile stimuli, the individual with ASD, or their caregiver, could be encouraged to bring a preferred blanket upon which the individual could sit during their visit. Touch coming from the healthcare provider should be delivered slowly and after preparatory activities (e.g., "tell, show, do"). For olfactory stimuli, most of which cannot be altered (e.g., disinfectant used for cleaning), staff should be encouraged to not wear perfume or cologne to help minimize extraneous olfactory stimuli in the environment or appointments could be scheduled not immediately following facility cleaning. Giving individuals with ASD a choice of tastes is helpful to mitigate the negative effects of unpleasant or unexpected gustatory stimuli. For example, a dentist or dental assistant could allow individuals to choose the cherry, orange, or tasteless cleaning product in order to make the choice perceived as the least noxious by that person. Lastly, for an individual who is overresponsive to vestibular (movement) stimuli, an individual with ASD could be asked to lay down on an already reclined chair, similar to the bed he or she has at home.

These strategies have the potential to be successful with individuals with ASD across the lifespan, taking into consideration that individualization and application of appropriate strategies is important for success. For example, tactile, vibratory, and visual adaptations were made for an adult with ASD during his stay in the intensive care unit to minimize distress and decrease sedation (Hsieh, Oh, Chellappa, Szeftel, & Jones, 2014). As stated above, communication with the individual with ASD and/or a caregiver can facilitate appropriate adaptation choices (see Box 4.1 for sample questions).

Moreover, adaptations that provide calming sensations in the environment include visual stimuli such as bubble tubes, fiber optic light sprays, or even an aquarium. Auditory stimuli could include soft, slow music such as nature/classical music or a sound machine. Tactile stimuli could include beanbag style chairs that would mold to the individual's body and provide tactile input, weighted blankets or lap pads, or vibrating pillows. Aromatherapy scents such as lavender could be introduced as a calming olfactory stimulus; however, these smells may be noxious to some individuals with ASD while calming to others, so they should be used sparingly. In regard to vestibular input, rocking chairs could be introduced to the healthcare environment, as slow linear movement can be calming. Lastly, we would like to emphasize the importance of the environment not only of the healthcare office, but also of the waiting room. Many of these adaptations (dim lighting, aquarium, calming music, bean bag or rocking chairs, specific aromatherapy scents) can also be helpful for those with ASD immediately prior to their healthcare visit.

The majority of the previous discussion relates to individuals who exhibit over-responsiveness to sensory stimuli. However, some individuals exhibit underresponsivity to stimuli and others a mixed representation of over- and underresponsivity; these individuals may require individualized adaptations. Additionally, professionals who care for individuals with ASD understand that each person is unique and the above strategies must be individualized before implemented and then systematically evaluated for effectiveness.

Social Strategies

Social strategies target the sensory factors that are commonly part of interactions within the healthcare environment. The sensory factors associated with the social environment in healthcare settings are often overwhelming and threatening for an individual with ASD. It is common for physical touch to be part of most medical interactions, which is distressing for an individual with over-responsivity to tactile (touch) input and can negatively impact his or her ability to attend to other, more pertinent, stimuli. There is a great deal of "sensory clutter," additional irrelevant sensory stimuli, in healthcare settings. Individuals with ASD have difficulty distinguishing relevant from irrelevant information in stimulating environments, resulting in the inability to attend to those interactions that are part of their individual care. An individual might need to process the auditory input of what a health care provider is saying while blocking out other multiple sources of auditory stimuli in the healthcare environment. There is also the need to visually interpret non-verbal communication and process multisensory stimuli throughout the communication process. These are challenging and complex tasks for people with sensory processing differences.

ADJUSTING THE INTERACTION. Social strategies often focus on the methods of interactions and the environment in which these interactions occur. For example, modifying the tone and volume of one's voice when talking to a patient with ASD might help him better process this auditory information. A healthcare provider may change the way in which they interact with the person physically. It is common for touch to occur when interacting with another person, especially when examining a patient. The amount of physical contact can be minimized for a person who is overly sensitive, or the type of touch can be changed. For a person with sensory over-responsivity, deep pressure touch is often perceived as less aversive than light touch. Some of the previous anticipatory and physical strategies discussed can also help improve the social environment for a person with ASD. For example, modifying the physical environment so that there is not as much competing sensory clutter can help the person better understand and process information conveyed verbally. Another example is preparing the individual for the touch associated with the social interaction in a procedure through either verbal or visual communication methods.

Educating Health Professions

It is essential that education for healthcare providers include information specifically about individuals with ASD, both during their initial training as well as throughout on-going continuing education. Healthcare providers need to have an understanding of the unique needs of individuals with ASD and knowledge of the evidence supporting best practices in order to provide integrated and effective health care for this population. This includes an understanding of the sensory needs and responses to stimuli in the health care environment that may impact the behavior and involvement of the individual with ASD during health care encounters. Swiezy, Stuart, and Korzekwa (2008) proposed levels of learning necessary for effective training of professionals working with individuals with ASD. These included entry-level learning experiences focused on awareness, traditional instruction at universities, as well as more specific learning experiences through workshops and observations.

It is highly suggested that hands-on experiences, mentoring, and coaching be included as components of training individuals working directly with those with ASD. Instructional workshops, observations, and hands-on practicums will allow the professional to observe first-hand the potential impact the sensory environment has on individuals with ASD. With the addition of mentor knowledge and suggestions, these experiences have high potential to lead to the application of strategies to modify the sensory factors present in the physical and social healthcare environments.

A process to screen patients for sensory processing difficulties may help the healthcare professional to plan the best approach to engaging the person during the healthcare encounter, as well as to reduce anxiety and maladaptive behaviors that interfere with therapeutic rapport. Physicians recently reported that "knowing the individual child's needs and challenges aids in preparation" prior to health care encounters and procedures (Davignon et al., 2014, pp. 210). See Box 4.1.

This could include a basic sensory screening completed upon intake to understand the sensory processing needs of the individual. The Short Sensory Profile (SSP) (Dunn, 1999) and Sensory Processing Measure (SPM) (Parham & Ecker, 2007) are quick parent-report screening measures to assess the behavioral responses to sensory stimuli in the environment. Both tools are available for pediatric age ranges (e.g., SSP for ages 3–10 years, SPM for ages 2–12 years) and are easily included in the intake paperwork traditionally completed by families/caregivers. The Adolescent/Adult Sensory Profile (Brown & Dunn, 2002) is an additional resource that is completed by the individual with ASD 11 years of age and older, if able, in order to provide similar information.

Another important area of consideration is communication and interactions styles. Researchers have identified challenges in multisensory processing as a common characteristic of individuals with ASD (Ben Sasson et al., 2009; Davidson, 2010; Marco et al., 2011). These characteristics warrant the modification of communication styles when interacting with this patient population. Communicating with a clear and quiet voice in a room adapted to minimize sensory stimuli may enhance comprehension of verbal communication for the individual with ASD. Another individual may benefit from the use of visual aids to assist with comprehension throughout the care process. Although modifications in communication styles may be necessary, it is especially important to communicate what will happen to the individual throughout the care process in order to enhance the perceived control and predictability for the person, which then helps to reduce anxious and maladaptive responses. For instance, preparing a person with significant tactile over-responsivity for the tactile stimuli associated with common medical exams and interventions could make the difference and allow for a successful interaction and the ability to provide effective care.

Conclusion

Individuals with ASD have unique sensory differences that can pose barriers to the effective provision of healthcare services. Interventions and strategies targeting the sensory factors in both the physical and social environments are important to consider prior to and throughout the care process. Anticipatory strategies such as social stories, pre-prepared materials, and preparatory activities can help increase the predictability and perceived control in potentially over-stimulating healthcare environments in order to reduce anxious responses. Physical strategies include adaptations and modifications of the physical environment to reduce distressing sensory stimuli or enhance calming sensory stimuli. Social strategies include adapting methods of communication and interactional styles to facilitate the successful interactions and increase participation of individuals with ASD in the care process. Finally, educating professionals about the unique sensory needs of individuals with ASD is essential for the successful provision of care.

There is a well-developed area of research identifying the sensory differences in individuals with ASD and a separate but emerging area of research on the provision of health care for individuals with ASD. There is a need for research to better understand the impact of sensory environmental factors from both the perspective of the healthcare provider, and more importantly from that of the patient. Additionally, there is a need for interdisciplinary research identifying effective interventions that target the sensory environment barriers to care for individuals with ASD. For additional resources see Box 4.2.

Box 4.2. Resources

- About Sensory Processing Disorder (Sensory Processing Disorder Foundation): http://spdfoundation.net/about-sensory-processing -disorder.html
- Dental Professionals' Tool Kit for Treating Children with ASD (Autism Speaks, Autism Treatment Network, Autism Intervention Research Network on Physical Health): http://www.autismspeaks .org/science/resources-programs/autism-treatment-network/tools -you-can-use/dental
- Taking the Work Out of Blood Work: Helping Your Patient with Autism–A Provider's Guide (Autism Speaks, Autism Treatment Network, Autism Intervention Research Network on Physical Health): http://www.autismspeaks.org/science/resources-programs/autism-treatment-network/tools-you-can-use/blood-draw-toolkits
- Visual Supports and Autism Spectrum Disorders (Autism Speaks, Autism Treatment Network): http://www.autismspeaks.org/science /resources-programs/autism-treatment-network/tools-you-can-use /visual-supports
- Center for Autism & Related Disabilities at University of South Florida (specifically the links for (1) Autism & The Hospital Emergency Room, (2) Your Next Patient has Autism): http://card-usf.fmhi.usf .edu/resources/materials/health.html
- HANDS in Autism–Interdisciplinary Training and Resource Center (Indiana University School of Medicine): https://handsinautism .iupui.edu/medical.html
- ASD Services Toolkits and Resources: http://autismscience foundation.org/sites/default/files/Autism%20Toolkits.pdf

References

American Psychiatric Association. (2013). *Diagnostic and statistical manual of mental disorders* (5th ed.). Washington, D.C.: American Psychiatric Association.

Ayres, A. J. (2005). Disorders involving the vestibular system: The sense of movement and how it influences the development of many skills. In *Sensory integration and the child: Understanding hidden sensory challenges* (pp. 61–85). California: Western Psychological Services.

Baker, A. E. Z., Lane, A., Angley, M. T., & Young, R. I. (2008). The relationship between sensory processing patterns and behavioural responsiveness in autistic disorder: A pilot study. *Journal of Autism and Developmental Disorders, 38,* 867–875.

Baranek, G. T. (2002). Efficacy of sensory and motor interventions for children with autism. *Journal of Autism & Developmental Disorders, 32,* 397–422.

Bedell, G. M., Cohn, E. S., & Dumas, H. M. (2005). Exploring parents' use of strategies to promote social participation of school-age children with acquired brain injuries. *American Journal of Occupational Therapy, 59,* 273–284.

Ben-Sasson, A., Hen, L., Fluss, R., Cermak, S., Engel-Yeger, B., & Gal, E. (2009). A meta-analysis of sensory modulation symptoms in individuals with autism spectrum disorders. *Journal of Autism & Developmental Disorders, 39,* 1–11.

Brown, C., & Dunn, W. (2002). *Adolescent/adult sensory profile user's manual.* San Antonio, TX: Psychological Corporation.

Carbone, P. S., Behl, D. D., Azor, V., & Murphy, N. A. (2010). The medical home for children with autism spectrum disorders: Parent and pediatrician perspectives. *Journal of Autism & Developmental Disorders, 40,* 317–324.

Cath, D. C., Ran, N., Smit, J. H., van Balkom, A. J. L. M., & Comijs, H. C. (2007). Symptom overlap between autism spectrum disorder, generalized social anxiety disorder and obsessive-compulsive disorder in adults: A preliminary case-controlled study. *Psychopathology, 41,* 101–110.

Cermak, S. A., Stein Duker, L. I., Williams, M. E., Dawson, M. E., Lane, C. J., & Polido, J. C. (2015). Sensory adapted dental environments to enhance oral care for children with autism spectrum disorders: A randomized controlled pilot study. *Journal of Autism & Developmental Disorders, 45,* 2876–2888.

Champagne, T., & Stromberg, N. (2004). Sensory approaches in inpatient psychiatric settings: Innovative alternatives to seclusion and restraint. *Journal of Psychiatric Nursing, 42*(9), 3544.

Chan, S. W., Thompson, D. R., Chau, J. P. C., Tam, W. W. S., Chiu, I. W. S., & Lo, S. H. S. (2010). The effects of multisensory therapy on behaviour of adult clients with developmental disabilities–A systematic review. *International Journal of Nursing Studies, 47,* 108–122.

Chang, M. C., Parham, L. D., Blanche, E. I., Schell, A., Chou, C., Dawson, M., & Clark, F. (2012). Autonomic and behavioral responses of children with autism to auditory stimuli. *American Journal of Occupational Therapy, 66,* 567–576.

Conelea, C. A., Carter, A. C., & Freeman, J. B. (2014). Sensory over-responsivity in a sample of children seeking treatment for anxiety. *Journal of Developmental and Behavioral Pediatrics, 35,* 510–521.

Corbett, B. A., Mendoza, S., Abdullah, M., Wegelin, J. A., & Levine, S. (2006). Cortisol circadian rhythms and response to stress in children with autism. *Psychoneuroendocrinology, 31,* 59–68.

Crane, L., Goddard, L., & Pring, L. (2009). Sensory processing in adults with autism spectrum disorders. *Autism, 13,* 215–228.

Davidson, J. (2010). 'It cuts both ways': A relational approach to access and accommodation for autism. *Social Science & Medicine, 70,* 305–312.

Davignon, M. N., Friedlaender, E., Cronholm, P. F., Paciotti, B., & Levy, S. E. (2014). Parent and provider perspectives on procedural care for children with autism spectrum disorders. *Journal of Developmental & Behavioral Pediatrics, 35,* 207–215.

Dunn, W. (1999). *The sensory profile: User's manual.* San Antonio, TX: Psychological Corporation.

Evans, D. W., Canavera, B. S., Kleinpeter, F. L., Maccubbin, E., & Taga, K. (2005). The fears, phobias, and anxieties of children with autism spectrum disorders and Down syndrome: Comparisons with developmentally and chronologically age-matched children. *Child Psychiatry and Human Development, 36,* 3–24.

Fava, L., & Strauss, K. (2010). Multi-sensory rooms: Comparing effects of the Snoezelen and the stimulus preference environment on the behavior of adults with profound mental retardation. *Research in Developmental Disabilities, 31,* 160–171.

Gessaroli, E., Santelli, E., di Pellegrino, G., & Frassinetti, F. (2013). Personal space regulation in childhood autism spectrum disorders. *PLoS ONE, 8*(9), e74959.

Gillis, J. M., Natof, T. H., Lockshin, S. B., & Romanczyk, R. G. (2009). Fear of routine physical exams in children with autism spectrum disorders: Prevalence and intervention effectiveness. *Focus on Autism and Other Developmental Disabilities, 24,* 156–168.

Gillott, A., & Standen, P. J. (2007). Levels of anxiety and sources of stress in adults with autism. *Journal of Intellectual Disabilities, 11,* 359–370.

Golnik, A., Scal, P., Wey, A., & Gaillard, P. (2012). Autism-specific primary care medical home intervention. *Journal of Autism & Developmental Disorders, 42,* 1087–1093.

Green, S. A., Rudie, J. D., Colich, N. L., Wood, J. J., Shirinyan, D., Hernandez, . . . Bookheimer, S. Y. (2013). Overreactive brain responses to sensory stimuli in youth with autism spectrum disorders. *Journal of the American Academy of Child and Adolescent Psychiatry, 52,* 1158–1172.

Hart, S., & Banda, D. R. (2010) Picture exchange communication system with individuals with developmental disabilities: A meta-analysis of single subject studies. *Remedial and Special Education, 31*(6), 476–488.

Hauck, M., Fein, D., Waterhouse, L., & Feinstein, C. (1995). Social initiations by autistic children to adults and other children. *Journal of Autism & Developmental Disorders, 25,* 579–595.

Hilton, C. L., Harper, J. D., Holmes Kueker, R., Runzi Lang, A., Abbacchi A. M., Todorov, A., & LaVesser, P. D. (2010). Sensory responsiveness as a predictor of social severity in children with high functioning autism spectrum disorders. *Journal of Autism & Developmental Disorders, 40,* 937–945.

Hogg, J., Cavet, J., Lambe, L., & Smeddle, M. (2001). The use of 'Snoezelen' as multisensory stimulation with people with intellectual disabilities: A review of the research. *Research in Developmental Disabilities, 22,* 353–372.

Hotz, G. A., Castelblanco, A., Lara, I. M., Weiss, A. D., Duncan, R., & Klutz, J. W. (2006). Snoezelen: A controlled multi-sensory stimulation therapy for children recovering from severe brain injury. *Brain Injury, 20*(8), 879–888.

Jansen, L. M. C., Gispen-de Wied, C. C., van der Gaag, R., & van Engeland, H. (2003). Differentiation between autism and multiple complex developmental disorder in response to psychosocial stress. *Neuropsychopharmacology, 28,* 582–590.

Joseph, R. M., Ehrman, K., McNally, R., & Keehn, B. (2008). Affective response to eye contact and face recognition ability in children with ASD. *Journal of the International Neuropsychological Society, 14,* 947–955.

Kaplan, H., Clopton, M., Kaplan, M., Messbauer, L., & McPherson, K. (2006). Snoezelen multi-sensory environments: Task engagement and generalization. *Research in Developmental Disabilities, 27,* 443–455.

Lane, A. E., Young, R. L., Baker, A. E. Z., & Angley, M.T . (2010). Sensory processing subtypes in autism: Association with adaptive behavior. *Journal of Autism and Developmental Disorders, 40,* 112–122.

Leekam, S. R., Nieto, C., Libby, S. J., Wing, L., & Gould, J. (2007). Describing the sensory abnormalities of children and adults with autism. *Journal of Autism & Developmental Disorders, 37,* 894–910.

Liptak, G. S., Orlando, M., Yingling, J. T., Theurer-Kaufman, K. L., Malay, D. P., Tompkins, L. A., & Flynn, J. R. (2006). Satisfaction with primary health care received by families of children with developmental disabilities. *Journal of Pediatric Health Care, 20,* 245–252.

Marco, E. J., Hinkley, L. B. N., Hill, S. S., & Nagarajan, S. S. (2011). Sensory processing in Autism: A review of physiological findings. *Pediatric Research, 69,* 48–54.

Norton-Westwood, D. (2012). The health-care environment through the eyes of a child–Does it soothe or provoke anxiety? *International Journal of Nursing Practice, 18,* 7–11.

Ozdemir, S. (2010). Social stories: An intervention technique for children with autism. *Procedia Social and Behavioral Sciences, 5,* 1827–1830.

Parham, L. D., & Ecker, C. (2007). *Sensory processing measure: Home edition.* Torrance, CA: WPS.

Pereira, A. I. F., Barros, L., & Mendonca, D. (2012). Perceived control and anxiety in Portuguese children. *Spanish Journal of Psychology, 15,* 631–637.

Perry, W., Minassian, A., Lopez, B., Maron, L., & Lincoln, A. (2007). Sensorimotor gating deficits in adults with autism. *Biological Psychiatry, 61,* 482–486.

Pfeiffer, B., & Kinnealey, M. (2003). Treatment of sensory defensiveness in adults. *Occupational Therapy International, 10,* 175–184.

Pfeiffer, B., Kinnealey, M., Reed, C., & Herzberg, G. (2005). Sensory modulation and affective disorders in children and adolescents with Asperger's disorder. *American Journal of Occupational Therapy, 59,* 335–345.

Poza, J., Gomez, C., Gutierrez, M. T., Mendoza, N., & Hornero, R. (2013). Effects of a multi-sensory environment on brain-injured patients: Assessment of spectral patterns. *Medical Engineering & Physics, 35,* 365–375.

Sachs, D., & Nasser, K. (2009). Facilitating family occupations: Family member perceptions of a specialized environment for children with mental retardation. *The American Journal of Occupational Therapy, 63*(4), 453–462.

Schofield, P. (2003). A pilot study into the use of a multi-sensory environment (Snoezelen) within a palliative day-care setting. *International Journal of Palliative Nursing, 9,* 124–129.

Schofield, P. A. (2005). A pilot study comparing environments in which relaxation is taught: Investigating the potential of Snoezelen for chronic pain management. *American Journal of Recreation Therapy, 4,* 17–27.

Shapiro, M., Roth, D., & Marcus, A. (2001). The effect of lighting on the behavior of children who are developmentally disabled. *Journal of International Special Needs Education, 4,* 19–23.

Shapiro, M. (2011). *Beit Issie Shapiro's approach to multi-sensory environments (Snoezleen): A handbook for practitioners.* Israel: Rotem Publishing & Productions LTD.

Sherman, S. A., Shepley, M. M., & Varni, J. W (2005). Children's environments and health-related quality of life: Evidence informing pediatric healthcare environmental design. *Children, Youth and Environments, 15,* 186–223.

Sherman-Bein, S. A., Malcarne, V. L., Roesch, S., Varni, J. W., & Katz, E. R. (2011). Quantifying the relationship among hospital design, satisfaction, and psychosocial functioning in a pediatric hematology-oncology inpatient unit. *Herd Journal, 4*(4), 34–59.

Stein, L. I., Polido, J. C., & Cermak, S. A. (2013). Oral care and sensory over-responsivity in children with autism spectrum disorders. *Pediatric Dentistry, 35,* 230–235.

Stein, L. I., Lane, C. J., Williams, M. E., Dawson, M. E., Polido, J. C., & Cermak, S. A. (2014). Physiological and behavioral stress and anxiety in children with autism spectrum disorders during routine oral care. *BioMed Research International,* epub Article ID 6948 76.

strategy. (n.d.). In *Merriam-Webster's online dictionary* (11th ed.). Retrieved from: www.merriam-webster.com/dictionary/strategy

Swiezy, N., Stuart, M., & Korzekwa, P. (2008). Bridging for success in autism: Training and collaboration across medical, education, and community systems. *Child and Adolescent Psychiatric Clinics of North America, 17,* 907–922.

Szatmari, P., & McConnell, B. (2011). Anxiety and mood disorders in individuals with autism spectrum disorder. In D. G. Amaral, G. Dawson, & D. H. Geschwind (Eds.), *Autism spectrum disorders* (pp. 330–338). New York: Oxford University Press.

Talay-Ongan, A., & Wood, K. (2000). Unusual sensory sensitivities in autism: A possible crossroads. *International Journal of Disability, Development and Education, 47,* 201–212.

Tavassoli, T., Miller, L. J., Schoen, S. A., Nielsen, D. M., & Baron-Cohen, S. (2014). Sensory over-responsivity in adults with autism spectrum disorder. *Autism, 18,* 428–432.

Tomchek, S. D. (2010). Sensory processing in individuals with an autism spectrum disorder. In H. Miller-Kuhaneck, & R. Watling (Eds.), *Autism: A comprehensive occupational therapy approach* (3rd ed., pp. 135–162). Maryland: AOTA Press.

Tomchek, S. D., & Dunn, W. (2007). Sensory processing in children with and without autism: A comparative study using the Short Sensory Profile. *American Journal of Occupational Therapy, 61,* 190–200.

Ulrich, R. S., Zimring, C., Zhu, X., DuBose, J., Seo, H., Choi, Y., . . . Joseph, A. (2008). A review of the research literature on evidence-based healthcare design. *Health Environments Research and Design Journal, 1,* 61–125.

Van Hecke, A. V., Lebow, J., Bal, E., Lamb, D., Harden, E., Kramer, A., . . . Porges, S. W. (2009). Electroencephalogram and heart rate regulation to familiar and unfamiliar people in children with autism spectrum disorders. *Child Development, 80,* 1118–1133.

White, S. W., Oswald, D., Ollendick, T., & Scahill, L. (2009). Anxiety in children and adolescents with autism spectrum disorder. *Clinical Psychology Review, 29,* 216–229.

Zvolensky, M. J., Eifert, G. H., Lejuez, C. W., Hopko, D. R., & Forsyth, J. P. (2000). Assessing the perceived predictability of anxiety-related events: A report on the perceived predictability index. *Journal of Behaviour Therapy, 31,* 201–218.

Chapter 5

MEDICATIONS FOR THE TREATMENT
OF THE PSYCHIATRIC COMORBIDITIES

PAUL A. KETTL

Few sets of data in public health are as astonishing as the growth of the diagnosis of autism spectrum disorders (ASD). When Leo Kanner, the first chief of child psychiatry at Johns Hopkins University, described the syndrome in the 1940s in his largely affluent set of young Caucasian patients, it was thought to be a relatively rare disorder. However, his descriptions and those that followed, initiated the knowledge base of the condition, and ASD became increasingly better described and recognized. ASD is a neurodevelopmental disorder of unknown etiology, which impacts an individual's cognition, emotional regulation, and causes problems in communication and social interactions. The severity on one's impairment varies widely across individuals with ASD and its effects are present across the lifespan (Roux, Shattuck, Rast, Rava, & Anderson, 2015).

While ASD has become better-recognized and diagnosed, pharmacotherapeutic treatments for the disorder have limited effectiveness. Current approaches to pharmacotherapy are borrowed from the treatment of other disorders, but the lack of a clear idea about the etiology of the disorder hampers a fuller exploration of treatment.

This chapter consists of three sections. The first section includes the prevalence of comorbid mental health conditions in ASD in an effort to set the background for treatment. The second section contains a review of the current range of medications used in treatment protocols. Finally, the third section outlines the new, investigational approaches and hopes for the treatment of ASD.

Introduction

The etiology of ASD is unknown for the more than 3.5 million Americans with an ASD (Ostrow, 2014). Genetics is believed to play a role in its development, but the rise in the numbers of individuals diagnosed with ASD cannot be attributed to genetics, alone. A population based survey conducted in Sweden of more than two million children born between 1982 and 2006 showed that in the sample, 14,416 children, were diagnosed with ASD, representing 0.07% of the total sample (Sandin et al., 2014). This is a much lower prevalence than hypothesized, as heritability of ASD in this group was postulated to be about 50% (Sandin et al., 2014). Recent studies have associated the age of the parent at conception with ASD in the child, such that incidence increases with parental age. In a review of over 400,000 Swedish children, increasing maternal and paternal age appeared to be a risk factor for ASD (Idring et al., 2014). Therefore, other factors, perhaps environmental, or development must be examined and much more research is needed to address the lifelong health, mental health, and service needs of persons with an ASD.

Comorbid Mental Health Conditions in ASD

Higher rates of psychiatric comorbidity are reported in persons with ASD compared to those in the general population, in national and international studies (Berjerot, Eriksson, & Mortberg, 2014; Garcia-Villamisar & Rohahn, 2015; Roux et al., 2015). The comorbid psychiatric conditions considered most relevant by ASD researchers include: Anxiety disorders, attention-deficit disorder (ADD), attention-deficit with hyperactivity disorder (ADHD), obsessive-compulsive disorders (OCD), and depression and mood disorders (Garcia-Villamisar & Rohahn, 2015; Roux et al., 2015).

Multiple comorbidities were identified (i.e., at least two health or mental health conditions) in 60% of youth ages 15–17 years, based on the 2011 nationwide survey, Pathways to Diagnosis and Services (Pathways) (Roux et al., 2015). Researchers found incidence of: ADD/ADHD (53%), anxiety (51%), behavioral problems (37%), depression (24%), and seizure disorder (13%), among 15–17 year olds with ASD. Not surprising were high rates of polypharmacy, and respondents (77%) consumed one or more medications routinely, which did not include vitamins. Antianxiety agents and mood stabilizers (40%), stimulants (31%), antidepressants (31%), antipsychotics (20%), and antiseizure (16%) drugs were used on a daily basis (Roux et al., 2015).

Research in ASD

Research in comorbid mental health disorders typically excludes non-verbal individuals, who are lower functioning. In addition, ASD research studies are skewed toward children and youth, hence, we know less about mental health concerns in adults with ASD. The dearth of studies and/or routinely updated useful indicators reporting on the health, mental health, service access and experiences of individuals with ASD is problematic and researchers report, "virtually ends at the age of 25" (Roux et al., 2015, p. 65).

A systematic review of published research on psychiatric comorbidity for the years 2000–2011 (Mazzone, Ruta, & Reale, 2012) identified 26 separate studies that explored depression and bipolar mood disorders, anxiety disorders, OCD, and ADHD in individuals with Asperger syndrome (AS) and high-functioning ASD. Fifty percent of the 26 studies utilized comparison or control group designs, and the majority of studies (73%) included children and adolescents between the ages of 6–19 years. There was only one study that explored anxiety and depression in young adults, i.e., between the ages of 23–30 years (Mazzone et al., 2012). Clearly, more research is needed, especially studies of psychiatric comorbidities in adults with ASD.

Mental Health Diagnostic Challenges in ASD

Diagnostic challenges for mental health disorders also exist, including appropriate utilization of psychometric tools and symptom presentations of psychopathology that may be expressed differently in persons with ASD as compared to the general population. An individual with ASD, for example, may have difficulty with internal reflection, have challenges with expressive communication, have difficulty making eye contact, have impaired cognitive and poor verbal abilities, resulting in the clinician's need to rely on observable behavior versus subjective reports of symptoms. Often a diagnosis of psychiatric disorders remains dependent on obtaining information about an individual's behavior from proxies; for example, caregivers, family members, or those who most frequently observe the behavior (Rubin & Crocker, 2006). Importantly, recognition and accurate diagnosis of psychopathology in ASD are critical for treatment interventions.

Anxiety Disorders in Children and Adolescents with ASD

Researchers found in a study of 112 children aged 10–14 years, at least one current psychiatric disorder (71%), with the most common comorbidities of social anxiety (29%), ADHD (28%), and oppositional defiant disorder (28%) (Simonoff et al., 2008). A number of clinical studies of children with AS identified high rates of anxiety disorders including: General anxiety, social anxiety, and OCD (Burnette et al., 2005; Green, Gilchrist, Burton, & Cox, 2000; Meyer, Mundy, Van Hecke, Durocher, 2006; Russell & Sofronoff, 2005); and significant correlation between sensory defensiveness and anxiety in children with AS (Pfeiffer, Kinnealey, Reed, & Herzberg, 2005). In one study of 171 children aged 6–11, pathological scores for at least one anxiety disorder were identified using the Child and Adolescent Symptom Inventory (CASI), where higher levels of anxiety were associated with higher IQ, functional language use, and stereotyped behaviors (Sukhodolsky et al., 2008). Clearly, children and adolescents with an ASD are prone to anxiety disorders.

Attention Deficit Hyperactivity Disorder

ADHD is characterized by inattention and a combination of impulsivity and hyperactivity. ADHD may be the most common comorbid mental health disorder, and has been identified in a number of ASD clinical studies (Holtmann, Bolte, & Poustka, 2007; Mattila et al., 2010; Roux et al., 2015; Simonoff et al., 2008). ADHD was the most common disorder reported when comparing rate and type of psychiatric comorbidity in children and adolescents with AS (N=30) and high functioning autism (N=30) (Mukaddes, Hergunner, & Tanidir, 2010).

Depression in Children and Adolescents with an ASD

Depressive disorders were also identified in children and adolescents with an ASD (Barnhill, 2001; Green et al., 2000; White, Oswald, Ollendick, & Scahill, 2009). In a study that explored the relationship between loneliness and depressive symptoms of 35 youth aged 13–15 years with AS, a control group was utilized and depression was measured with the Center for Epidemiological Studies Depression Scale for Children (CES-DC). Almost two-thirds of the AS group (N=23), self-reported significantly higher levels of depressive symptoms when compared to the control group (Whitehouse, Durkin, Jacquet, & Ziatas, 2009).

The physical, mental health, behavioral challenges, and service needs for many with ASD will continue into adulthood and older age. Research is needed to address these continuing needs, especially as services decrease precipitously when one loses eligibility for education services, reportedly around age 25 years (Roux et al., 2015), and to evaluate the transferability of findings from AS to the entire autism spectrum.

Treating Adults with ASD

Few clinical studies have addressed the persistent impairments–including psychiatric problems–or effectiveness of psychotropic medication prescribed for adults with ASD despite the known need for ongoing services and treatment, including psychiatric treatment (Esbensen, Greenberg, Seltzer, & Aman, 2009). These individuals should be treated in psychiatric clinics, but the number of those with ASD in adult psychiatric clinics is small. One explanation is that adults with ASD lack the ability to pay for services, or lack insurance coverage, or simply do not have access to a treatment facility. Another explanation for the small number of adults in treatment is that some adults on the autism spectrum are receiving treatments in psychiatric clinics, but are misdiagnosed. Additionally, some suspect that clinic rosters may increase as the population of children diagnosed with ASD transition to adult care. Findings from a nationwide survey identify that over one-half million youth with ASD will age out of special education eligibility services over the next decade (Roux et al, 2015), suggesting to others that an "autism tsunami" is to be expected (Khan, 2015).

Traditionally, there has been a split between child psychiatry and adult psychiatry, with the idea that the disorders which affected children were "neurodevelopmental" and different than the disorders which emerged in teens and young adults. Yet, ASD is a chronic disorder in which symptoms may improve but persist and often require lifelong care.

Prevalence of Comorbid Mental Health Conditions in Adults with ASD

Mental health conditions, including depression, mood disorder, and anxiety, were measured using the Structured Clinical Interview for DSM-IV Axis I Disorders (SCID) in 54 AS adults between the ages of 23–30 (Lugnegard, Hallerback, & Gillberg, 2011). Researchers identified 70% with at least one episode of depression, and 50% of those had recurrent major depressive illness. Bipolar mood disorders were identified in five participants (9%). Anxiety disorder was present in 56% of the total group, and 11 of those had two or more anxiety disorders, which included social anxiety (22%), generalized anxiety (22%), panic disorder (13%), agoraphobia (15%), and OCD (7%).

A case-controlled electronic health record (EHR) review of 108 adults with ASD to a matched control cohort of 206 patients for chronic diseases and treatments for psychiatric disorders was completed for the years 2005–2008 at the Cleveland Clinic (Tyler, Schramm, Karafa, Tang, & Jain, 2011). Researchers identified high rates of obesity (34.9%), hyperlipidemia (31.5%), and treatment for psychiatric disorders and polypharmacy. Persons with

ASD were prescribed antidepressants (53%) and antipsychotic medications (36%) at significantly higher rates when compared to the control group. Antipsychotics were more than twice as often prescribed for persons with ASD (Tyler et al., 2011).

Misdiagnosed Adults with ASD

Adults with ASD have been diagnosed as schizotypal or schizoid personality disorder. Those with schizotypal or schizoid personality disorder exhibit many of the same symptoms as those with ASD. The clinical tradition of these personality disorders holds they may be a more minor form of schizophrenia or an incompletely expressed version of the disease.

In the US in the 1940s and 1950s, it was thought that schizophrenia was widespread, and was likely overdiagnosed. The Freudian tradition of seeing disorders as being on a continuum from health to neuroses to psychoses influenced this view. It was not until the late 1960s that ASD was identified as a separate syndrome distinguishing it from schizophrenia (Gewin, 2008) and Freudian traditions.

Leo Kanner distinguished autism from childhood schizophrenia in 1943 (Fischbach, 2007), but autism continued to be considered childhood schizophrenia for much of the twentieth century (Gewin, 2008). Kanner described the symptoms of 11 children with behavioral similarities. These descriptors of autistic aloneness, insistence on sameness, and innate inability to form relationships corresponds with contemporary diagnostic indicators (Gewin, 2008).

SCHIZOID PERSONALITY DISORDER OR ASD? According to the American Psychiatric Association's (APA) fifth edition of the Diagnostic and Statistical Manual of Mental Disorders (DSM-5), those with schizoid personality disorder have a pervasive pattern of detachment from social relationships and a restricted expression of emotions (APA, 2013). They do not desire or enjoy close relationships, and seem to choose solitary activities. They have difficulty establishing close friendships, and show some emotional detachment or flattened affect. This set of symptoms is remarkably similar to that of ASD, and there may be diagnostic overlap (Konstantareas & Hewitt, 2001), with difficulty differentiating individuals with schizoid personality disorder from those with milder forms of ASD (APA, 2013). Approximately, 3% to 5% of the population is thought to suffer from schizoid personality disorder (APA, 2013). Since symptoms of schizoid personality disorder mimic those of ASD, the obvious question is whether adults who are labeled as being schizoid were in fact, autistic children now grown to adulthood?

SCHIZOTYPAL PERSONALITY DISORDER OR ASD? Another category in the DSM-5 is the schizotypal personality disorder. Individuals with this condition also have a pervasive pattern of social and interpersonal deficits but they also have cognitive or perceptual distortions and eccentricities of behavior. They may have special, odd beliefs or behavior or appearance that is odd. These individuals also, though, have restricted affect and a lack of close friends and may show excessive social anxiety (APA, 2013). These descriptions seem remarkably similar to ASD. Some clinicians wonder whether schizoid personality disorder or schizotypal personality disorder may simply be adults with ASD.

ASD represents a syndrome, or a collection of disorders with overlapping symptomatology, which has been growing with psychiatric nomenclatures. Mired in the traditions of the past, these attempts have not been able to explain the condition. Clinicians hypothesized that medications used for symptoms in one psychiatric disorder could be used therapeutically across disorders with similar symptoms. This led to clinicians experimenting with a variety of medications.

Medications Prescribed for Patients with ASD

Many children and adults with ASD suffer from agitation, which further inhibits normal social interaction. Clinicians presumed that antipsychotic medications helpful in treating agitation could also be used to treat ASD. The hope was that the antipsychotic drugs might free a child or adult with the disorder from overreacting to internal stimuli, or overreacting in general.

Antipsychotic Medications

Antipsychotic medications were tried in these individuals in the hope they would help both the agitation these children and adults experience, as well as help them in some way freeing them from the internal stimuli that may be distracting them. As the atypical antipsychotics emerged at the end of the twentieth century, they were tried in increasing frequency in children, and have been somewhat helpful. They carry less of a side effect burden of extrapyramidal or muscle side effects, like irregular spasms, rigidity or jerky movements, and a lower rate of tardive dyskinesia. However, other side effects such as weight gain and altered glucose metabolism shadowed their use, and research is needed to assess the long-term safety of these medications in treating children and adults with ASD (Almandil et al., 2013).

RISPERIDONE. Clinical trials of antipsychotic medications, such as risperidone were helpful in reducing agitation as well as irritability in children with ASD (Dove et al., 2012; Doyle & McDougle, 2012; Mohiuddin & Ghaziuddin, 2013). In addition, risperidone was helpful in the overall reduction of symptoms of ASD as measured by the clinical global impressions inventory (Mohiuddin & Ghaziuddin, 2013). While there have been a limited number of double-blind studies, those conducted generated consistent evidence that risperidone and similar drugs are helpful (Nagaraj, Singhi, & Malki, 2006; McDougle et al., 2005; McDougle et al., 1998). The exact reason why these drugs are helpful is not clear. But, these medications block dopamine in the brain, and the assumption is that blocking dopamine, especially the developing brain, leads to a reduction in agitation and accompanying symptoms in ASD.

While risperidone is helpful, it is not without its problems. Side effects include sedation and weight gain which leads to an increased risk of hyperglycemia. Risperidone causes a lower risk of muscle tremor and extrapyramidal (or Parkinsonian) side effects, and lower risks of tardive dyskinesia than older antipsychotic drugs. Older medications such as haloperidol have proven somewhat useful over the years but are burdened with a greater risk of extrapyramidal, or muscle stiffness symptoms, and a higher risk of tardive dyskinesia.

With the risk of these side effects, the overall efficacy of risperidone must be examined. One review of children and adolescents with ASD showed that children who were more likely to have received antipsychotics and also antidepressants did better, overall and had a higher functional outcome than those who did not (Orinstein et al., 2014).

ARIPIPRAZOLE. Another antipsychotic medication, aripiprazole, has also been effectively used to treat irritability in both children and adolescents with ASD (Marcus et al., 2009; Owen et al., 2009). However, again, along with the positive effects of the medications, come the side effects as well. Those on aripiprazole were more likely to get muscle symptoms, or extrapyramidal side effects compared to placebo, and weight gain was more common (Owen et al., 2009).

Other antipsychotics have been investigated to see if they would be of help, and there is little reason to think that they would not have similar results. Thus, the use of antipsychotic medications has led to some improvements in not only symptoms of ASD and also in a small way in the functional outcomes in years later.

Postulated reason for efficacy. While a child is still developing, he or she must practice all social interactions and social skills to develop them fully. More practice leads to better social skills. Those with better social skills can have other, broader opportunities, leading to further experience and further improvement. So, reducing agitation or irritability early in life can reduce barriers to and facilitate social interaction, leading to some growth in skills, which can continue to develop across the lifespan. While antipsychotics do not cure ASD, they seem to limit agitation leading to opportunities for greater social interaction and increase the potential for social success.

Stimulants

Other medications have been tried as well, including stimulants, such as methylphenidate or dextroamphetamine. A review of the scant literature on the subject (Doyle & McDougle, 2012; Mohiuddin, & Ghaziuddin, 2013) showed that stimulant medications could be helpful. In one study, methylphenidate reduced hyperactivity and impulsivity (Posey et al., 2007). Newer treatments for ADD/ADHD may also be helpful. Atomoxetine, one such newer drug, carries a lower side effect burden can also be helpful for the symptoms of ASD (Aman et al., 2014).

Stimulant medications generally are not as helpful as the antipsychotic medications in the treatment of ASD. The side effect burden of the stimulants includes the possibility of some increased risk of irritability, sleeplessness, and decreased appetite. These side effects need to be brought into consideration in examining the use of these drugs. So, they can be helpful in some individuals, but the effect is typically smaller than preferred.

Antidepressants

Children and adults with ASD are often withdrawn from social stimuli, and depression is a comorbid psychiatric disorder among this cohort (Levy et al., 2010). Reviews of the use of antidepressant medications show that they also are generally helpful for the treatment of this withdrawn behavior in ASD (Mohiuddin & Ghaziuddin, 2013); however, the effect is usually small, and generally not as effective as the antipsychotic medications (Doyle & McDougle, 2012). Follow-up studies of children who had received antidepressant medications in childhood show generally better outcome in adolescence (Orinstein et al., 2014).

Depression and associated symptoms can continue to be a major problem in the individual with ASD, as they age. Significant depressive symptoms are reported in 31% of adults with AS (Cassidy et al., 2014) and, depression can also be fatal. In two separate reviews, 35% of adults with AS reported plans or attempts at suicide (Cassidy et al., 2014; Paquette-Smith, Weiss, & Lunsky, 2014). Therefore, the presence of depression is common in adults with AS. Trials of antidepressant medication can be attempted, although the database for their effectiveness in this group is lacking. A review of suicidal ideation and suicide attempts must be done in every individual with ASD. Interventions for these thoughts and activities include antidepressant medications, psychotherapy, and crisis interventions through hotlines and emergency services.

Antidepressants, especially the selective serotonin reuptake inhibitors (SSRIs) are used to treat obsessive-compulsive disorder. In this disorder, sufferers present with repetitive worries, as well as repetitive behaviors seeking to control the anxiety associated with the condition. Individuals with ASD also present commonly with repetitive behaviors, and when these behaviors are interrupted, anxiety, irritability, or aggression can be the result (APA, 2013).

SSRI medications may be helpful to treat the repetitive behaviors in ASD. A trial of fluoxetine identified improvement for these repetitive behaviors in 35% of the group receiving the medication. No one in the placebo group in the same study showed any significant improvement (Hollander et al., 2012). Fluoxetine has been available for decades in this country. The medication is also in phase III clinical trials in the US to further investigate its usefulness in repetitive behaviors in those with ASD (Carrasco, Volkmar, & Bloch, 2012).

A reduction in repetitive behaviors can be important for the social growth of those with ASD. Those who had decreases in repetitive behaviors as children had more positive outcomes as young adults (Anderson, Liang, & Lord, 2014). Decreasing this symptom allows opportunities for social growth and experiences, which then multiply as time goes on in development for these young people.

Memantine

Yet another available medication being investigated for the treatment of symptoms of ASD is memantine, which is approved for use for advanced Alzheimer's disease. Memantine is a moderate affinity antagonist of the *N*-methylD-aspartic acid (NMDA) glutamate receptor (MedlinePlus, 2015). Glutamate is the main excitatory neurotransmitter in the brain, and it is feared that an overactivity of glutamate could lead to over excitation or even inflammation in the brain. Too much glutamate may lead to agitation, hyperfocusing on one set of stimuli, or other changes in the developing brain.

A trial of memantine in an open-label study showed significant improvements in language function, social behavior, and self-stimulatory behaviors. It should be emphasized that this was an open label, unblended study where both the parents and researchers were looking for changes after initiating treatment with memantine. Still, the results were positive (Chez et al., 2007). Another, open label retrospective study of memantine showed that 61% of children and adolescents improved, using the Clinical Global Impressions Scale (Erickson et al., 2007).

Sedatives

Sleep problems are also common in those with ASD. Many sedating medications, including the antipsychotic medications, or sedating antidepressants have been tried. However, another interesting approach also yielded some success. Melatonin is a hormone released by the pineal gland shortly before sleep initiation. Some studies show some abnormalities in melatonin functioning in those with ASD. A review of melatonin use in these individuals showed that melatonin was associated with better sleep, but also better daytime behavior. The two may well be linked. Melatonin was also well tolerated in this group (Rossingol & Frye, 2011).

Even with the available medication and other treatment for individuals with ASD, the outcome is generally not good. While those who receive optimal treatment do better, only about 20% of children followed for a period of 17 years showed enough improvement in the core symptoms of ASD to no longer fit the criteria for the diagnosis (Anderson et al., 2014).

Generally, risperidone and other antipsychotic medications are thought to be first-line treatments for ASD. Other medications, such as the stimulants to help attention, and perhaps antidepressant medications, which may help mood as well as repetitive behaviors, have been tried (Carrasco et al., 2012; Chez et al., 2007). Clinicians are optimistic about the value of memantine and melatonin.

Medications and Treatments under Investigation

Brain development in those with ASD is not normal as the child moves from infancy and into childhood. Normally, when an infant and child begin to mature, the neural tree in the brain grows rapidly with a dramatic growth in synapses or connections within the brain. During later childhood, there is a pruning or limiting of these brain synapses or connections, so parts of the brain can develop specialized functions, and not be overwhelmed with large amounts of sensory data (Tang et al., 2014).

Tang and colleagues (2014) proposed that natural pruning of synaptic connections does not occur in the brain of the child with ASD and so the child and then the adult is overwhelmed by neuronal input, leading the person with ASD to withdraw to avoid overstimulation, or to specialize in a couple of specific interests. Some evidence has now accumulated to show that there is a lack of pruning or eliminating synapses in the brains in those who suffer from ASD (Tang et al., 2014).

This hypothesis also brings with it a potential treatment for ASD. Rapamycin, an immunosuppressant drug that is currently used to prevent rejection in organ transplants, can also restore normal synaptic pruning in the developing mouse brain, and can improve autistic-like behaviors in mice. The hope is that this medication may also do the same in humans, and effectively treat ASD (Sato et al., 2012).

Stem Cell Research

Stem cell research holds promise for people with ASD. At the Sutter Neuroscience Institute in Sacramento, California, along with the Cord Blood Registry, umbilical cord blood is collected from newborns, which contains stem cells. This blood is then stored, and later is infused in the children who develop signs of ASD. Researchers hypothesized that children with ASD may suffer from abnormal immune systems, which delay the development or damage the development of the central nervous system. The infusion of umbilical cord stem cells later hopefully would offer a way to repair the damage done leading to autistic behaviors (Cord Blood Registry, 2014).

Oxytocin

An idea offered as a possible treatment is the use of oxytocin, which is released immediately postpartum, and stimulates uterine contraction to prevent bleeding. It is also released with the stimulation of nipples during breast-feeding. Oxytocin binds to receptors in the brain, and may help to initiate maternal and social behaviors, such as mother-infant bonding and oxytocin may help in the development of socially meaningful stimuli in children. There is some evidence to suggest that oxytocin is deficient, or at least functions differently, in children with ASD (Gordon et al., 2013). Another way of delivering oxytocin-like compounds is through the use of oxytonin nasal spray. This is now being investigated to see if this would help in social interaction in those with ASD. A double-blind, placebo-controlled crossover trial of an oxytocin nasal spray in 20 males with ASD lead to an improved ability to recognize others' social emotions (Aoki et al., 2014). Moreover, following oxytocin infusion, 15 adults with autism or AS in another study showed a reduction in repetitive behaviors (Hollander et al., 2003).

This use of oxytonin was approved by the FDA in 1960 to help with breast milk ejection but was withdrawn by its manufacturer in 1997 for economic reasons. It is currently in Phase II trials for ASD in the US (Skitch, 2014). Long-acting oxytocin receptor agonists are available and used to help stimulate the body's production of oxytocin (Feifel, Shilling, & Belcher, 2012).

RG7314 is a vasopressin -1 receptor antagonist, and is currently in Phase II trials in the US. Both vasopressin as well as oxytocin are thought to be involved in the regulation of maternal-infant attachment and the processing of social stimuli. It is hoped that this vasopressin receptor antagonist would also help in the development of socialization in those suffering from ASD (Febo & Ferris, 2014).

A variety of hypotheses have been presented, and some are yielding clear treatment strategies. All of these strategies have a theoretical base, and some are less traditional. However, traditional treatments have been disappointing. While none of the suggested reasons and treatments for ASD has a large body of evidence, having a wide range of potential treatments is at least promising.

Altering the Microbiome

One idea proposed to explain the growth of ASD involves the microbiome, or the large number of bacteria, which inhabit the human body. Researchers estimate that over 100 trillion bacterial cells inhabit our bodies and may outnumber human body cells (Mulle, Sharpe, & Cubells, 2013). These bacteria are active participants in their host. It seems that the vagus nerve is able to differentiate between pathogenic bacteria and nonpathogenic bacteria in this transmission of responses from the gut to the central nervous system (Forsythe, Bienenstock, & Kunze, 2014). Gut bacteria can therefore affect the enteric neuronal or afferent signaling to the brain.

It has long been postulated with fairly good evidence that the communication between the gut and the brain can affect behavior, and some wonder if changes in the microbiome or changes in the bacteria in the gut and body may be related to the growing prevalence of ASD (Kang et al., 2013; Mulle et al., 2013). If the body and bowel are exposed early in life to antibiotics, which kill a set of bacteria, and it is not allowed to develop normal flora, or an array of bacteria, the set of bacteria in the body is limited. The body may become more hypersensitive to any new stimulus, and become more reactive to this stimulus as well. The concern is that this hyper-reaction can affect the developing brain in the young child and that a less diverse microbiome, or set of gut bacteria, could lead to a hyper-reaction to any new stimuli. This hyper-reaction could then lead to different afferent signaling from the gut to the brain, causing brain changes, leading to ASD. If this theory is at all correct, one way of treating the disorder could be to make the load of bacteria in those suffering from ASD more diverse. This would allow the body to accept a more diverse group of bacteria and allow the body to be less reactive, and less likely to affect the developing brain.

Use of Parasites for Inflammatory Response

To add a more diverse microbiome, studies are underway to introduce *trichuris suis ova,* the eggs of a pig-based whipworm, into adults with ASD (Hollander, 2014). These eggs do not multiply in the host, and are not transmissible. However the presence of these whipworm eggs in the bowel seems to decrease the inflammatory response in the body. The theory holds that this parasite decreases the immune response in the body in an effort to increase its own survival within the host's body. If ASD is partially caused by an overreaction, or hyper-response to remaining stimuli or bacteria or "dirt" in the body, this may decrease it, and serve as a potential treatment (Friedrich, 2014). The study introducing *trichuris suis ova* to adults is currently in phase II trials in the US (Hollander, 2014).

Similarly, to support the idea that the introduction of pathogens into the body may be helpful, it also has been observed that children with ASD show some improvement when they have fevers. A study where children were exposed to higher temperatures through use of a hot tub led to better prosocial behaviors on the days of heat exposure (Friedrich, 2014).

Probiotics

Some parents have insisted over time that their children with the disorder have a variety of gastrointestinal symptoms, and have sought to treat these symptoms with a special or restrictive diet. But, another treatment possibility could be delivering a probiotic, the process of introducing new bacteria into the gut to treat ASD. The idea is that if gut bacteria are different, then behavior could also be different because of afferent pathways or links from the gut to the brain. There is an ever-widening appreciation of the role the gut microbiome may play in behavior (Kang et al., 2013; Mulle et al., 2013), and it leads to another potential search of medication or probiotic treatment for the symptoms of ASD.

Environmental Toxins

Exposure to toxins and heavy metals in the environment also has been suggested as a cause of ASD, which could affect the developing brain. This idea holds that the increase in ASD is due to the increasing use of pesticides and exposure to toxins in an industrial developing area. The theory is that with modernity the number and amount of toxins we are exposed to increase as well. A survey of 970 women showed that living within a mile of exposure to organophosphate pesticides was associated with a 60% increased risk for ASD. This was even higher if the mother was exposed during the third trimester when the brain is further developing in utero (Shelton et al., 2014).

Summary of Current Approaches to Medication Treatment

The increasing risk for ASD in the population demands better treatment. Pharmacotherapy for ASD is not optimal, but will continue to have a role in the treatment of ASD. Medications are the second best treatment, behind behavioral approaches that seek to broaden and strengthen social interaction for the developing child, and the developing brain. While this may well be true, it also needs to be remembered that types of behavioral approaches in themselves also have a limited database.

Antipsychotic medications are helpful in reducing agitation, and perhaps can even improve sociability. This improvement does not come without cost since the medications such as risperidone or aripiprazole also bring side effects, which need to be evaluated and monitored. Stimulant medications may be of some use in those with clear problems with attention. There are ongoing trials testing the usefulness of SSRIs such as fluoxetine to decrease repetitive behaviors (Hagerman, 2015; Hollander et al., 2005; King et al., 2009).

Finally, depression and suicidal ideation is a large problem for the growing number of adults with ASD. While there are scant data on the subject, it makes sense to use existing antidepressant medications, including fluoxetine to help the symptoms of depression. Routine and comprehensive clinical practice should include screening for suicidal ideation for all individuals with ASD.

Newer treatments under investigation include changing the biome, or gut bacteria, protecting the developing brain from toxins, or in some way use of medications to better prune an overactive neuronal connecting system in the brain. Even collecting umbilical cord blood to store stem cells for potential use in these children or their siblings is being done. These approaches offer hope, but not enough data or conclusive evidence of efficacy currently.

More research is needed to provide better treatments for those with ASD. The growth of adults with this condition will make consent for research and the research projects themselves easier to undertake. It must be remembered that those who suffer from ASD are our partners in these investigations, and they should be treated as full partners in the process of research (Fisher & Kettl, 2009). We hope the future will bring better medications, and better medication treatments for those with ASD.

References

Almandil, N. B., Liu, Y., Murray, M. L., Besag, F. M., Aitchison, K. J., & Wong, I. C. (2013). Weight gain and other metabolic adverse effects associated with atypical antipsychotic treatment of children and adolescents: A systematic review and meta-analysis. *Paediatric Drugs, 15*(2), 139–150.

Aman, M. G., Smith, T., Arnold, L. E., Corbett-Dick, P., Tumuluru, R., Hollway, J. A., . . . Handen, B. (2014). A review of atomoxetine effects in young people with developmental disabilities. *Research in Developmental Disabilities, 35*(6), 1412–1424.

American Psychiatric Association. (2013). *Diagnostic and statistical manual of mental disorders* (5th edition). Washington, DC: Author.

Anderson, D. K., Liang, J. W., & Lord, C. (2014). Predicting young adult outcome among more and less cognitively able individuals with autism spectrum disorders. *Journal of Child Psychology and Psychiatry, 55*(5), 485–494.

Aoki, Y., Yahata, N., Watanabe, T., Takano, Y., Kawakubo, Y., Kuwabara, H., . . . Yamasue, H. (2014). Oxytocin improves behavioural and neural deficits in inferring others' social emotions in autism. *Brain.* Retrieved from http://brain.oxford journals.org/content/early/2014/08/22/brain.awu231

Barnhill, G. P. (2001). Social attributes and depression in adolescents with Asperger syndrome. *Focus on Autism and Other Developmental Disabilities, 16*(1), 46–53.

Berjerot, S., Eriksson, J. M., & Mortberg, E. (2014). Social anxiety in adult autism spectrum disorder. *Psychiatry Research, 220,* 705–707.

Burnette, C. P., Mundy, P. C., Meyer, J. A., Sutton, S. K., Vaughan, A. E., & Charak, D. (2005). Weak central coherence and its relations to theory of mind and anxiety in autism. *Journal of Autism & Developmental Disorders, 35*(1), 63–73.

Carrasco, M., Volkmar, F. R., & Bloch, M. H. (2012). Pharmacologic treatment of repetitive behaviors in autism spectrum disorders: Evidence of publication bias. *Pediatrics, 1*(2), 142–147.

Cassidy, S., Bradley, P., Robinson, J., Allison, C., McHugh, M., & Baron-Cohen, S. (2014). Suicidal ideation and suicide plans or attempts in adults with Asperger's syndrome attending a specialist diagnostic clinic: A clinical cohort study. *The Lancet Psychiatry, 1*(2), 142–147.

Chez, M. G., Burton, Q., Dowling, T., Chang, M., Khanna, P., & Kramer, C. (2007). Memantine as adjunctive therapy in children diagnosed with autism spectrum disorders: An observation of initial clinical response and maintenance tolerability. *Journal of Child Neurology, 22*(5), 574–579.

Cord Blood Registry. (2014). Autism clinical trial. Retrieved from http://www .cordblood.com/stem-cell-research/cord-blood-research/autism

Dove, D., Warren, Z., McPheeters M. L., Taylor, J. L., Sathe, N. A., & Veenstra-VanderWeele, J. (2012). Medications for adolescents and young adults with autism spectrum disorders: A systematic review. *Pediatrics, 130*(4), 717–726.

Doyle, C. A., & McDougle, C. J. (2012). Pharmacotherapy to control behavioral symptoms in children with autism. *Expert Opinion Pharmacotherapy, 13*(11), 1615–1629.

Erickson, C. A., Posey, D. J., Stigler, K. A., Mullett, J., Katschke, A. R., & McDougle, C. J. (2007). A retrospective study of memantine in children and adolescents with pervasive developmental disorders. *Psychopharmacology, 191*(1), 141–147.

Esbensen, A. J., Greenberg, J. S., Seltzer, M. M., & Aman, M. G. (2009). A longitudinal investigation of psychotropic and non-psychotropic medication use among adolescents and adults with autism spectrum disorders. *Journal of Autism & Developmental Disorders, 39*(9), 1339–1340.

Febo, M., & Ferris, C. F. (2014). Oxytocin and vasopressin modulation of the neural correlates of motivation and emotion: Results from functional MRI studies in awake rats. *Brain Research,* 1580–1588.

Feifel, D., Shilling, P. D., & Belcher, A. M. (2012). The effects of oxytocin and its analog, carbetocin, on genetic deficits in sensorimotor gating. *European Neuropsychopharmacoloy, 22*(5), 374–378.

Fischbach, G. D. (2007). Leo Kanner's 1943 paper on autism. *Simons Foundation on Autism Research.* Retrieved from http://sfari.org/news-and-opinion/classic-paper-reviews/2007/leo-kanners-1943-paper-on-autism-commentary-by-gerald-fischbach

Fisher, K., & Kettl, P. (2009). Examining problems in informed consent for the growing population of elders with intellectual disability. *American Journal of Forensic Psychiatry, 30*(4), 17–29.

Forsythe, P., Bienenstock, J., & Kunze, W. A. (2014). Vagal pathways for microbiome-brain-gut axis communication. *Advances in Experimental Medicine and Biology, 817,* 115–133.

Friedrich, M. J. (2014). Research on psychiatric disorders targets inflammation. *Journal of the American Medical Association, 312*(4), 474–476.

Garcia-Villamisar, D., & Rojahn, J. (2015). Comorbid psychopathology and stress mediate the relationship between autistic traits and repetitive behaviors in adults with autism. *Journal of Intellectual Disability Research, 59*(Part 2), 116–124.

Gewin, V. (2008). Autism and schizophrenia: A tale of two disorders. *Simons Foundation on Autism Research.* Retrieved from http://sfari.org/news-and opinion/news/2008/autism-and-schizophrenia-a-tale-of-two-disorders

Gillott, A., Furniss, F., & Walter, A. (2001). Anxiety in high-functioning children with autism. *Autism, 5*(3), 277–286.

Gordon, I., VanderWyk, B. C., Bennett, R. H., Cordeaux, C., Lucas, M. V., Eilbott, J. A., . . . Pelphrey, K. A. (2013). Oxytocin enhances brain function in children with autism. *Proceedings of the National Academy of Sciences of the United States of America.* Retrieved from http://www.ncbi.nlm.nih.gov/pmc/articles/PMC 3876263/

Green, J., Gilchrist, A., Burton, D., & Cox, A. (2000). Social and psychiatric functioning in adolescents with Asperger syndrome compared with conduct disorder. *Journal of Autism & Developmental Disorders, 30*(4), 279–293.

Hagerman, R. J., (2015). A trial of sertraline in young children with autism spectrum disorder (Sert 2). *Clinical trials.gov.* Identifier NCT02385799. Retrieved from https://clinicaltrials.gov/ct2/show/results/NCT02385799

Hollander, E. (2014). *Trichuris suis ova* in autism spectrum disorders (TSO) *ClinicalTrials.gov.* Identifier NCT01040221. Retrieved from https://clinicaltrials .gov/ct2/show/NCT01040221

Hollander, E., Novotny, S., Hanratty, M., Yaffe, R., DeCaria, C. M., Aronowitz, B. R., . . . Mosovich, S. (2003). Oxytocin infusion reduces repetitive behaviors in adults with autistic and Asperger's disorders. *Neuropsychopharmacology, 28*(1), 193–198.

Hollander, E., Soorya, L., Chaplin, W., Anagnostou, E., Taylor, B. P., Ferretti, C. J., . . . Settipani, C. (2012). A double-blind-controlled trial of fluoxetine for repetitive behaviors and global severity in adult autism spectrum disorder. *American Journal of Psychiatry, 169*(3), 292–299.

Holtmann, M., Bolte, S., & Poustka, F. (2007). Attention deficit hyperactivity disorder symptoms in pervasive developmental disorders: Association with autistic behavior domains and coexisting psychopathology. *Psychopathology, 40*(3), 172–177.

Idring, S., Magnusson, C., Lundberg, M., Ek, M., Rai, D., & Lee, B. K. (2014). Parental age and the risk of autism spectrum disorders: Findings from a Swedish population-based cohort. *International Journal of Epidemiology, 43*(1), 107–115.

Kang, D. W., Park, J. G., Ilhan, Z. E., Wallstrom, G., LaBaer, J., Adams, J. B., . . . Krajmalnik-Brown, R. (2013). Reduced incidence of *prevotella* and other fermenters in intestinal microflora of autistic children. Retrieved from http: //journals.plos.org/plosone/article?id=10.1371/journal.pone.0068322

Khan, A. (2015, January). The US is on the verge of an "Autism Tsunami." *US News & World Report.* Retrieved from http://www.businessinsider.com/increasing -numbers-of-autistic-adults-2015-1

King, B. H., Hollander, E., Sikich, L., McCracken, J. T., Scahill, L., Bregman, J. D., . . . Ritz, L. (2009). Lack of efficacy of citalopram in children with autism spectrum disorders and high levels of repetitive behavior. *Archives of General Psychiatry, 66*(6), 583–590.

Konstantareas, M. M., & Hewitt, T. (2001). Autistic disorder and schizophrenia: Diagnostic overlaps. *Journal of Autism & Developmental Disorders, 31*(1), 19–28.

Levy, S. E., Giarelli, E., Lee, L. C., Schieve, L. S., Kirby, R. S., Cunniff, C., . . . Rice, C. (2010). Autism spectrum disorder and co-occurring developmental, psychiatric, and medical conditions among children in multiple populations in the United States. *Journal of Developmental & Behavioral Problems, 31*(3), 1–9.

Lugengard, T., Hallerback, M. U., & Gillberg, C. (2011). Psychiatric comorbidity in young adults with a clinical diagnosis of Asperger syndrome. *Research in Developmental Disabilities, 32,* 1910–1917.

Marcus, R. N., Owen, R., Kamen, L., Manos, G., McQuade, R. D., Carson, W. H., . . . Aman, M. G. (2009). A placebo-controlled, fixed-dose study of aripiprazole in children and adolescents with irritability associated with autistic disorder. *Journal of the American Academy of Child & Adolescent Psychiatry, 48,* 1110–1119.

Mattila, M.L., Hurtig, T., Haapsamo, H., Jussila, K., Kuusikko-Gauffin, S., Kielinen, M., . . . Moilanen, I. (2010). Comorbid psychiatric disorders associated with

Asperger syndrome/high-functioning autism: A community and clinic-based study. *Journal of Autism & Developmental Disorder, 40*(9), 1080–1093.

Mazzone, L., Ruta, L., & Reale, L. (2012). Psychiatric comorbidities in Asperger syndrome and high functioning autism: Diagnostic challenges. *Annals of General Psychiatry, 25,* 11–16.

McDougle, C. J., Holmes, J. P., Carlson, D. C., Pelton, G. H., Cohen, D. J., & Price, L.H. (2005). A double-blind, placebo-controlled study of risperidone in adults with autistic disorder and other pervasive developmental disorders. *American Journal of Psychiatry, 162*(6), 1142–1148.

McDougle, C. J., Scahill, L., Aman, M. G., McCracken, J. T., Tierney, E., Davies, M., . . . Vitiello, B. (1998). Risperidone for the core symptom domains of autism: Results from the study by the autism network of the research units on pediatric psychopharmacology. *Archives of General Psychiatry, 55*(7), 633–641.

MedlinePlus. (2015). Memantine. National Institutes of Health, US National Library of Medicine. Retrieved from http://www.nlm.nih.gov/medlineplus/druginfo/meds/a604006.html

Meyer, J. A., Mundy, P. C., Van Hecke, A.V., & Durocher, J. S. (2006). Social attribution processes and comorbid psychiatric symptoms in children with Asperger syndrome. *Autism, 10*(4), 383–402.

Mohiuddin, S., & Ghaziuddin, M. (2013). Psychopharmacology of autism spectrum disorders: A selective review. *Autism, 17,* 645–654.

Muhle, R., Trentacoste, S. V., & Rapin, I. (2004). The genetics of autism. *Pediatrics, 113*(5), e472–e486. Retrieved from http://www.ncbi.nlm.nih.gov/pubmed/15121991

Mukaddes, N. M., Herguner, S., & Tanidir, C. (2010). Psychiatric disorders in individuals with high-functioning autism and Asperger's disorder: Similarities and differences. *World Journal of Biological Psychiatry, 11*(8), 964–971.

Mulle, W. G., Sharp, J. F., & Cubells, J. F. (2013). The gut microbiome: A new frontier in autism research. *Current Psychiatry Reports, 15*(2), 337–345.

Nagaraj, R., Singhi, P., & Malki, P. (2006). Risperidone in children with autism: Randomized, placebo-controlled, double-blind study. *Journal of Child Neurology, 21*(6), 450–455.

Orinstein, A. J., Helt, M., Troyb, E., Tyson, K. E., Barton, M. L., Eigsti, I. M. . . . Fein, D. A. (2014). Intervention for optimal outcome in children and adolescents with a history of autism. *Journal of Developmental & Behavioral Pediatrics, 35*(4), 247–256.

Ostrow, N. (2014, June). Autism costs more than $2 million over patient's life. Bloomberg Business News. Retrieved from http://www.bloomberg.com/news/articles/2014-06-09/autism-costs-more-than-2-million-over-patient-s-life

Owen, R., Sikich L., Marcus, R. N., Corey-Lisle, P., Manos, G., McQuade, R. D., . . . Findling, R. L. (2009). Aripiprazole in the treatment of irritability in children and adolescents with autistic disorder. *Pediatrics, 124*(6), 1533–1540.

Paquette-Smith, M., Weiss, J., & Lunsky, Y. (2014). History of suicide attempts in adults with Asperger's syndrome. *Crisis: The Journal of Crisis Intervention and Suicide Prevention, 35*(4), 273–277.

Pfeiffer, B., Kinnealey, M., Reed, C., & Herzberg, G. (2005). Sensory modulation and affective disorders in children and adolescents with Asperger's disorder. *American Journal of Occupational Therapy, 59*(3), 335–345.

Posey, D. J., Aman, M. G., McCracken, J. T., Scahill, L., Tierney, E., Arnold, L. E., . . . McDougle, C. J. (2007). Positive effects of methylphenidate on inattention and hyperactivity on inattention and hyperactivity in pervasive developmental disorders: An analysis of secondary measures. *Biological Psychiatry, 61*(4), 538–544.

Rossignol, D. A., & Frye, R. E. (2011). Melatonin in autism spectrum disorders: A systematic review and meta-analysis. *Developmental Medicine and Child Neurology, 53*(9), 783–792.

Roux, A. M., Shattuck, P. T., Rast, J. E., Rava, J. A., & Anderson, K. A. (2015). *National autism indicators report: Transition into young adulthood.* Philadelphia, PA: Life Course Outcomes Research Program, A. J. Drexel Autism Institute, Drexel University.

Rubin, I. L., & Crocker, A. C. (2006). *Medical care for children & adults with developmental disabilities* (2nd edition). Baltimore, MD: Paul H Brookes.

Russell, E., & Sofronoff, K. (2005). Anxiety and social worries in children with Asperger syndrome. *The Australian and New Zealand Journal of Psychiatry, 39*(7), 633–638.

Sandin, S., Lichtenstein, P., Kuja-Halkola, R., Larsson, H., Hultman, C. M., & Reichenberg, A. (2014). The familial risk of autism. *Journal of the American Medical Association, 311*(17), 1770–1777.

Sato, A., Kasai, S., Kobayashi, T., Takamatsu, Y., Hino, O., Ikeda, K., . . . Mizuguchi, M. (2012). Rapamycin reverses impaired social interaction in mouse models of tuberous sclerosis complex. *Nature Communications, 3,* 1292. Retrieved from http://www.ncbi.nlm.nih.gov/pubmed/23250422

Shelton, J. F., Geraghty, E. M., Tancredi, D. J., Delwiche, L. D., Schmidt, R. J., Ritz, B., . . . Hertz-Picciotto, I. (2014). *Environmental Health Perspectives, 122*(10), 1103–1109.

Simonoff, E., Pickles, A. C., Chandler, S., Loucas, T., & Baird, G. (2008). Psychiatric disorders in children with autism spectrum disorders: Prevalence, comorbidity, and associated factors in a population-derived sample. *Journal of the American Academy of Child and Adolescent Psychiatry, 47,* 921–929.

Skitch, L. (2014). Phase II study of oxytocin in autism to improve reciprocal social behaviors. *ClinicalTrials.gov Identifier: NCT01944046.* Retrieved from https://clinicaltrials.gov/ct2/show/NCT01944046

Sukhodolsky, D. G., Scahill, L., Gadow, K. D, Arnold, L. E., Aman, M. G., McDougle, C. J., . . . Vitiello B. (2008). Parent-rated anxiety symptoms in children with pervasive developmental disorders: Frequency and association with core autism symptoms and cognitive functioning. *Journal of Abnormal Child Psychology, 36*(1), 117–128.

Tang, G., Gudsnuk K., Kuo, S-H., Cotrina, M.L., Rosoklija, G., Sosunov, . . . Sulzer, D. (2014). Loss of motor-dependent macroautophagy causes autistic-like synaptic pruning deficits. *Neuron, 83*(5), 1131–1143.

Tyler, C., Schramm, C., Karafa, M., Tang, A., & Jain, A. (2011). Chronic disease risk in young adults with ASD: Forewarned is forearmed. *American Journal of Intellectual and Developmental Disability, 116*(5), 371–380.

White, S. W., Oswald, D., Ollendick, T., & Scahill, L. (2009). Anxiety in children and adolescents with autism spectrum disorders. *Clinical Psychology Review, 29*(3), 216–229.

Whitehouse, A. J., Durkin, K., Jacquet, E., & Ziatas, K. (2009) Friendship, loneliness, and depression in adolescents with Asperger's syndrome. *Journal of Adolescence, 32*(2), 309–322.

Section 2

THE SOLUTIONS: EFFECTIVE, SAFE, COORDINATED CARE

Chapter 6

FRAMEWORK TO GUIDE PRACTICE AND RESEARCH WITH PATIENTS

JOAN ROSEN BLOCH

The role healthcare systems play in promoting optimal health for people with autism spectrum disorder (ASD) is surprisingly understudied. Implementing and evaluating best practices of healthcare delivery to people with ASD necessitates a broad conceptualization that goes beyond individual-level biomedical services, towards developing, implementing, and evaluating integrated healthcare delivery models designed to optimize outcomes in health promotion and disease prevention for this population with special needs.

ASD is a lifelong neurodevelopmental disability, for which there is no cure, and for which patients require long-term treatment to help them manage their most challenging characteristics (Giarelli, 2012). Treatments for ASD are expensive and require intensive time commitments across the life span (Liptak, Stuart, & Auinger, 2006; Mandell, 2013; Wang, Mandell, Lawer, Cidav, & Leslie, 2013). People with ASD and their families face a wide range of complex, and often confusing, choices when deciding which healthcare services promote optimal health and wellness.

Benchmarked standards for interventions and treatments that promote healthy outcomes in people with ASD have yet to be established. At this juncture in the overall research agenda for ASD, there is a need for a systematic framework to guide rigorous ASD health services research and translation. Such a framework can help practitioners design and deliver care that is equitable, appropriately utilized, effective, and efficient. When carefully designed care is delivered, outcomes for people with autism will improve.

Conceptual Approach

This chapter addresses how healthcare delivery systems can optimize overall physical, psychological, and social health outcomes of people with ASD throughout their lifespan. It provides a framework to guide advancing knowledge that can be translated into developing and implementing efficient and effective healthcare services for those with ASD. This chapter is guided by the integration of concepts from two classic theoretical approaches to evaluating healthcare systems and health services. These are (a) the approach of Aday, which is used by those who study the equity of access to health care and use among vulnerable patient populations (Aday, 2001; Aday & Anderson, 1981; Anderson & Aday, 1978); and (b) the concepts presented by Donabedian, which are used to evaluate the quality of health care (Aday, Begley, Lairson, & Slater, 1998; Donabedian, 2005). The first section addresses access and utilization of healthcare services for people with ASD. The second section addresses integrated healthcare systems for people with ASD and includes a discussion of benchmarking for evaluating and implementing healthcare system improvements for this population. The last section discusses health services research, concluding with an ASD-specific health care services research framework to guide the advancement of knowledge needed for implementing high performing infrastructures and processes of health care that optimize health and health outcomes for people with ASD.

Access and Utilization of Health Care Services

To ensure equity of health care for vulnerable populations it is necessary to study access and utilization of healthcare services by the population of concern. Over the last several decades the literature on access to and utilization by high-risk or vulnerable populations has grown. Improving efficiencies and health outcomes of those using the American healthcare system has been a research priority since the 1980s when the insurmountable rising costs of the healthcare system was identified as a critical problem (Bard & Nugent, 2011). Research specifically studying healthcare service to those with ASD has been conducted primarily on subjects that were mostly children, with a few focused on adolescents. Studies of adults with ASD are rare. Considering that prior to the 1990s, few patients were given formal diagnoses of ASD (Hollander, Kolevzon, & Coye, 2011), it is understandable that the research on adults with ASD is scant. However, now that the cohorts of children diagnosed during the 1990s have aged to adulthood, research on adults is not only warranted, but urgently needed. Unknown are the specific healthcare needs of aging individuals with ASD, and how health care usage influences their well-being and function. To guide expanding this field of research, the major categories of research are summarized below.

Category: Disparities in Access and Utilization of Healthcare Services

Accessing medical and other healthcare services for acute and chronic illnesses can be particularly challenging to those with ASD or their family caregivers, who must navigate primary and specialty care for their acute and chronic illnesses in addition to accessing treatment for ASD (Golden & Nageswaran, 2012; Lobar, 2014). People with ASD have unique needs that may present barriers to their ability to access and use the array of regimens of health care available to make a diagnosis of ASD and to evaluate medical problems (Lobar, 2014; Barker et al., 2010).

OBTAINING THE DIAGNOSIS. Obtaining the initial formal diagnosis of ASD may be problematic. To secure an early diagnosis, parents must be cognizant of early warning signs and bring these to the attention of a primary care physician or nurse practitioner. Bloch and Gardner (2007) found in their qualitative study that seeking a formal diagnosis of autism for a preschool child required that parents be persistent and knowledgeable. The parents, mostly the mother, had to navigate a confusing and often unfriendly healthcare system in order to find the most appropriate diagnostician (Bloch & Gardner, 2007). Russel, Steer, and Golding (2011) work supported this finding. They reported that maternal factors were instrumental in obtaining a formal ASD diagnosis for a child. Among younger mothers in their study, mothers of first-born children, and for mothers who had depression, formal diagnoses were delayed in their children. Documented delays in diagnosing autism were also found based on sex (Giarelli et al., 2010), race and ethnicity (Liptak et al., 2008; Mandell et al., 2009), and where families resided and the age of the child (Daniels & Mandell, 2013). Girls, especially those without cognitive impairment, were diagnosed at later ages than boys (Giarelli et al., 2010). This remained true for adults (Begeer et al., 2013).

Where families live matters for timely early diagnoses of ASD. Observed patterns in geographical variations in the early diagnosis of autism are best explained by community resources and state policies that create environments that are either more or less conducive to having the necessary healthcare services accessible for early identification and management of autism in children (Daniels & Mandell, 2013; Thomas, Parish, Rose, & Kilany, 2012). Delaying the initial early diagnosis of ASD translated into missed opportunities for providing intervention during the most critical developmental period of early childhood.

ACCESSING ONGOING TREATMENT. Even after a diagnosis is obtained, children with ASD continue to have problems accessing healthcare services for their ASD-related and non ASD-related conditions, resulting in many unmet healthcare needs (Acef & Aubrun, 2010; Gourdine, Baffour, & Teasley, 2011; Thomas et al., 2012). In particular, Thomas and colleagues (2007) studied the autism-related healthcare services most frequently used by families in North Carolina who had a child 11 years old or younger with ASD (n=383). The most frequently used medical specialty provider was a neurologist followed by a developmental pediatrician. But, less than one-third of the families actually reported receiving healthcare services by these medical specialists (Thomas et al., 2007). By age eight, more than half of the children were receiving medications for their ASD. By age 11, over two-thirds of the children used medication (Thomas et al., 2007). The exact medications, their costs, and the type of healthcare provider managing this medical treatment were not described. Clearly medical management is a core component of treatment for ASD.

Moreover, variation in accessing healthcare services exists across the United States (US). When families live in states with higher Medicaid reimbursement rates, they are less likely to have problems accessing autism-related care (Thomas et al., 2012).

Using a nationally represented sample, the 2005–2006 National Survey of Children with Special Health Care Needs, Kogan and colleagues (2008) examined the healthcare experiences of children with ASD. Overall, they found inadequate access and utilization of needed ongoing health care among children with ASD. Compared to other children with special healthcare needs without emotional, developmental, or behavioral problems, children with ASD were more likely to have unmet needs for specific healthcare services, family support services, delayed or foregone care, difficulty receiving referrals, and care that was not family centered. Their results corroborated results from other researchers that children with ASD were significantly more likely to have problems regarding access to care and that their families had greater financial, employment, and time burdens than those of other children with special healthcare needs (Charles, 2010; Kogan et al., 2008; Leslie & Martin, 2007; Liptak et al., 2008). It is unknown if problems with access to care extends across the lifespan as children go forth into adulthood and then into their elderly years.

Furthermore, compared to families that have children with other diagnosed special needs, families of children with ASD have greater financial, employment, and time burdens (Kogan et al., 2008). The additional family-specific challenges or inadequacies in finances or employment compete with the added burdens of caring for the special needs child or adult who resides in the household. Even more problematic is the adult with ASD who is not capable of independent living and does not have a family home in which to reside. Safe, comfortable housing arrangements may not be so easy to find, especially if the adult with ASD has challenging behaviors and demanding health care use.

RACIAL AND ETHNIC DISPARITIES. Documented racial and ethnic disparities exist in the access and utilization of quality healthcare services for black and Latino children with ASD (Gourdine et al., 2011; Liptak et al., 2008; Mandell et al., 2009; Parish, Magana, Rose, Timberlake, & Swaine, 2012; Thomas et al., 2007). According to the Centers for Disease Control and Prevention (2014), white children are more likely to be given an ASD diagnosis than black children; black children are more likely to be to be given an ASD diagnosis than Hispanic children; and Hispanic children are more likely to be given an ASD diagnosis than Asian children. The diagnosis of ASD is made at later ages for black children than for white children. Consequently, black children often may require more intensive interventions for longer periods because the most opportune time for the most effective intervention of early childhood is missed if the initial diagnosis is delayed (Gourdine et al., 2011).

Intense commitment of the parent in searching for medical care to determine if their child really has a medical problem is the critical factor in early diagnosis. Low income, marginalized minority groups of parents may not have the time or financial resources to persevere to obtain diagnosis for their young toddlers. Additionally, healthcare providers may lack the requisite cultural sensitivity to understand how parents from diverse ethnic backgrounds perceive the meaning and severity of ASD symptoms, such as avoidance of eye contact, social avoidance, and communication deficits. Moreover, we do not fully understand how parents access and use services when English is not their primary language.

Parish and colleagues (2012) examined access and utilization of health care by parents of Latino children with ASD and other developmental disabilities using data from the National Survey of Children with Special Health Care Needs. They found these children had less access to and utilization of quality health care than white children. The researchers specifically identified that provider-related issues adversely mediated the relationship between ethnicity and poor quality of health care associated with inadequate utilization of health care. Three significant provider-related indicators of poor health care quality were: (1) Not enough time was spent with the child; (2) the provider was perceived as not culturally sensitive; and (3) the parent did not feel that the provider made the parent feel like a partner. These researchers concluded that interventions are needed to target improving the cultural sensitivity and behavior of providers during the clinical encounter as a means of reducing these ethnic disparities in the use and quality of healthcare services to Latinos with ASD (Parish et al., 2012).

Overall, optimizing well-being and functioning is the goal for all children and adults with ASD. Barriers to ASD health care among marginalized ethnic groups must be eliminated. Special consideration is needed to understand and integrate the diverse cultural beliefs, attitudes, and practices of families when tailoring health care.

Category: Health Care Insurance Coverage

In the US, Medicaid (the government insurance program) is probably the largest payer of medically necessary services for children with ASD. As such, it is likely that Medicaid provides coverage for more comprehensive services than most commercial health insurance providers (Semansky, Xie, Lawer, & Mandell, 2013). To delineate the extent of Medicaid's coverage of the array of services needed to promote optimal health for children with ASD, Semansky et al. (2013) reviewed the national Medicaid outpatient claims for 2005. To organize the massive amount of data that had so many different Current Procedural Terminology (CPT) codes in the claims data for paid services from 48 states, the researchers created categories of health services. Their choice of broad service categories was guided by their extensive review of the literature of evidence-based and effective community-based therapies used to treat deficits associated with autism (Semansky et al., 2013). The authors created 16 categories of healthcare services (see Table 6.1). They found a marked variation in coverage of these services among the 48 states for children aged 3 to 17 years who had a primary diagnosis code (i.e., ICD-9 code: 299.0) indicating an ASD. Because each state has the right to determine what their state Medicaid insurance will or will not cover, it is not surprising that they found variations. However, the extent of the variations for health care for people with ASD across the nation is surprising. For example, Table 6.1 illustrates the percentage of US states among 48 that reported having services that are utilized by patients with ASD. As seen in Table 6.1, some states could be classified as being more ASD "friendly" such that they provided more comprehensive coverage. The most ASD "friendly" states are the two states Maryland and Missouri, where their Medicaid covered the highest number of services (n=11) (Semansky et al., 2013, p. 1054). The average number of services covered by Medicaid among the states was seven.

It is important to replicate in future studies the categories of healthcare services identified by these researchers to enhance comparability across studies, thereby maximizing knowledge about the healthcare services needed for

Table 6.1
VARIATION IN UTILIZATION OF HEALTH CARE SERVICES
AMONG CHILDREN WITH A PRIMARY DIAGNOSIS OF
AUTISM THAT WERE PAID FOR BY MEDICAID DURING 2005

Health Care Service Category	Percentage of the 48 States (%)*
Individual Therapy	96
Physical and Occupational Therapy	89
In-home Supports	89
Speech Therapy	79
Diagnostic Assessment	66
Behavior Modification	62
Family Therapy	57
Case Management	55
Targeted Case Management	38
Respite	32
Day Treatment	23
Social Skills Training	19
Habilitation services	17
Treatment planning	15
Family education and training	15
Assistive communication device	9
Non-autism related medical care	?

*This table illustrates the overall percentage of the 48 states that paid for the specific service category. Table was compiled with data from Semansky et al. (2013).

people with ASD. Semansky and colleagues (2013) provided the data dictionary for their list of 2,775 procedure codes (CPT codes) retrieved from the 2005 Medicaid data claims (http://www.med.upenn.edu/cmhpsr/resources .html). The list is long because it includes Medicaid CPT codes that were paid for in each state for services provided to children with ASD. Actual CPT codes vary for some who received the same services. For example, there are slightly different CPT codes used across the states for what appears to be similar services, such as case management, respite care, and speech therapy. This may account for variations in state-specific nuances in securing payment through Medicaid.

To examine how utilization of health care services among those with ASDs changes over time as a child ages, Cidav and colleagues (2013) used the same dataset as Semansky et al. (2013). The services they examined are the same as those listed in Table 6.1. They found that the use of long-term care, psychiatric medications, case management, medication management, day treatment/partial hospitalization, and respite services increased with age.

In contrast, the use of occupational/physical therapy, speech therapy, mental health services, diagnostic/assessment services, and family therapy declined as children grew older (Cidav et al., 2013).

In another study, Shimabukuro, Grosse, and Rice (2008) examined medical expenditures in a large, national sample of privately insured children and adolescents with ASD. They found, on average, that medical expenditures for those with an ASD were 4.1 to 6.2 times greater than those without an ASD. Their findings concurred with a growing body of evidence that children and adolescents with ASD have greater utilization of medical care (Mandell, 2013; Shimabukuro, Grosse, & Rice, 2008; Wu, Kung, Li, & Tsai, 2014). Elucidating the reasons why medical expenditures are greater among those with ASD is important for the development of efficient, integrated, and coordinated delivery sytems for pediatric patients and those transitioning to adult services.

How use of these services changes as people with ASD transition into adulthood is unknown. Most of the research has been limited primarily to studies of children and their families. It is, however, expected that health care utilization and costs will increase as adults experience the increased morbidity that is as expected with the aging process. Yet, as the prevalence of autism dramatically increased in the last two decades, and as many of the children diagnosed in the 1990s with ASD have transitioning into adulthood, more attention is being paid to the adult population with ASD. Autism is becoming a recognized disorder for adults, not just children (Mandell, 2013; Tavassoli, Miller, Schoen, & Nielson, 2014; Wick & Zanni, 2009). There are newly released guidelines for autism screening and diagnosis in adults (National Guideline Clearinghouse, 2012). Future research assessing adequate access and utilization of quality healthcare services for adults with ASD is warranted.

Category: Using Tailored Adaptations of Health Care Services

Another unexamined area is the tailoring of healthcare services to the specific needs of people with ASD. It is especially important that healthcare providers at all points of care, in nonautism health settings be educated about ASD so they can appreciate and anticipate the unique needs of patients with the diagnosis. Sensitivity and awareness are needed while interacting with the patient and family members. No assumptions should be made about the needs and behaviors of the individual with ASD seeking medical care. Only after conducting comprehensive assessments of the individual's medical and psychiatric comorbidities and symptoms should the intervention plan be developed. The reader is referred to the book edited by Giarelli and Gardner

(2012) for more information about potential challenges of providing evidence-based health care that meets the special needs of ASD patients across their life span and in multiple healthcare clinical settings.

Because of the nature of ASD and associated sensitivities, not much is known about what types of medical services during the life course best promote health. Specifically, what is the best practice for emergency care for children with an ASD? What is the best way to treat a woman with Asperger's syndrome during childbearing? Do adults with an ASD access and utilize adequate care for their chronic illnesses (e.g., cancer, diabetes, epilepsy)? These are all areas that warrant further investigation and may become exemplars for integrated health care.

Healthcare service research that tracks access and utilization of healthcare services for people with ASD is critically important in planning and developing efficient and effective integrated healthcare delivery systems for people with ASD across the lifespan. Tracking CPT codes for medical services paid for by public and private insurance is a robust research strategy. Extending this research approach to the adult population with ASD is needed.

The Content and Process of Quality Care for ASD

The ideal model of healthcare services for those with ASD is one that is comprehensive, coordinated, and integrated. By design, the administrative, physical, and electronic infrastructure of the healthcare system should allow for comprehensive coordination of care and sharing of all information among the multiple healthcare providers who serve the individual with ASD. As seen in Table 6.1, categories of healthcare services are available to treat patients with ASD. In the current policy environment with legislated mandates for widespread use of electronic medical records (EMR), meaningful use and interoperability of all necessary patient-protected health information must exist to optimize efficient and effective use of the healthcare services.

The recent support of the Institute of Medicine for integrated systems (IOM, 2012), justifies our efforts to redesign models of care for ASD that are patient-centered and integrated. Figure 6.1 illustrates a proposed integrated model of interventions and treatments for ASD for patient-centered care with linkages between the patient and providers. The model could be expanded to include other educational and social support (e.g., housing) services. The structure and process of how to create and sustain effective and efficient linkages are important areas for future development. The proposed model can be used as a conceptual blueprint to guide development of integrated EMR that enable information to flow among categories of treatment

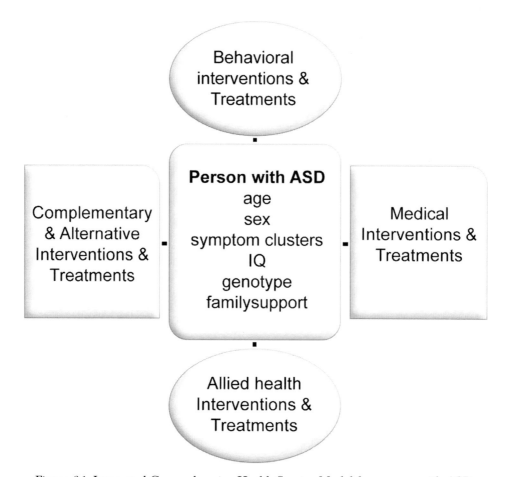

Figure 6.1. Integrated Comprehensive Health Service Model for persons with ASD.

and interventions for the patient. Linkages also are created between all providers so that information and communication can be optimized for the sake of the patient with ASD. In the center of the model is pertinant demographic and medical information about the patient with ASD. Capturing the comprehensive and holistic approaches used by many with ASD is needed to more fully describe the content and processes of care for ASD. This knowledge is fundamentally needed in order to answer questions about health outcomes of ASD treatments and interventions.

Unfortunately, integrated, comprehensive health service models for persons with an ASD are almost nonexistent because of the fragmentation and inefficiencies found in aspects of the current health care system. The fee-for-service reimbursement system does not encourage the time intensive aspects that are needed to collaborate for integrated approaches for health care (Barnes, Unruh, Chukmaitov, & van Ginneken, 2014; IOM, 2012). Healthcare providers are paid based on the basis of the services they provide. Except for case-management services, which are unclear, the reimbursement system encourages providers to be efficient with their time when they see their patients. They are paid for the services they provide directly to the patient, not for the time and effort to coordinate and integrate their management plans across different intervention domains. Systematic changes are needed to create mechanisms for retrieving reliable information and providing communication to the multiple providers caring for patients with ASD.

Moving from Isolated to Integrated Health Care Systems

Integration of health services is now a buzzword associated with the increased attention to improving the American health care system. The Institute of Medicine (IOM) defined integration of healthcare services as the "linkage of programs and activities to promote overall efficiency and effectiveness to achieve gains in population health" (IOM, 2012, p.3). The authors conceptualized integration in terms of multiple variables with different levels and partners and as a continuum ranging from systems in which all healthcare services are isolated to one in which all health care services are merged (IOM, 2012). Key differentiating characteristics that distinguish a fragmented system from an integrated system are illustrated in Figure 6.2. Isolated systems are autonomous without formal infrastructures for communication, health information, and coordination of care.

Integrated systems have linkages horizontally and vertically for maximal co-ordination and cooperation. The horizontal linkage of integrated systems refers to linkage of providers across different specialties. An example of integration at the horizontal level would be linkages among dental, pediatric, and behavioral health. The vertical level refers to linkages between and among primary, secondary, and tertiary care levels. An example would be a link between primary care and specialist. Patient care is integrated (coordinated and comanaged) during transitions from the community to the hospital and back to the community.

CASE EXAMPLE. The following fictitious clinical scenario serves as an example of an integrated system. Imagine an adult patient with ASD who sought medical care because he noticed blood in his urine (hematuria). After a series of appointments and medical procedures by his urologist, the diagnosis of bladder cancer was determined to be the cause of his hematuria. Throughout this period, all information about his care (e.g., office visits, biopsy and radiology reports, medication lists) was part of an integrated health

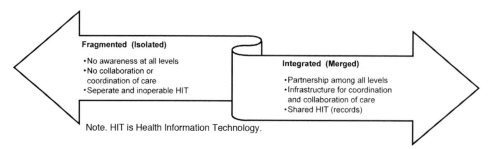

Figure 6.2. Key differences between a Fragmented verses an Integrated Healthcare System.

information system that was transparent to his entire health care team. His health care team included all those treating his bladder cancer, ASD (e.g., neurologist, behavioral therapist, case manager), and other primary health care needs. The patient's team that managed the patient's ASD-related health care would all have had real time information with abilities to coordinate and comanage all aspects of care from an initial office visit for bladder biopsies to the hospital for a radical cystectomy (surgical removal of bladder), and then back home for recovery. While this is an extreme example, it illustrates the complexity of issues when the patient with ASD must receive health care for serious medical conditions.

Striving for a more effective and efficient health care system, the Affordable Care Act, which was passed in 2010, has incentivized landmark changes by creating accountable care organizations (ACOs) (Barnes, Unruh, Chukmaitov, & van Giet al., 2014). Three key aims of the Affordable Care Act (2010) are to: (1) Improve the experience of care, (2) improve the health of populations, and (3) reduce per capita costs (Barnes et al., 2014). These are laudable aims for the population with ASD. However, the need is great for well-designed health services research projects to ensure that these aims are met for the ASD population. Achieving this goal is critical because different iterations of ACOs are likely to roll out soon in communities throughout the US. Best practices in developing and implementing ACOs have yet to be determined.

Barnes and colleagues (2014) stressed the importance of including the following three key components in integrated models of healthcare systems. *First,* needed is a formal legal and governance structure to overcome fragmentation. Rewards or incentives for cooperation and collaboration among providers for attaining quality and cost benchmarks must be built in. *Second,* linkage must be in place through the care continuum between providers and settings (e.g., inpatient and outpatient). *Third,* integrated health information technology systems must be in place to facilitate effective care coordination and disease management to monitor and analyze quality, cost, and patient outcomes. Measurable outcomes are a legislative mandate for ACOs. Thus, the ASD community must identify and define salient outcomes with benchmarking quality metrics for comprehensive, integrated service delivery.

Although no one organizational structure has been determined as the best model for an ACO, Kaiser Permanente, a traditional health maintenance organization has sustained itself as a fully integrated health delivery system for over 70 years and should be considered as an exemplary model for an ACO (Feachem, Sekhri, & White, 2002). In 1945, Kaiser was formed just after the Great Depression years, in the Western US, as both the payer (insurer) and provider of health care delivery services (Feachem et al., 2002). A much closer study of Kaiser is warranted for those who are interested in the study of healthcare systems and how to create an integrated ACO. Kaiser's track record of integrated coordinated care and use of clinical data (Clift, Scott, Johnson, & Gonzalez, 2014) collected through their integrated health record system (even before conversion to electronic health records) have been instrumental in their ability to develop one of this nation's leading programs of autism research. They are investigating genetic and environmental risk factors for ASD and patterns of detection, diagnosis, and utilization of health services for ASD. More information can be found on their website dedicated just to autism research (http://www.dor.kaiser.org/external /dorexternal/autism/index.aspx, retrieved September 14, 2014). Kaiser's sustainability over many decades as an integrated system of care underscores how their maximized collaboration, coordination, and use of integrated health data to generate knowledge, and its research contributions underscore its value as a type of ACO model (Clift et al., 2014; Feachem et al., 2002).

Benchmarking Quality and Integrative Services for People with ASD

Creating benchmarks for best practices is necessary to improve the quality of healthcare services for those with ASD. Although establishing *best-practices* for effective, safe, coordinated patient-centered care, integrated care across the life span of people with ASD makes sense. The Joint Commission, a not-for-profit organization that accredits and certifies health care organizations and programs in the US, has now published the second edition of its detailed guide to benchmarking in health care (Joint Commission, 2012).

The Joint Commission (2012) defined benchmarking as "a systematic, data-driven process of continuous improvement that involves internally and externally comparing performance to identify, achieve, and sustain best practices" (Joint Commission, 2012, p. 1). A key premise underlying benchmarking is the feasibility of implementing and evaluating healthcare practices. Benchmarking is data driven with specified process and outcome variables that are measurable. When carefully planned and used accordingly, benchmarking serves as an indispensable tool in a healthcare organization's approach to achieving and sustaining clinical effectiveness and superior performance (Joint Commission, 2012). Collaboration within and across organizations and major stakeholders is key to successful benchmarking and serves as an important step in benchmarking in order to generate the necessary knowledge to identify best practices.

Because benchmarking is a process intended to produce change, support and involvement from the highest levels of management are critical for success (Joint Commission, 2012). Management support means allocating resources to support standardized data collection and reporting to ensure that they meet the requirements of the databases, and providing adequate time to carry out activities related to benchmarking projects. Successful benchmarking of best practices for health care for people with ASD requires careful planning, investigation, implementation, and continuous evaluation. Adequate allocation of time is necessary to identify the many additional steps within and across organizations needed to develop effective benchmarking process to improve care.

Best practices need to be identified before one can use benchmarking processes to improve integrated health care for those with an ASD. Once benchmarks are established for integrated, coordinated, and comprehensive health care, then the quality of the processes and integrated healthcare services for people with ASD can be measured and evaluated with salient health care outcomes.

Although different benchmarking approaches are used, the approach used for benchmarking by the Dartmouth Collaborative, a collaboration of six organizations, is highlighted as an exemplar by the Joint Commission (2012). To demonstrate how benchmarking can be applied to improve integrated high-quality healthcare for people with ASD, Table 6.2 provides an outline of the key steps to plan for during the benchmarking process. Best practice benchmarks are needed for specific clinical scenarios. Some examples include the diabetic patient with ASD or emergency room admissions for the patient with ASD.

Health Services Research

The field of health services research evolved in the 1970s with conceptual and methodological approaches to generate knowledge necessary to help improve people's health and the health care delivery systems (Aday, 2001).

Table 6.2
PROPOSED OBJECTIVES AND STEPS TO IMPLEMENT
THE BENCHMARKING PROCESSES FOR INTEGRATED
HEALTHCARE DELIVERY FOR PEOPLE WITH ASDs

Main Objective	*Steps*
Share current processes of fragmented vs. integrated healthcare delivery	• Convene key stakeholders. • Everyone needs to understand how others are currently delivering care. • Begin critical conversations to foster a rapid learning process around effective practices.
Clearly define the problems	• Use skilled trained group facilitators to make sure consensus is reached because much work lies ahead. • Without trained facilitators it is easy to get off track and jeopardize attaining a collegial and collaborative group process.
Seek out evidence and gaps	• Use a variety of sources that may or may not begin with the published literature to understand the current evidence and gaps in integrated health care for people with ASD. • Be sure to reach out to a variety of key stakeholders, including interdisciplinary clinicians, people with ASD, advocacy groups, and researchers.
Standardize definitions so data can be combined and compared	• Conceptualize and operationalize definitions of key constructs. • Criteria for defining measures need to be standardized and measurable. For example, how is integrated health care defined and measured. What data will be used? Will qualitative and quantitative data be used?
Perform analyses to identify improvements towards integrated health care	• Use a well defined process for data collection that is clearly replicable. • Conduct comparative analyses to determine performance in terms of quality, outcomes, and costs.
Collaborate to develop best practice models	• Establish benchmarks.

The conceptual models of Donabedian and Aday and colleagues continue to guide active programs of health services research. They are relevant today for those concerned about planning, implementing, and evaluating health care delivery models that promote optimal health outcomes for people with ASD.

Aday wrote, "Health services research is a multidisciplinary field of inquiry, both basic and applied, that examines the use, costs, quality, accessibility, delivery, organization, financing, and effects of health care services to increase knowledge and understanding of the structure, processes, and effects [outcomes] of health care services for individuals and populations" (Aday et al., 1998, p. 4). Whereas clinical research focuses on the patient, and public health research focuses on communities and their environments and populations, health service research focuses on healthcare systems and institutions (Aday et al., 1998). The Donabedian model is described below.

Donabedian's Quality Care Model

The Quality Care Model of Avedis Donabedian, a physician and health service researcher, is perhaps the founding conceptual model from which the field of health services research evolved. His landmark paper was published in 1966 by the *Milbank Memorial Fund Quarterly* (Donabedian, 2005). Donabedian posited that to evaluate the quality of medical/health care, the structure in which the processes of care occur must be fully assessed along with outcomes of care. This, in essence, is the integration of health care. His model has three main interrelated concepts: Structure, process, and outcome.

Health service researchers further elaborated on Donadedian's conceptual model to operationalize the three key concepts for the field of health service research. According to Aday et al., (1998), *structure* is defined as the characteristics of the context in which health care takes place. This structure includes multiple dimensions of the delivery system, such as organizational structure (e.g., integrated vs. isolated), health policy financing and economics, workload (e.g., nurse/patient ratios), physical space and location, providers of health care (e.g., medical doctors vs. nurse practitioners), and other factors related to the structure of the healthcare delivery system (Aday et al., 1998). The healthcare delivery system is defined by the researcher and their focus of study. They may focus on a large-scale healthcare system or a smaller, specific delivery system of health care. An example of a smaller, specific focus would be the study of *case management delivery services* for the ASD population. Because little standardization exists, this is an important area for future research to advance knowledge about what *structure* of case management is associated with best outcomes for people with ASD. Some important unanswered questions relate to who is providing case management? What is the required training? Who pays for case management? What is the ratio of ASD patients for each case manager? This knowledge is important for the field of health service research pertaining to developing and implementing integrated models of care.

Process is defined as all the activities that go on within and between health care professionals and patients that occur during the use of the services obtained from the healthcare system (Aday et al., 1998). Examples of process variables include specific aspects of healthcare visits (Aday et al., 1998) such as the process to gain access to care (e.g., electronic or paper referrals vs. no referrals); interpersonal interactions among the patients and healthcare professionals (e.g., time spent, counseling, communication level of patients and healthcare professionals); and specific processes of health care rendered during the received healthcare services (e.g., antenatal breastfeeding health education); Chlamydia (a sexually transmitted infection) testing by getting vaginal samples vs. urine samples; and counseling conducted before HIV testing).

Lastly, *outcomes* are broadly defined as the "consequences to the health and welfare of individuals and of society" (as cited in Aday, 1998, p. 50). Many patient-oriented health outcomes research programs are guided by this Quality Care Model. The model lends itself to the study of broad, holistic health outcomes that include biological, psychological, and social dimensions of health and wellbeing.

Aday's Framework for Health Equity, Effectiveness, and Efficiency Research

Aday and Anderson developed a conceptual model of equity of access to medical care by measuring access and utilization of health care (Aday & Anderson, 1981). Whereas, Donabedian focused on outcomes of health care based on the structure and processes of health care services, Aday and Anderson focused on health equity. They defined equity as the concern with health disparities and the fairness and effectiveness of what is being done to address them (Aday et al., 1998). Fairness with respect to one's access to health care is achieved when services and healthcare goods are distributed on the basis of need. Inequity occurs when services are distributed on the basis of demographic variables such as race, income, and where people live (Aday & Anderson, 1981). They posited that variations in a patient's access to and utilization of health care occur as a function of the availability and the organizational structure of healthcare services. Predisposing or enabling characteristics of the individuals are also considered important factors that could hinder or facilitate individuals' health behaviors in seeking healthcare services (Aday & Anderson, 1981). An example of a *predisposing factor* that may hinder a pregnant woman with Asperger's syndrome attendance at childbirth classes may be her intense social anxiety about being in group situations.

Broadening their original framework, Aday and colleagues (Aday, 1994, 2001; Aday & Anderson, 1981; Aday et al., 1998) added the constructs of effectiveness, and efficiency to their original health equity model. Effectiveness is defined as the benefits of using health care by measuring health outcomes (Aday et al., 1998). Efficiency is defined as determining the benefits of using health care by measuring health outcomes. Efficiency is often measured through cost variables in health services research.

The conceptual models of Donabedian and Aday and colleagues continue to guide active programs of health services research. They are relevant today for those concerned about planning, implementing, and evaluating healthcare delivery models that promote optimal health outcomes for people with ASD. While the term "integrated health care" is used as an ideal for people with ASD, research is needed to further identify and delineate the structures and processes of integrated care that best serve the health and well-being of those with ASD when they undergo treatments for other healthcare needs. Aforementioned clinical situations such as the patient with ASD who is diagnosed with bladder cancer or the patient with Asperger's syndrome who is pregnant illustrate some examples. Unknown is exactly what integrated care for people with ASD should look like. In order to implement best practices, health service research is needed.

A New Conceptual Framework for ASD

A new conceptual framework can guide a robust research agenda to generate the knowledge needed to uncover the structures and processes of healthcare services that promote optimal health outcomes for people with ASD (see Figure 6.3). This new framework synthesizes the systems perspective and key constructs of Aday et al. (1998), and the core constructs of structure, process, and outcomes proposed by Donabedian (2005).

The framework created by the nexus of economics, ethnicity, and disability with issues of vulnerability and health disparities for those with ASD who must access health care services for health promotion and disease prevention, can guide appropriate choices of a wide variety of empirical indicators to fully study multilevel factors.

As shown in the framework, even federal, state, and local health policies are important. Contextual factors (i.e., delivery system, environment) and individual factors (i.e., ASD patients and their families) are important when investigating and evaluating barriers and facilitators to equitable access and utilization of healthcare services. Individual-level factors that flow directly from the person with ASD, and his or her caretaker and family, are (a) real and perceived need for health care and health beliefs; and (b) family income,

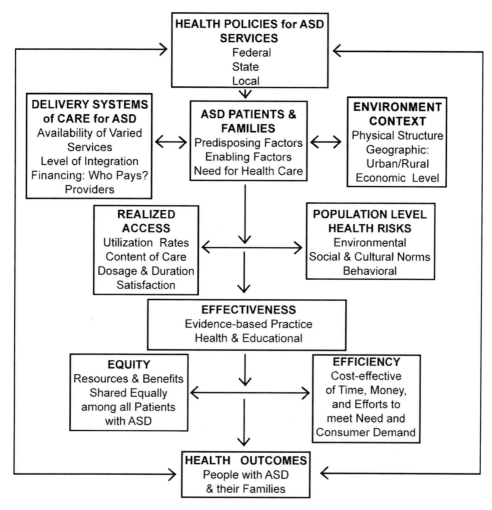

Figure 6.3. Synthesis of Donabedian and Aday frameworks to evaluate effectiveness, efficiency, and equity of delivery systems of care for peope with ASD and associated health outcomes.

health insurance coverage, and social support. Other individual-level factors are the patient's age, age of the family caregiver, sex of the patient and family caregiver, and race.

Identifying the salient patient-centered outcomes for ASD remains an important and understudied area of research and policy development. Measureable patient-centered outcomes specific to people with ASD that reflect optimal biological, psychological, social, and spiritual health wellness are of utmost importance. These measures will form the basis of wise and effective health policy to guide the development of quality, safe, efficient, and effective health care for people with ASD.

Conclusions

Implementing and evaluating best practices for the delivery of health care to people with ASD necessitates looking beyond individual-level biomedical services but to a broader holistic and patient-centered healthcare delivery model that aims to optimize outcomes in health promotion and disease prevention. How healthcare delivery systems for people with ASD are structured and how and when services are offered to patients will ultimately impact health outcomes. While attempting to implement and evaluating models of integrated, comprehensive care for people with ASD, we must continue to study health outcomes in a systematic way that promises to inform practice and policy.

References

Acef, S., & Aubrun, P. (2010). Somatic care and autism: Removal of barriers to reducing inequalities. *Sante Publique (Vandoeuvre-Les-Nancey), 22*(5), 529–539.

Aday, L. (1994). Health status of vulnerable populations. *Annual Review of Public Health, 15,* 487–509.

Aday, L. (2001). Establishment of a conceptual base for health services research. *Journal of Health Services Research, 6*(3), 183–185.

Aday, L., & Anderson, R. (1981). Equity of access to medical care: A conceptual and empirical overview. *Medical Care, 19*(12), 4–27.

Aday, L., Begley, C. E., Lairson, D. R., & Slater, C. H. (1998). *Evaluating the healthcare system: Effectiveness, efficiency, and equity.* Chicago, IL: Health Administration Press.

Affordable Care Act of 2010, 42 U.S.C., 111th Congress. Retrieved from http://housedocs.house.gov/energycommerce/ppacacon.pdf

Anderson, R., & Aday, L. (1978). Access to medical care in the U.S.: Realized and potential. *Medical Care, 16*(7), 533–546.

Bard, M., & Nugent, M. (2011). *Accountable care organizations: Your guide to strategy, design, and implementation.* Chicago, IL: Health Administration Press.

Barker, E. T., Hartley, S. L., Seltzer, S. L., Floyd, F. J., Greenberg, J. S., & Orsmond, G. I. (2011). Trajectories of emothional well-being in mothers of adolescents and adults with autism. *Developmental Psychology, 47*(2), 551–561.

Barnes, A. J., Unruh, L., Chukmaitov, A., & van Ginneken, E. (2014). Accountable care organizations in the USA: Types, developments and challenges. *Health Policy, 118*(1), 1–7.

Begeer, S., Mandell, D., Winjker-Holmes, B., Venderbosch, S., Rem, D., Stekelenburg, F., & Koot, H. M. (2013). Sex differences in the timing and identification among children and adults with autism spectrum disorders. *Journal of Autism & Developmental Disorders, 43*(5), 1151–1156.

Bloch, J. R., & Gardner, M. (2007). Accessing a diagnosis for a child with an autism spectrum disorder: The burden is on the caregiver. *American Journal for Nurse Practitioners, 11*(8), 10–17.

Centers for Disease Control and Prevention. (2014). Prevalence of autism spectrum disorder among children aged 8 years: Autism and Developmental Disabilities Monitoring Network, 11 sites, United States, 2010. *Mortality and Morbidity Weekly Report, 63*(SS 2), 1–21.

Charles, J. M. (2010). Dental care in children with developmental disabilities: Attention deficit disorder, intellectual disabilities, and autism. *Journal of Dentistry for Children (Chicago, Ill.), 77*(2), 84–91.

Cidav, Z., Lawer, L., Marcus, S. C., & Mandell, D. S. (2013). Age-related variation in health service use and associated expenditures among children with autism. *Journal of Autism & Developmental Disorders, 43*(4), 924–931.

Clift, K., Scott, L., Johnson, M., & Gonzalez, C. (2014). Leveraging geographic information systems in an integrated health care delivery organization. *The Permanente Journal, 18*(2), 71–75.

Daniels, A. M., & Mandell, D. S. (2013). Explaining differences in age at autism spectrum disorder diagnosis: A critical review. *Autism, 18*(5), 583–597.

Donabedian, A. (2005). Evaluating the quality of medical care. 1966. *Milbank Quarterly, 83*(4), 691–729.

Feachem, R., Sekhri, N. K., & White, K. L. (2002). Getting more for their dollar: A comparison of the NHS with California's Kaiser Permanente. *British Medical Journal, 324*(7330), 135–141.

Giarelli, E. (2012). Introduction and background: Core features, autism spectrum disorder prevalence, and the role of nursing. In E. Giarelli & M. R. Gardner (Eds.), *Nursing of autism spectrum disorder: Evidence-based integrated care across the lifespan* (pp. 1–4). New York: Springer.

Giarelli, E., Wiggins, L. D., Rice, C. E., Levy, S. E., Kirby, R. S., Pinto-Martin, J., & Mandell, D. (2010). Sex differences in the evaluation and diagnosis of autism spectrum disorders among children. *Disability and Health Journal, 3*(2), 107–116.

Golden, S. L., & Nageswaran, S. (2012). Caregiver voices: Coordinating care for children with complex chronic conditions. *Clinical Pediatrics, 51*(8), 723–729.

Gourdine, R. M., Baffour, T. D., & Teasley, M. (2011). Autism and the African American community. *Social Work in Public Health, 26*(4), 454–470.

Hollander, E., Kolevzon, A., & Coyle, J. T. (Eds.). (2011). T*extbook of autism spectrum disorders.* Washington, DC: American Psychiatric Publishing.

Institute of Medicine (IOM). (2012). *Primary care and public health.* Washington, DC: The National Academies Press.

Joint Commission. (2012). *Benchmarking in health care* (2nd ed.). Oakbrook Terrace, IL: Joint Commission Resources, Inc.

Kogan, M. D., Strickland, B. B., Blumberg, S. J., Singh, G. K., Perrin, J. M., & van Dyck, P. C. (2008). A national profile of the health care experiences and family impact of autism spectrum disorder among children in the United States, 2005–2006. *Pediatrics, 122*(6), e1149–e1158.

Leslie, D. L., & Martin, A. (2007). Health care expenditures associated with autism spectrum disorders. *Archives of Pediatrics & Adolescent Medicine, 161*(4), 350–355.

Liptak, G. S., Benzoni, L. B., Mruzek, D. W., Nolan, K. W., Thingvoll, M. A., Wade, C. M., & Fryer, G. E. (2008). Disparities in diagnosis and access to health services for children with autism: Data from the National Survey of Children's Health. *Journal of Developmental & Behavioral Pediatrics, 29*(3), 152–160.

Liptak, G. S., Stuart, T., & Auinger, P. (2006). Health care utilization and expenditures for children with autism: Data from US National Samples. *Journal of Autism & Developmental Disorders, 36*(7), 871–879.

Lobar, S. (2014). Family adjustment across cultural groups in autistic spectrum disorders. *Advances in Nursing Science, 37*(2), 174–186.

Mandell, D. S. (2013). Adults with autism–a new minority. *Journal of General Intern Medicine, 28*(6), 751–752.

Mandell, D. S., Wiggins, L. D., Carpenter, L. A., Daniels, J., DiGuiseppi, C., Durkin, M. S., . . . Kirby, R. S. (2009). Racial/ethnic disparities in the identification of children with autism spectrum disorders. *American Journal of Public Health, 99*(3), 493–498.

National Guideline Clearinghouse (NGC). (2012). Guideline: Autism: recognition, referral, diagnosis and management of adults on the autism spectrum. In *National guideline clearinghouse (NGC)* [website]. Rockville, MD: Agency for Healthcare Research and Quality (AHRQ). Available from: http://www .guideline.gov

Parish, S., Magana, S., Rose, R., Timberlake, M., & Swaine, J. G. (2012). Health care of Latino children with autism and other developmental disabilities: Quality of provider interaction mediates utilization. *American Journal on Intellectual & Developmental Disabilities, 117*(4), 304–315.

Semansky, R. M., Xie, M., Lawer, L. J., & Mandell, D. S. (2013). How states use Medicaid to fund community-based services to children with autism spectrum disorders. *Psychiatric Serices, 64*(10), 1051–1055.

Tavassoli, T., Miller, L. J., Schoen, S. A., Nielson, D. M., & Baron-Cohen, S. (2014). Sensory over-responsivity in adults with autism spectrum conditions. *Autism, 18*(4), 428–432.

Thomas, K. C., Ellis, A. R., McLaurin, C., Daniels, J., & Morrissey, J. P. (2007). Access to care for autism-related services. *Journal of Autism & Developmental Disorders, 37*(10), 1902–1912.

Thomas, K. C., Parish, S. L., Rose, R. A., & Kilany, M. (2012). Access to care for children with autism in the context of state Medicaid reimbursement. *Maternal & Child Health Journal, 16*(8), 1636–1644.

Wang, L., Mandell, D. S., Lawer, L., Cidav, Z., & Leslie, D. L. (2013). Healthcare service use and costs for autism spectrum disorder: A comparison between medicaid and private insurance. *Journal of Autism & Developmental Disorders, 43*(5), 1057–1064.

Wick, J. Y., & Zanni, G. R. (2009). Autism and aging: Hardly out of the woods. *Consultant Pharmacist, 24*(9), 653–660.

Chapter 7

BUILDING A MEDICAL HOME FOR CHILDREN AND YOUTH WITH ACUTE CARE NEEDS

RENEE TURCHI

Introduction

The growing population of children with autism spectrum disorders (ASD) requires that clinicians caring for children with ASD provide optimal healthcare delivery for this vulnerable population. Children with ASD, by definition, face many challenges in their lives, including but not limited to: Social adjustment, emotional and mental health maintenance, education, accessing comprehensive medical care, achieving financial maintenance, and transitioning to adult-oriented systems. A patient and family-centered medical home for children with ASD can foster integration, coordination, and comprehensive planning for children with ASD and their families.

The Medical Home Model

The medical home is the standard of care in healthcare delivery systems for children and youth (Turchi, Gatto, & Antonelli, 2007). First introduced by the American Academy of Pediatrics in 1967 (American Academy of Pediatrics, 1967) as a central repository for children's medical records, the medical home has evolved over time and core tenets are contained in the description of the primary care workforce in the test of the Affordable Care Act (US Department of Health and Human Services, 2010). While it is not necessarily a building, it does connote a location that is easily accessible for families and delivers care that is coordinated, family/patient-centered, culturally ef-

fective, and comprehensive (American Academy of Pediatrics, 2002; Kellerman & Kirk, 2007). In principle, the contemporary medical home is a partnership among the patient, family, and primary provider that, when needed,
solicits input from specialists, and support from the community. The patient
and his or her family are at the center of the model. A key aspect of the medical home is that the focus has shifted to include all children and adults, not
just children with special health care needs.

While pediatric and adult primary care providers agree on core constructs of the medical home (Kellerman & Kirk, 2007), there are fundamental principles intrinsic to pediatrics warranting further consideration (Stille,
Turchi, Cheng, Antonelli, Cabana, & Perrinet, 2010). Among these differences is including the family as an integral component of care and an essential element of medical home. See Figure 7.1 for a model of a community-
based system of services.

Evidence in support of the medical home suggests that care provided in
a medical home is associated with: Decreases in health disparities, fewer
unmet needs, improved health care utilization, and favorable impacts on pa-
tient/family-centered care (Homer et al., 2008). However, in a study of factors associated with the use of the medical home, Knapp and colleagues (2013)
reported a lower use among families of children with a behavioral health
condition. This is a particularly concerning given the impact a diagnosis of
ASD can have on a child and his or her family and the need for ongoing access to comprehensive and coordinated care. Thus, it is imperative the goal
for children with ASD is provision of a high quality, integrated, patient/fam-
ily-centered, and coordinated medical home.

Application to Any Community

The medical home fosters a process of care delivery that is coordinated
and comprehensive beyond just medical settings. For example, children with
an ASD need support and advocacy in school, educational, and therapeutic
settings. The medical home model and team is intricately linked to the community and policies and thus would support families in nonmedical sectors.
Moreover, the tenants of medical home extend throughout the life course, so
it applies to youth with ASD grow older and require support transitioning to
adult-oriented systems with vocational, education, and medical care. Patient
and family-centered care are central pillars in the medical home model, and
it is critical these principles extend into any provider, service, or settings
serving children with ASD.

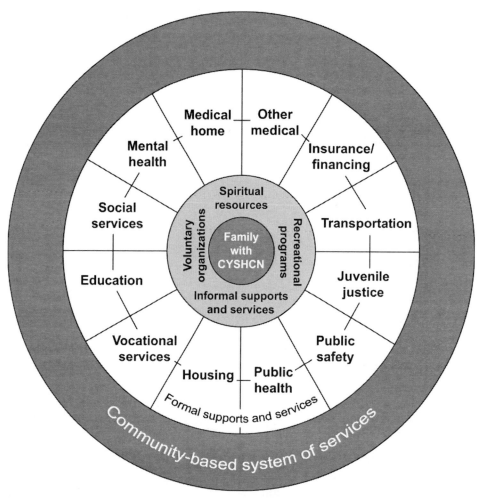

Figure 7.1. Community Systems and Services for Children with Special Health Care Needs. Permission to reprint from: Perrin et al. (2007). Services for children and youth with special care needs. *Archives of Pediatric Medicine, 161*(10), 933–936.

Medical Home for Children and Youth with ASD

Children and youth with special healthcare needs are defined as, children who have or are at risk for chronic physical, developmental, behavioral, or emotional conditions. These are children who require health and other services beyond that needed by children, in general (McPherson et al., 1998). Children with ASD are characterized as having special healthcare needs that warrant special consideration and can be best addressed in the medical home environment. The major components of the medical home are care provision and care coordination.

Care Provision

Care provision in a medical home is paramount for children with ASD. Typically they usually require mental health services, educational supports, medical care, and community partnerships across a variety of settings given their impaired social interactions, behaviors, and social skills. The patient and family-centered medical home fosters effective integration and coordination of these supports and services maximizing potential for children with ASD and their families. A high quality, functioning medical home does not need to provide every service alone, but does require effective partnerships across various settings and the community via coordination across systems (Turchi & Antonelli, 2014).

Care Coordination

Care coordination is also a hallmark of the medical home in practice. It takes many forms and can be individualized. Considering the availability of resources, supports, and services required in caring for children with ASD, information sharing will improve coordination of care for this population. For example, a child diagnosed with ASD as a toddler will benefit from coordination of care across multiple care settings (i.e., primary, specialty, family support network, etc.). Linking the family with another parent with a child of the same age with ASD provides another source of support. In addition, the parents' access to therapeutic services provided through early intervention programs will improve the likelihood or the delivery of timely and effective treatments. Care planning with the specialists needed to manage this child is paramount to ensure effective care and avoid duplication of services. Lasting care can be coordinated to assure that it makes full and fair use of available local, regional, and national resources and maximizes use of the insurance and other benefits to which the child is entitled.

Improved Use of Services

Families caring for children with ASD are often faced with the difficult task of navigating a complex array of services and professionals who are assigned to assist in care. Families of children with special needs are at the center of an array of services. There are spiritual, recreational, informational, and volunteer services directly connected to them that facilitate the linkages to the next layer—like spokes on the wheel—for accessing medical, mental, health, educational, vocational, insurance, and other needed services.

OBSTACLES TO USE OF SERVICES. Often families with children with ASD without a medical home find themselves attempting to integrate necessary services without a roadmap or guidelines while attempting to manage the care of their child (Carbone, Beh, Azor, & Murphy, 2010). Often each service or system has its own coordinator or point of contact. Without a medical home, no one is facilitating communication and ensuring there is not service duplication. Farmer and colleagues (2014) found in their analyses of this population that less than one in five children with ASD had a medical home. In this study the authors found, after controlling for sociodemographic variables, that while most families with children with ASD had a usual source of care, less than one-half received family-centered care and less than one-third felt their care was coordinated. By contrast, having a medical home was associated with fewer unmet needs. For example, those with a medical home were more likely to have had a usual source of care, sufficient behavioral therapy, and a personal doctor/nurse for specialty care (Farmer et al., 2014). These findings support the needs for ensuring children with ASD have access to this form of care (Cheak-Zamora & Farmer, 2014).

Family Satisfaction and Stress

The family as a whole benefits from the medical home. A study comparing children with ASD receiving an autism-specific medical home intervention to children with ASD (controls) receiving standard primary care found families receiving the medical home intervention reported improved satisfaction and greater shared decision making. However, there were no statistically significant differences in family stress (Golnik, Scal, Wey, & Gaillard, 2012). Family stress is a complex construct with many intrinsic and extrinsic variables that need further study in this population to parse out the factors that might be mitigated with the medical home model. This still needs to be evaluated and would be important to study in the future evaluation of family issues. Pediatricians endeavor to improve services for children with ASD, but report the lack of time, training, and resources as barriers to this outcome (Carbone et al., 2010). More research is needed on the role, adoption, and implementation of medical homes for children with ASD and their families (Cheak-Zamora & Farmer, 2014.)

Adapting the Medical Model for Specific Service Settings

There are several tools available to assist in adopting and implementing the medical home in practice settings. In pediatrics, some practices employ the Medical Home Index (Cooley, McAllister, Sherrieb, & Clark, 2003), a nationally validated instrument designed to assess measurement of medical home constructs in the outpatient practice setting. This index is a needs assessment for practice team members to complete which identifies areas of strength, gaps, and opportunities in medical home implementation like care coordination/planning, data systems and management, and care partnership and support.

Patient registries are critical to managing patients with chronic conditions (McAllister, Presler, Turchi, & Antonelli, 2009). These registries can be developed as part of an electronic healthcare record/spreadsheet including but not limited to information such as: Name, date of birth, height and weight measurements, immunizations, diagnoses, severity indices, need for home nursing and or equipment, specialists, community partners, and benchmarks related to clinical practice guidelines, such as studies and laboratory results.

The American Academy of Pediatrics has developed a medical home toolkit that can be found at the National Center for Medical Home Implementation (APA, 2015). The toolkit has materials to assist practitioners with assessments, preparation, and step-by-step guides on medical home implementation. Clinicians may employ quality improvement during practice transformation in medical home efforts. Ongoing practice reassessment, targeting goals for improvement, employing *Plan-Do-Study-Act* cycles are a few strategies practitioners can engage with their team as they implement the medical home. During these cycles team members identify an area needing improvement and develop an action plan to address or fix an issue. For example, a team might study patient wait times and identify when the longest wait times existed and why, then pilot a test solution and track if the intervention was effective. The major components of implementing medical home are establishing: Care partnership supports, a clinical care organization, care delivery management, resources and linkages, practice performance measurements, and approaches to payment and finance. Clear communication between the medical home and patients and families is critical to quality care. In a medical home, it is essential to have good, quick resources for patients and their families.

Care Coordination-Expanded View

Care coordination has been characterized as the set of activities that occur in the spaces between providers, visits, and entities (Turchi & Antonelli, 2014). In a recent Commonwealth Fund report, Antonelli, McAllister, and Popp (2009) defined pediatric care coordination as a "patient and family-centered, assessment driven, team based activity designed to meet the needs of children and youth while enhancing the caregiving capabilities of families" (p. 760). Ultimately, coordination of care enables the achievement of the "triple aim" described as: Better *care,* better *health,* and lower *cost.* These are principal outcomes for health system transformation (Berwick, Nolan, & Whittington, 2008).

An analysis of data from the 2005–2006 National Survey of Children with Special Health Care Needs (Maternal and Child Health Bureau, 2009) demonstrated positive associations among care coordination, family-provider relations, and family/child outcomes. Specifically, the provision of care coordination was positively associated with patient- and family-reported "receipt of family-centered care," resulting in partnerships with professionals, satisfaction with services, ease of getting referrals, less out-of-pocket expenses and family financial burden, fewer hours per week spent coordinating care, less impact on parental employment, and fewer school absences and emergency department (ED) visits (Turchi, Berhane, Bethell, Pomponio, Antonelli, & Minkovitz, 2009).

The effective coordination of a child's health services is critical to providing high quality efficient care, particularly for children with ASD and their families (McAllister et al. 2007). Successful care coordination takes into consideration the continuum of health, education, early childcare, and social services needed to improve the quality of care for children with ASD. It is to be distinguished from disease or case management that primarily focuses on health needs of the patients. The fundamental goals of care coordination are to: Develop an anticipatory/proactive plan for appropriate services for the child and family, integrate the recommendations of multiple professionals and service systems and the preferences of the child and family, assist the family in accessing needed services, share information, facilitate communication, avoid duplication of services and unnecessary costs, establish accountability, and optimize health and well-being of the child (Turchi & Antonelli, 2014). Coordinated care is characterized by system-focused activities. These are listed in Box 7.1.

Figure 7.2 depicts the care coordination framework exemplifying a family-centered approach with the focus on health systems with interdisciplinary and environmental structures, processes, and the outcomes required to best serve children and families. Optimal care coordination is provided best in the context of a team with effective working relationships with families, specialists, service providers, clinicians, community partners, and other professionals.

Box 7.1. Activities that Characterize Coordinated Care in the Medical Home

- Assess and update coordination needs;
- Create and update with families an individualized plan of care that includes a medical summary;
- Create and update with families an individualized plan of care that includes an action plan;
- Create and update with families an individualized plan of care that includes an emergency/contingency plan;
- Promote communication with families and among health team members;
- Communicate integrated information among the members of the health team, between health team and patients/family, and between the medical and nonmedical teams;
- Communicate integrated information and across settings;
- Manage/track tests, referrals, and outcomes;
- Facilitate transition across healthcare settings, from acute episode of care to chronic disease management
- Facilitate transition across healthcare settings from pediatric to an adult system of care; and
- Connect with community resources (Antonelli et al. 2009).

Using Actionable Plans

Care planning includes the use of an "actionable" care plan with assigned tasks/roles, a care plan document, emergency information form, and/or a medical summary, including past medical history and salient specialist information. These care plans are developed and implemented with input from members of the team caring for a child with ASD, including mental health providers, therapists, community partners, educational specialists, primary care providers, dental providers, medical subspecialists and surgical specialists, and most importantly, the family and patient themselves.

Coordinated care plans are used across the continuum of care by including medical, educational, mental health, community, and home care providers (Taylor, Lizzi, Marx, Chilkatowsky, Trachtenberg, & Ogle, 2012). These plans should state explicitly goals including early intervention, educational/vocational and family interventions that are therapeutically optimal

PEDIATRIC CARE COORDINATION FRAMEWORK

Care Coordination Definition:
Pediatric care coordination is a patient- and family-centered, assessment-driven, team-based activity designed to meet the needs of children and youth while enhancing the care giving capabilities of families. Care coordination addresses interrelated medical, social, developmental, behavioral, educational and financial needs to achieve optimal health and wellness outcomes.

Defining Characteristics of Care Coordination

1. Patient and family-centered (PFC)	3. Promotes self-care skills and independence
2. Proactive, planned, and comprehensive	4. Emphasizes cross-organizational relationships

Care Coordination Competencies:

1) Develops partnerships
2) Proficient communicator
3) Uses assessments for intervention
4) Facile in care planning skills (PFC)
5) Integrates all resource knowledge
6) Possesses goal/outcome orientation
7) Approach is adaptable and flexible
8) Desires continuous learning
9) Applies solid team/building skills
10) Adept with information technology

Care Coordination Functions:

1) Provide separate visits and CC interactions
2) Manage continuous communications
3) Complete/analyze assessments
4) Develop care plans (with family)
5) Manage/track tests, referrals, and outcomes
6) Coach patient/family skills learning
7) Integrate critical care information
8) Support/facilitate all care transitions
9) Facilitate PFC team meetings
10) Use health information technology for CC

Figure 7.2. The figure illustrates the care coordination (CC) including the interrelated medical, social, developmental, behavioral, educational, and financial needs that must be addressed to achieve optimal health and wellness. Permission to reprint from: Antonelli, R., McAllister, J., & Popp, J. (2009). *Developing Care Coordination as a Critical Component of a High Performance Pediatric Health Care System: Forging a Multidisciplinary Framework for Pediatric Care Coordination.* Washington, DC: The Commonwealth Fund.

and likely to maximize outcomes for children with ASD. These plans drive successful transitions to adult systems of care.

The care plans are dynamic in nature and shared among practitioners. Yet, caregivers of children with ASD reported receiving written information or having their physician plan with other providers less than 50% of the time (Williams, Tomchek, Grau, Bundy, Davis, & Kleinert, 2012). It is essential that plans are maintained and updated with timely and salient information from all partners to avoid duplication of services and to optimize care for patients. Resource and education about implementation of care planning for children with ASD is a crucial component of care coordination.

Cultural and Organizational Change

The increasing prevalence of ASD necessitates the need for early and continuous screening. Screening children for ASD and partnering with early intervention supports are integral to successfully caring for this population. The Act Early Project demonstrated the critical role of partnering with state agencies, provider groups, autism and disability agencies, and academic centers in early identification and intervention of children with ASD (Peacock & Lin, 2012).

Cultural and organizational changes must occur for effective care coordination. McDonald and colleagues (2014) developed an atlas for care coordination described as the Care Coordination Measures Atlas and is available from the Agency of Health Care Research and Quality (AHRQ). The atlas provides tools and an approach to a care coordination framework for children and their families. This is an excellent resource.

The medical home practice that attends to cultural and organizational change must engage a collaborative teamwork approach and transform work processes to:

- Accommodate the needs of diverse patients/families that require more time;
- Share culturally relevant information and knowledge with patients/ families;
- Create registries of children with ASD to identify those with unique needs, and facilitate communication and monitoring;
- Develop individualized evidence-based care plans;
- Engage in quality improvement activities around practice transformation;
- Designate a team member to carry out the essential care coordination functions, including tracking of referrals; and
- Provide access and linkage to community-based resources (Turchi & Mann, 2012).

Technology in Care Coordination

Health information technology can play a pivotal role in care coordination. Electronic tools facilitate information sharing among patients/families and their health care teams, and, subsequently among health care teams, community partners, and medical and nonmedical providers. For example, previsit summaries, comprehensive health care plans, medical summaries, and personal health records can be shared among partners and health care teams caring for patients thus fostering optimal health care and communication for children with ASD (Turchi & Antonelli, 2014).

Health information systems ensure successful transfer of information, and establishing and monitoring accountability. Interoperable electronic health records (EHR) within integrated systems support private collaborative communications between patients, families, and the care team and facilitate shared decision-making for children with ASD and their families. EHRs can bridge information gaps among clinicians serving as the medical home team with therapists and mental health providers. The use of registries can support tracking and monitoring functions. Other health information technology tools like telemedicine, remote monitoring, online patient and caregiver assessments, and personal health records may enable improved workflow and process changes improving experiences for families of children with ASD.

Internet-based tools, patient portal, which are a part of meaningful use, and social media can foster communication between families and providers, provide information, support skills training, allow networking among families, facilitate connections between health care providers and community partners, and elicit patient feedback on care (McDonald et al., 2014).

Relational Coordination

Coordination is not merely management of the interdependence between tasks. Rather, "relational coordination" is an emerging topic that addresses the management of the people who are performing tasks. Gittell and colleagues defined it as a mutually reinforcing process of interaction between communication and relationships carried out for the purpose of task integration (Gittell, Seidner, & Wimbush, 2010). This concept is particularly relevant to care for children with ASD, as care coordination "activities" such as accessing therapeutic services, coordinating services among specialists, and working with community partners, like the educational system, are as important as the team which may include physicians, nurses, mental health providers, social workers, therapists, as well as community partners and family members. Relational coordination values the quality of interpersonal communications and the quality of therapeutic relationships among families, patients, health care providers, and community partners.

Provision of Patient and Family-Centered Care

A family-centered medical home implies a commitment to seeking and valuing the voice of the family caregivers in care decisions; acknowledging they are usually the experts in the individual strengths and needs of the child.

Family-centered care occurs when the health professional assists the family in decision-making that honors and respects families' preferences (Institute for Patient and Family-Centered Care, 2015). Such issues as identifying the family's concerns, setting goals, and choosing treatment options are part of the decision-making process accompanying family-centered care. The degree to which families serve as the ultimate decision makers in this process is one measure of family centeredness.

Central to delivering care in the medical home is a team-based approach to care. The team consists of the patient/family, community partners/ agencies, educational systems, mental health teams, and medical and health care professionals. In the office, "teamlets" of physicians and ancillary staff (medical assistants or nurses) work with patients, families, and communities to coach patients/families to optimize their health care and management of chronic conditions (Chen et al., 2010).

Delivering high quality, patient/family-centered, and efficient care is the cornerstone of primary care. The team-based model collects and utilizes data from electronic health records, patient/family feedback, and benchmarks across various settings to achieve continuous quality improvement. The American Academy of Pediatrics has developed a website called Bright Futures (APA, 2015b; Hagan, 2007). This source provides nationally recognized clinical practice guidelines and standards for the provision of primary care for children. This includes routine developmental screening utilizing a validated developmental screener, and regular surveillance for autism. For example, the Modified Checklist for Autism in Toddlers (MCHAT) can be used to screen low-risk toddlers for autism at recommended intervals in practice (Robins, Casagrande, Barton, Chen, Dumont-Mathieu, & Fein, 2014). There is evidence that children with a medical home are more likely to receive health screening and anticipatory guidance than children not receiving care in the context of a medical home (Romaire & Bell, 2010).

Importance of Family

Family-centered care is distinguished by the recognition that the family is the constant in a child's life, while the service systems and support personnel within those systems changes (Shelton & Stepanek, 1994). A central theme is the respectful partnership between the child's family and the healthcare professional who allows for family/professional collaboration; exchange of complete and unbiased information; recognition of family diversity; and provision of appropriate, flexible, and accessible services and supports (Denboba, McPherson, Kenny, Strickland, & Newacheck, 2006). However, parents of children with ASD report frustrations and lack of family-centered care services for administrative supports for their children (Hodgetts, Nicholas, Zwaigenbaum, & McConnell, 2013). Fostering settings where family-centered care and shared decision making are achieved is paramount in health care delivery for children with ASD and worth the concerted effort.

SHARED DECISION-MAKING. Patient- and family-centered care involves shared decision-making (SDM), where families and patients partner with providers. Shared decision-making refers to a formal process in which patients, or their family caregivers, review evidence-based decision aids to understand the likely outcome of different treatment options, think about and discuss with a health care provider what is personally important about the risks and benefits of different options, and then decide jointly on a treatment or course of action that best reflects the patients' and parents' preferences, needs, and values. The essential elements of SDM include recognizing and acknowledging a decision is required; knowing and understanding the best available evidence; and incorporating patient/family values and preferences into decisions. Incorporating feedback also includes eliciting family feedback regarding the practice's performance as a patient and family-centered medical home to best meet the needs of patient/families (Barratt, 2008; Fiks, Mayne, Localio, Alessandrini, & Guevara, 2012; Perrin et al, 2007).

The Institute for Healthcare Improvement stated:

> Health care financing is an overriding issue; others include overcoming disparities in access to care, improving health literacy, meeting the needs of a burgeoning population of older Americans and of the increasing numbers of people living with chronic conditions, improving patient safety, overcoming workforce shortages, and ensuring the appropriate use of technology. There is growing awareness that to achieve the best outcomes, patients and families must be more actively engaged in decisions about their health care and must have enhanced access to information and support. (Johnson et al., 2008, p. v)

This statement was followed by an extensive and comprehensive set of recommendations and guidelines for partnering with parents (Johnson et al., 2008). The recommendations are relevant for and easily translated to the parent and providers of care to children with ASD.

Role of Community Partners

A high-quality, functioning medical home does not need to provide every service alone, but does require effective partnerships across various settings and the community (McAlllister et al., 2009). Sixty-nine percent of parents of children with ASD reported physicians not providing adequate information about services in the community (Williams et al., 2012).

High-functioning community services and partnerships are key for children with ASD and their families. Care coordination is the hallmark to achieving these community partnerships. The Institute of Medicine (IOM) described a healthcare system for the twenty-first century as care coordination and cross-cutting system intervention fostering improved health care quality for adults and children (The Institute of Medicine, 2001). Primary care clinicians also need to communicate and collaborate with community-based educational, mental health clinicians, therapists, and social service agencies and programs in their support of children with ASD and their families (Turchi & Antonelli, 2014). This may involve working together to develop forms and checklists that clinicians can utilize to communicate the needed information for a particular program, such as eligibility information. Knowledge of the type of information needed by community service agencies and mental health/behavioral programs enhances the ability of the clinicians to communicate effectively and efficiently with those entities and assist families of children with ASD.

Comanagement with Specialist and Behavior Management Partners

Children with ASD often require more hospitalizations, more prescribed medications, and more healthcare visits (Johnson & Rodriguez, 2013). Information sharing improves coordination of care. Families need information about the ASD diagnosis, treatment options, and probable outcomes; information in the child's medical records; and information about community resources. There is evidence that well-designed information, whether paper- or Web-based, can help to improve patient knowledge and experiences of care as well as have positive effects on self-efficacy and health behavior (Coulter & Ellins, 2007). While some families are comfortable handling communication among primary care and specialty care physicians, others are uncomfortable serving as the intermediary (Stille, 2009).

Comanagement, communication, and collaboration among specialists and primary care providers are integral to managing patients with ASD (Turchi & Antonelli 2014). Ideally, relationships between primary care providers and specialists are reciprocal, and require bidirectional communication via various modes, including email, phone call, postal mail, and facsimile (Stille, 2009). Electronic health records provide automated systems and interfaces, but this does not mitigate the need for communication among the healthcare professionals and children with ASD.

According to Turchi and Mann (2012), when a patient with ASD and his or her family is referred to a specialist, the following needs to occur:

- The family is adequately prepared for the initial visit and know what to expect;
- There is timely and ongoing communication between the primary care clinician and the specialist;
- The consulting specialist receives the appropriate clinical information, including the reason for the consultation and any relevant laboratory and radiological results, before the initial visit;
- The primary care clinician follow-ups with patient/families after the visit with the specialist to review any recommendations;
- The primary care clinician assists the family in making decisions when multiple specialists may offer divergent points of view about the treatment regimen or the process; and
- The primary care clinician assists the family with obtaining the referral when there are financial barriers.

It is important that responsibilities for management be specifically delineated and families with children with ASD are given care plans delineating roles between mental health, specialty clinician, and the primary care team. In addition, children with ASD and their families' views, concerns, and needs must be taken into account, with open reciprocal communication among all involved parties. In order to successfully implement the medical home model, primary and specialty care teams need to pay close attention to coordination of roles and to identify a general process for communication that is efficient and that provides a structure for a rapid response.

Medical Home for the Adult with ASD

Youth with ASD transitioning to adult-oriented systems require additional supports medically, educationally, and vocationally to ensure a healthy and successful transition to adult-oriented systems (Schidlow & Fiel, 1990). The policies, training, and resources necessary to provide appropriate care to these patients has not kept pace with their growth in numbers making the transition process more challenging for all involved. Youth and young adults with ASD need additional support with adult mental health services, transportation, vocational services, educational services, self-management, and support services when transitioning successfully to adult systems and adult medical homes. This requires scaffolding, or temporary support structures, from pediatric to adult services that includes the coordination of family-centered care. This is essential for establishing high-quality medical homes for adults with ASD.

Conclusion

Children with ASD represent a growing and fragile population of children with special health care needs. Their needs are complex and best-practice care is resource intensive. This population will benefit from a high-quality, integrated, family-centered, coordinated medical home. Continued efforts of training and education for healthcare practitioners related to ASD should continue, including early identification, screening, referral supports, interventions, care coordination among specialist and community partners caring for children with ASD, and family professional partnerships (Hyman & Johnson, 2012). Clinicians, community agencies, mental health, social services, educational systems, and therapists in the medical home neighborhood can effectively partner, working together to maximize the potential of children with ASD.

References

American Academy of Pediatrics, Council on Pediatric Practice. (1967). Pediatric Records and a "medical home." In *Standards of child care* (pp. 77–79). Evanston, IL: American Academy of Pediatrics.

American Academy of Pediatrics. (2002). Medical Home Initiatives for children with Special Health Care Needs Advisory Committee. Policy statement: The medical home. *Pediatrics, 110,* 184–186.

American Academy of Pediatrics. (2015a). *Center for medical home implementation.* Available at http://www.medicalhomeinfo.org/

American Academy of Pediatrics. (2015b). *Bright futures.* Available at http://brightfutures.aap.org/index.html

Antonelli, R., McAllister, J., & Popp, J. (2009). *Developing care coordination as a critical component of a high performance pediatric health care system: Forging a multidisciplinary framework for pediatric care coordination.* Washington, DC: The Commonwealth Fund.

Barratt, A. (2008). Evidence based medicine and shared decision making: The challenge of getting both evidence and preferences into health care. *Patient Education and Counseling, 73,* 407–412.

Berwick, D. M., Nolan, T. W., & Whittington, J. (2008). The triple aim: Care, health and cost. *Health Affairs (Milwood), 27*(3), 759–769.

Carbone, P. S., Beh, D. D., Azor, V., & Murphy, N. A. (2010). The medical home for children with autism spectrum disorders: Parent and physician perspectives. *Journal of Autism & Developmental Disorders, 40,* 317–324.

Cheak-Zamora, N. C., & Farmer, J. E. (2015). The impact of the medical home on access to care for children with autism spectrum disorders. *Journal of Autism & Developmental Disorders, 45*(3), 636–644.

Chen, E. H., Thorn, D. H., Hessler, D. M., LaPhengrasamy, L., Hammer, H., Saba, G., & Bodenheimer, T. (2010). Using the teamlet model to improve chronic care in an academic primary care practice. *Journal of General Internal Medicine, 25*(Suppl 4), S610–S614.

Cooley, C., McAllister, J. W., Sherrieb, K., & Clark, R. E. (2003). The Medical Home Index: Development and validation of a new practice-level measure of implementation of the medical home model. *Academic Pediatrics, 3*(4), 173–180.

Coulter, A., & Ellins. J. (2007). Effectiveness of strategies for informing, educating, and involving patients. *British Medical Journal, 335,* 24–27.

Denboba, D., McPherson, M. G., Kenney, M. K., Strickland, B., & Newacheck P. W. (2006). Achieving family and provider partnerships for children with special health care needs. *Pediatrics, 118*(4), 1607–1615.

Fiks, A. G., Mayne, S., Localio, A. R., Alessandrini, E. A., & Guevara, J. P. (2012). Shared decision-making and health care expenditures among children with special health care needs. *Pediatrics, 129*(1), 99–107.

Farmer, J. E., Clark, M. J., Mayfield, W. A., Cheak-Zamora, N., Marvin, A. R., Law, J. K., & Law, P. A. (2014). The relationship between the medical home and unmet needs for children with autism spectrum disorders. *Maternal Child Health Journal, 18,* 672–680.

Gittell, J. H., Seidner, R., & Wimbush, J. (2010) A relational model of how high-performance work systems work. *Organizational Science, 21*(2), 490–506.

Golnik, A., Scal, P., Wey, A., & Gaillard, P. (2012). Autism-specific primary care medical home intervention. *Journal of Autism & Developmental Disorders, 42,* 1087–1093.

Hagan, J. (2007). *Bright futures: Guidelines for health supervision of infants, children and adolescents.* Evanston, IL: American Academy of Pediatrics.

Hodgetts, S., Nicholas, D., Zwaigenbaum, L., & McConnell, D. (2013). Parents' and professionals' perceptions of family-centered care for children with autism spectrum disorder across service sectors. *Social Science & Medicine, 96,* 138–146.

Hyman, S. L., & Johnson, J. K. (2012). Autism and pediatric practice: Toward a medical home. *Journal of Autism & Developmental Disorders, 42,* 1156–1164.

Homer, C. J., Klatka, K., Romm, D., Kuhlthau, K., Bloom, S., Newacheck, P., Van Cleave, J., & Perrin, J. M. (2008). A review of the evidence for the medical home for children with special health care needs. *Pediatrics, 122*(4), e922–e937.

Institute of Medicine, Committee on Quality of Health Care in America. (2001). *Crossing the quality chasm: A new health system for the 21st Century.* Washington, DC: National Academy Press.

Institute for Patient and Family-Centered Care. (2015). What is patient- and family-centered health care? Available at http://www.ipfcc.org/faq.html

Johnson, B., Abraham, M., Conway, J., Simmons, L., Edgman-Levitan, S., Sodomka, P., . . . Ford, D. (2008). *Partnering with patients and families to design a patient and family-centered health care system: Recommendations and promising practices.* Cambridge, MA: Institute for Healthcare Improvement. Available at: www.ipfcc .org/pdf/PartneringwithPatientsandFamilies.pdf

Johnson, N. L., & Rodriguez, D. (2013). Children with autism spectrum disorders at a pediatric hospital: A systematic review of the literature. *Pediatric Nursing, 39*(3), 131–142.

Kellerman, R., & Kirk, L. (2007). Principles of the patient-centered medical home. *American Family Physician.* Available at: http://www.aafp.org/afp/2007/0915/p774 .html

Knapp, C., Woodworth, L., Fernandez-Baca, D., Baron-Lee, J., Thompson, L., & Hinojosa, M. (2013). Factors associated with a patient centered medial home among children with behavioral health conditions. *Maternal and Child Health Journal, 17,* 1658–1664.

Maternal and Child Health Bureau, Health Resources and Services Administration, US Department of Health and Human Services. (2009, December 29). *The National Survey of Children with Special Health Care Needs Chartbook 2005–2006.* Rockville, Maryland: US Department of Health and Human Services, 2008. Available at: http://mchb.hrsa.gov/cshcn05.

McAllister, J. W., Presler, E., Turchi, R. M., & Antonelli, R. C. (2009). Achieving effective care coordination in the medical home. *Pediatric Annals, 38*(9), 491–497.

McDonald, K. M., Schultz, E., Albin, L., Pineda, N., Lonhart, J., Sundaram, V., . . . Davies, S. (2014). *Care Coordination Atlas Version 4 (Prepared by Stanford University under subcontract to American Institutes for Research on Contract No. HHSA290-2010-000051). AHRQ Publication No.14-0037-EF.* Rockville, MD: NIH/Agency for Healthcare Research and Quality.

Newacheck, P. W., & Kim, S. E. (2005). A national profile of health care utilization and expenditures for children with special health care needs. *Archives of Pediatric and Adolescent Medicine, 159*(1), 10–17.

Peacock, G., & Lin, S. C. (2012). Enhancing early identification and coordination of intervention services for young children with autism spectrum disorders: Report from the Act Early Regional Summit Project. *Disability and Health Journal, 5*(1), 55–59.

Perrin, J. M., Romm, D., Bloom, S. R., Homer, C. J., Kuhlthau, K. A., Cooley, C., . . . Newacheck, P. (2007). Family-centered, community-based system of services for children and youth with special health care needs. *Archives of Pediatric & Adolescent Medicine, 161*(10), 933–936.

Robins, D. L., Casagrande, K., Barton, M., Chen, C. M., Dumont-Mathieu, T., & Fein, D. (2014). Validation of the Modified Checklist for Autism in Toddlers, Revised with follow-up (M-CHAT-R/F). *Pediatrics, 133*(1), 37–45.

Romaire, M. A., & Bell, J. F. (2010). The medical home, preventive care screenings, and counseling for children: Evidence from the Medical Expenditure Panel Survey. *Academy of Pediatrics, 10*(5), 338–345.

Schidlow, D. V., & Fiel, S. B. (1990). Life beyond pediatrics: Transition of chronically ill adolescents from pediatric to adult health care systems. *Medical Clinics of North America, 74*(5), 1113–1120.

Shelton, T. L., & Stepanek J. S. (1994). *Family-centered care for children needing specialized health and developmental services.* Bethesda, MD: Association for the Care of Children's Health.

Stille, C. J. (2009). Communication, co-management and collaborative care for children and youth with special health care needs. *Pediatric Annals, 38*(9), 498–504.

Stille, C., Turchi, R. M., Cheng, T., Antonelli, R. C., Cabana, M., & Perrin, J. (2010). The family centered medical home (FCMH): Specific considerations for child health research and policy–Academic Pediatric Association Task Force on the Family Centered Medical Home. *Academic Pediatrics, 10*(4), 211–217.

Taylor, A., Lizzi, M., Marx, A., Chilkatowsky, M., Trachtenberg, S., & Ogle, S. (2013). Implementing a care coordination program for children with special healthcare needs: Partnering with families and providers. *Journal of Healthcare Quality, 35*(5), 70–77.

Turchi, R. M., & Antonelli, R. (2014). Council on Children with Disabilities. Policy statement-patient and family centered care coordination: Integrating care for children and youth across multiple systems. *Pediatrics, 133*(5), 1451–1460.

Turchi, R. M., Berhane, Z., Bethell, C., Pomponio, A., Antonelli, R., & Minkovitz, C. S. (2009). Care coordination for CSHCN: Associations with family-provider relations and family/child outcomes. *Pediatrics, 124*(Suppl 4), S428–S434.

Turchi, R. M., Gatto, M., & Antonelli, R. (2007). Children and youth with special healthcare needs: There is no place like (a medical) home. *Current Opinions in Pediatrics, 19*(4), 503–508.

Turchi, R. M., & Mann, M. (2012). *Handbook for children with special health care needs: Building medical home for children and youth with special health care needs.* Philadelphia: Springer Publishing.

US Department of Health and Human Services. (2010). Affordable Care Act and Title X Program. Available at http://www.hhs.gov/healthcare/facts/factsheets /2013/06/jobs06212012.html

Williams, P. G., Tomchek, S., Grau, R., Bundy, M. B., Davis, D. W., & Kleinert, H. (2012). Parent and physician perceptions of medical home care for children with autism spectrum disorders in the state of Kentucky. *Clinical Pediatrics, 51,* 1071–1078.

Chapter 8

THE ADULT MEDICAL HOME

James E. Connell, Margaret C. Souders and Connor M. Kerns

Introduction

The need for evidence-based services for adults with autism spectrum disorder (ASD) grows greater with each new cohort aging out of the education system. It is estimated that nationwide, almost 50,000 individuals with ASD turn 18 each year and enter the adult services system (Shattuck, Roux, Hudson, Taylor, Maenner, & Trani, 2012). There are known treatments (National Autism Center, 2009; McPheeters, Warren, Sathe, Bruzek, Krishnaswami, Jerome, & Veenstra-VanderWeele, 2011) and consultative approaches to deliver those treatments (Connell, 2010; Noell et al., 2005; Pellecchia et al., 2011; Solomon, Klein, & Politylo, 2012) that will help mental and behavioral health provider agencies respond more effectively to the diverse and complex needs of the adult population. Research, however, suggests that the current healthcare system is unprepared to support the complex medical and behavioral needs of this maturing population.

The paucity of services available to adults and their families is a challenge that many adults with ASD face. Changes in financial revenue streams, health policy, and models of care will be critical in order to provide comprehensive evidence-based care for this population.

The present chapter reviews our current understanding regarding the dearth of services currently available to adults with ASD, and the direct and indirect consequences of this service gap–for the individual, family, and community. It then considers a potential solution to the problem–a means to efficiently and effectively reduce this gap by integrating behavioral health services into medical home settings–the Provider Agency Consultation Therapy (PACT) model. A collaborative case consultative model (Erchul & Martens, 2002) can be used by a multidisciplinary team of experts in ASD to advise the treatment and service delivery for adults with ASD. Within this model, hospitals, clinics, community mental health centers (CMHCs), and mental and behavioral health care agencies can maximize organizational and individual outcomes.

The Demand for Adult ASD Services

In 2004, Pennsylvania created a new bureau in its Department of Public Welfare (now the Department of Human Services), the Bureau of Autism Services (BAS). The BAS, a first of its kind in the nation, was in response to the recommendations made by the Pennsylvania Autism Task Force, which consisted of a group of state legislators, individuals with autism, and family members concerned about the lack of services for individuals on the spectrum, especially as they grew older. Indeed, Pennsylvania, like many other states, had waves of children moving through the education system, entering their late teens, and getting ready to "age out" of all the services provided by IDEA. In 2009, when the first Pennsylvania Autism Census data were released (Lawer & Mandell, 2009), there were approximately 20,000 individuals with ASD in Pennsylvania, 4,000 of whom were adults. However, the first Pennsylvania Autism Census was flawed in its attempt to capture a close estimate of the total number of individuals on the spectrum, and thus a second census was initiated (Lawer, 2014).

Access to agency data was unprecedented and a much closer estimate to the true number was obtained by a record review of Medicaid claims and data from the education and justice systems, from multiple agencies. The agencies were: Office of Medical Assistance Programs, Office of Children, Youth and Families, Office of Developmental Programs, Autism & Intellectual Disability Services, Office of Mental Health and Substance Abuse Services, Department of Education, Office of Vocational Rehabilitation, Department of Corrections and the PA Commission on Crime and Delinquency. The results indicated that there were over 55,000 individuals with autism living in the state, and the adult population was estimated to be more than 17,000 in 2015 (Lawer, 2014).

Because of the Individuals with Disabilities Education Act, young adults are eligible for supports through the public education system until age 21; however, services and supports rapidly decrease through secondary school, and fall off dramatically after age 21 (Shattuck, Narendorf, & Cooper, 2012). In most US communities, including Philadelphia, there are few ongoing educational programs, clinical services, employment training or opportunities, social skill development, and residential support options specifically tailored to the population of adults with ASD. The limited programs that focus more generally on disabled adults tend not to provide services designed to build the competencies, skills, or behavioral domains that promote independence for this population. For example, the data generated from the Pennsylvania Census data project indicated a decrease in mental health, behavioral health, occupational therapy, speech, language, and the use of evidence-based practices to reduce the occurrence of problem behaviors, and increase communication, adaptive living, and social skills. The need for these services was highlighted in the Pennsylvania needs assessment and is consistent with other data showing a significant drop-off of health-related services for problem behavior reduction and skill acquisition (Gerhardt, 2009; Shattuck, Roux et al., 2012).

Adult Needs Assessment

The Pennsylvania BAS recently published the ASD Needs Assessment (BAS DPW, 2011), a survey of over 3,500 youth and adults on the autism spectrum. This survey was distributed to adults with ASD, and their parents and caregivers in Pennsylvania. The survey solicited information about the types of services currently available and utilized, as well as satisfaction with those services. Data were collected by asking adults and their parents about the type and amount of service they currently received in critical health areas including: Behavioral and mental health, medication management, sleep disorders, physical health functional and occupational therapy, employment services, and postsecondary education support. Individuals and their parents were invited to respond that they were either receiving these services, or that they were an unmet need. The findings clearly indicated that individuals and parents of adults with ASD had significant unmet needs across all service domains. The PA BAS Needs Assessment data mirrored what Shattuck and colleagues (Shattuck, Roux, Hudson, Taylor, Maenner, & Trani, 2012) found in their study.

Among the needs for adults on the autism spectrum, the greatest are for mental and behavioral health care services, as well as employment services. Comorbid psychiatric disorders are highly prevalent in this population, with estimates tending to cluster in the 70% range (Mattila et al., 2010; Simonoff, Pickles, Charman, Chandler, Loucas, & Biard, 2008). The presence of a comorbid disorder often complicates the assessment of the amount and type of services needed for the patient. For example, anxiety and depression are among the most commonly diagnosed psychiatric comorbidities in adults with ASD. They are also associated with increased self-injurious behavior, suicidality, social difficulties, and somatic symptoms in individuals with ASD

(Cassidy, Bradley, Robinson, McHugh, & Baron-Cohen, 2014; Kerns, Kendall, Zickgraf, Franklin, Miller, & Herrington, 2015; Mazurek, Kanne, & Wodka, 2013; Storch, Sulkowski, & Jacob, 2013). Despite the seriousness of these comorbidities, the Pennsylvania Autism Needs Assessment (BAS DPW, 2011) found that every age group of individuals with ASD struggled to access mental health services. Service gaps were greatest after childhood, with almost half of older adolescents, and three out of five adults reporting unmet mental health needs. Further, of those adults receiving mental health supports, over 30% were dissatisfied, and described their care as ineffective.

PATHWAYS TO EMPLOYMENT. Employment services and pathways toward successful vocational training, postsecondary education, and job placement are also a key area of need. National-level data show that over 50% of young adults on the autism spectrum are completely disconnected from any employment or education opportunities during the first two years after high school (Shattuck, Narendorf, Cooper, Sterzing, Wagner, & Taylor, 2012). Compared with youth who have other types of disabilities, they are also less likely to socialize with friends, to participate in community social activities with peers, and to live away from their parents' home (Howlin & Moss, 2012; Anderson, Shattuck, Cooper, Roux, & Wagner, 2013; Shattuck, Orsmond, Wagner, & Cooper, 2011). Only about half have had a position that provided payment in these first years. Even fewer (35%) attended college (Shattuck et al., 2012). The Pennsylvania Needs Assessment indicated similar trends. Employment was a desired adult outcome, and yet an ongoing unmet need. Lack of employment is a great concern for many reasons. Work-ready and capable adults who are not employed miss opportunities to socialize with peers, develop a social network, acquire social capital, and contribute to the economy. Lack of employment may also lead to lower self-esteem, and result in comorbid disorders and other health issues such as anxiety, depression, and obesity. As a result of this cascading debilitating trend, those adults ready and able to work are often sedentary, have significant mental health concerns that are largely treated with antipsychotic medications that exacerbate the obesity, and do nothing to solve the problem.

Direct and Indirect Consequences of the Service Gap

Research suggests that the paucity of services has a number of direct and indirect negative consequences for individuals with ASD, their families, and the country. The vast majority of individuals with ASD have limited independence, and encounter a number of adverse outcomes in adulthood, including: Decreased physical activity, poor physical health, loss of employment opportunities, and loss of social contact (BAS DPW, 2009; Shattuck et al., 2012). Some adults with ASD come into contact with the judicial system, homelessness, violent crime victimization, and illicit drug use, and many experience long-term institutional placements (PA, BAS Needs Assessment, 2011). Two specific consequences from the service gap that directly affect the health and wellbeing of people with ASD are use of multiple medication (polypharmacy) and costs of care.

POLYPHARMACY. Due to limited behavioral and mental health services for adults on the spectrum, treatment with polypharmacy is common. A state-wide autism prevalence study in Utah conducted from 2006 to 2011 found that approximately 60% of adults on the spectrum took one or more psycho-tropic medications regularly, with over a quarter of adults taking three or more (Buck et al., 2014). For a discussion of these medications see Chapter 5.

COST OF CARE. The service gap for adults with ASD is also associated with a significant financial burden at an individual and national level. The national estimated average cost to the nation's taxpayers for each person with an ASD has been estimated to fall between $1.4 million and $2.3 million (across the lifespan). This includes potentially avoidable costs such as expensive long-term housing, emergency health care, and inpatient behavioral health treatments, and lost tax revenue due to underemployment. A study conducted by Ariane, Buescher, Zuleyha, Knapp, and Mandell (2014). estimated that nonmedical (e.g., behavioral health, special education, interventions, childcare, and residential placement) and medical costs (e.g., medications, hospitalizations, outpatient services) absorbed by the nation's taxpayers may be close to $137 billion per year.

Further, because of the increase in prevalence rates of ASD and the high cost of associated care, per person health care expenditures are substantial and will continue to increase. For example, Medicaid data showed that total health care expenditures for ASD (per 10,000 covered lives) went from $1,270,435 in 2000 to $1,686,983 in 2003 [accounting for inflation](Wang & Leslie, 2010). That totals a 32.8% increase in Medicaid-reimbursed health care expenditures alone in only a three-year timeframe.

If more effective preventative and comprehensive treatment packages for adults with ASD were available, and were to include the use of evidence-based interventions for many of the behavioral concerns, it is likely that costs could be lowered and quality of life improved. For example, treatment packages that include known and effective interventions derived from the field of applied behavior analysis with an integrated care plan that includes physical health and medication management from qualified and experienced nursing can and will support community inclusion. That is, treatment packages that include evidence-based behavioral interventions, attention to physical health needs, and effective medication management using an interdisciplinary care model, with an integrated health plan will address a majority of the unmet needs, build skills for success in the community leading to less time spent sedentary at home, and increase physical health functioning.

Such treatment packages can become an essential component of integrated health care for this population.

Toward a Model for Integrated Care

The need for evidence-based services grows greater with each new cohort aging out of the education system. Fortunately, there are known treatments (National Autism Center, 2009; McPheeters et al., 2011) and consultative approaches (Connell, 2010; Noell et al., 2005; Pellecchia et al., 2011; Solomon, Klein, & Politylo, 2012) that will help physical, mental, and behavioral health agencies respond more effectively to the diverse and complex needs of this population. A collaborative case consultative model (Erchul & Martens, 2002) can be used by an interdisciplinary team of experts in ASD to advise the treatment and service delivery for adults with ASD. Within this model community, healthcare agencies can maximize organizational and individual outcomes.

Case Consultation Models

Case consultation has been used in community settings for decades with a significant amount of success. In most forms, consultation is a process whereby an expert transfers skill and knowledge to another person who is working on behalf of a client or an agency. The use of consultation to support skill and knowledge acquisition has been used in school settings since the passage of the Individuals with Disabilities Education Act (IDEA) and the development of the eco-behavioral model (Bergan, 1977), and in noneducational community settings supporting the needs of those with mental and behavioral health needs (Caplan, 1970). The use of consultation in community settings has many advantages, including the transfer of knowledge, skill, and expertise such that larger numbers of individuals and agencies can be effectively supported. Additionally, consultation to improve individual or agency functioning is highly cost-effective for the consumer.

COST EFFECTIVENESS. The cost effectiveness of consultation is proven in mental health and medical settings. In a sequence of studies by Smith and colleagues (1986, 1995), the authors demonstrated that case consultation can reduce the cost of care immediately and over time. Their first randomized control trial conducted at the University of Arkansas for Medical Sciences used a psychiatric consultation model to treat somatization disorder (now known as somatic symptom disorder) (Smith, Monson, & Ray, 1986). In this study, psychiatrists provided consultation services to physicians treating patients with somatization disorder. A group of patients received no treatment as comparison. The authors reported a 49% decrease in health care charges in the group receiving the psychiatric consultation intervention whereas group receiving no intervention has no significant change in health care charges. The researchers found that the collaborative consultation efforts resulted in an effective treatment plan which resulted in a reduction in health care costs (Smith et al., 1986). A follow-up to this study a decade later showed consistent results. The use of the intervention for patients resulted in a 32.9% reduction in the annual median cost of their medical care, as well as improved health outcomes for the patients (Smith, Rost, & Kasher, 1995).

More recently, the Doctor-Office Collaborative Care (DOCC) model (Kolko, Campo, Kilbourne, & Kelleher, 2012) was compared to standard clinical practice in pediatric waiting rooms for children with behavioral health needs. The DOCC model created an evidence-based, multidisciplinary, collaborative care approach to direct service provision that included training, consultation, and sustainability components, and technologies to monitor processes, outcomes, and communication. The data overwhelmingly supported the use of experts, consulting with pediatric office staff–including physicians–in the effective treatment of children with behavioral health needs.

The use of consultation to offer expert knowledge in a specific area (i.e., ASD) to those providing treatment plans (e.g., physicians or clinical staff in CHMC's) is a promising model for appropriately crafting and implementing treatment plans and interventions that will, in turn, reduce the costs of health care paid by individual and by the taxpayer. Over time, service delivery and treatment that is advised through a collaborative consultation model can reduce the societal healthcare expenditures that are attributed to lifelong care of people with ASD.

Case Consultation Model: Provider Agency Consultation Therapy (PACT)

One successful solution for coordinated care for individuals with ASD is the Provider Agency Consultation Therapy Model (PACT) developed by the first author as part of a Pennsylvania statewide initiative to develop services for adults with an ASD. PACT is an interdisciplinary care model that provides expert consultative support to provider agency administration and staff. Developed and tested over a three-year period, the model has demonstrated both clinical and cost effectiveness. In its fourth year, it became clear that the interdisciplinary consultative team must include: (a) A behavioral psychologist with extensive experience implementing effective, and evidence-based antecedent and consequent-based treatment packages; (b) an adult ASD-focused psychiatric nurse practitioner or psychiatrist; and (c) a social worker or case manager that supports coordination and access to services including a primary care nurse liaison. Other team members could include drug and alcohol therapists, sex therapists, CBT-focused psychologists, parents, and community members. One of the team members must have a background in mental health and/or behavioral consultation with extensive, successful experience implementing comprehensive treatment plans in community settings.

The interdisciplinary team approach ensures that the mental, physical, and behavioral health care needs are considered when evaluating the patients' concerns and for comprehensive treatment package recommendations. Consultative recommendations take a holistic approach to health management, and focus on the relationship between physical health and primary care, and behavioral health. Examples of case consultation include medication titration in coordination with the behavioral psychologist who provides graphs of targeted behaviors that monitor the effect of the medication, and potential side effects. Other examples include attention to physical health care needs such as dental care, routine health screening, blood laboratory work, diet modification, exercise program, transportation, and safety. The overarching goal is to provide systems-level consultation that informs the treatment approaches and services used by physical, mental, and behavioral health staff. The model described below borrows from clinical consultation models used in primary care and specialty mental, behavioral, and physical health care settings.

The PACT model was first developed and tested during the 2012–2013 fiscal year by the first author, with initial grant funding by the PA Bureau of Autism Services. Over the past three years, an interdisciplinary team (behavioral psychologist, adult-focused psychiatrist, nurse practitioner, and social worker) worked with health care agencies on high-cost, high utilization clients, and successfully supported the agency staff in developing comprehensive and effective treatment plans. The model was field-tested with two Philadelphia area service providers, and to date, has served more than 50 adults on the autism spectrum. The overwhelming response from the provider agencies was extremely positive, with one of the providers creating a line of employment within the organization to continue this work and build internal capacity. The multidisciplinary approach demonstrated cost savings associated with the standard of care, reduced medication requirements, decreased crisis intervention needs, and inpatient placements (see Figure 8.1).

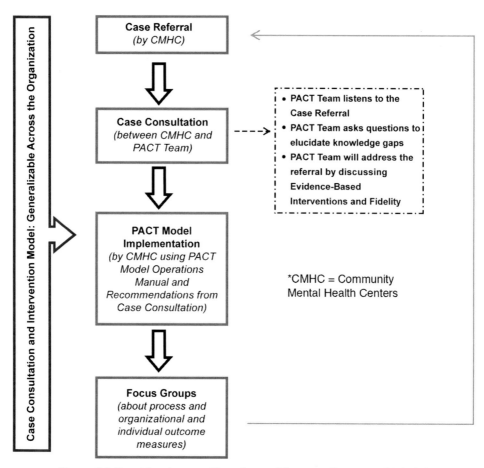

Figure 8.1. Provider Agency Consultative Therapy Conceptual Model.

Multidisciplinary Approach

The model uses an interdisciplinary approach that focuses on the implementation and dissemination of evidence-based medical and behavioral treatments (derived from the field of applied behavior analysis) in community settings. This team comprises individuals with expertise that can develop and execute an evidence-based medical and behavioral treatment package with fidelity, and has the capacity, with social work and nursing professionals, to facilitate seamless communication with the individual with ASD and their family and community.

Additionally, the use of expert case-consultation as an organizational intervention can easily be expanded to include telemedicine consultation. Consultation can be easily delivered with the incredible advances in technology, web-based interfaces, and secure servers to protect health information across the Internet. Finally, the model is easily replicable and portable through telemedicine capabilities.

The consultation is intended to educate staff from provider agencies about the use of evidence-based therapies for adults on the autism spectrum, which include behavioral supports and medication selection and effects. The consultation also assists the providers to integrate evidence on treatments from multiple disciplines when planning patient care. The interdisciplinary team guides the agencies in the selection and use of procedures and processes that promote treatment implementation fidelity and monitor the effects of treatments.

CONSULTATION PROCESS. The process begins with the consultative team reviewing the agency referral. A battery of initial referral forms is sent to the agency for completion by direct-care staff and then sent back to the consultation team. After reviewing the nature of the referral; medical history; current and past treatments; other medical, physical, and behavioral diagnoses, the team meets with the primary stakeholders from the referring agency, asks follow-up questions, and begins to conceptualize the nature of the referral and potential solutions, taking into account agency capacity, ability to implement interventions and monitor their progress. The team then offers a set of recommendations that addresses gaps in the staff knowledge about medications, antecedent and consequent behavioral interventions, data presentation and analysis, and consultation to direct care staff designed to increase treatment fidelity through the use of performance feedback. Consultation to the primary care staff implementing those interventions can include *in vivo* coaching, feedback, and follow-up consultative support. These processes are completed in cooperation with the agency staff (i.e., nursing, case management, behavior specialists, residential care staff, psychiatry), and allow both knowledge transfer and skill transfer to the primary care staff (see Box 8.1. Steps in the Case Consultation Process).

The process is easy to implement. Each week, the behavioral psychologist discusses the cases to be presented with the primary contact person at the agency. During that meeting, a brief review of the case is followed by recommendations from the PACT team about who should be at the meeting (e.g., psychiatrist, behavior specialist, social worker, dietician, nurse, substance abuse counselor). The agency then prepares the case for presentation. Case preparation includes referring to the assessment battery sent earlier by the PACT team which includes a case/developmental history form, reason for referral form, adaptive functioning scale, social communication scale, and an ASD adult screening tool. The agency contact person gathers this information from the appropriate sources, and then adds IQ and performance

---

Box 8.1. Steps in the Case Consultation Process.

1. Agency contacts the consultation team
2. Consultation team accepts case, emails document packet to the agency
3. Agency completes document packet, emails back to consultation team
4. A date is scheduled to discuss the case
5. Consultation team reviews the document packet
6. Agency and consultation team meet to conceptualize the case
7. Medical, physical health, behavioral health, and mental health concerns are presented. Also presented are agency staff capacity, training, and motivation
8. Intervention recommendations are offered across disciplines, but in coordination with each consultation team member adding to the recommendations in a coordinated approach
9. Agency discusses the capacity to implement any one, or more of the interventions, and discusses staff capacity to implement with fidelity
10. Consultation team helps troubleshoot potential barriers to implementation
11. Plan is agreed upon, agency and individual outcome measures are identified
12. Follow-up meeting is scheduled to assess the effectiveness of the plan
13. Follow-up consultation meeting follows one of three paths:
    (a) Plan worked well–maintain plan
    (b) Plan worked but not optimal–plan modification needed
    (c) Plan had no effect–problem solve case conceptualization–present intervention recommendations

---

assessments, necessary medical information, history of the concern, and other relevant chart information. These documents are then discussed in detail during the case-conceptualization meeting. The case-conceptualization meeting is designed to help the team to understand how the agency staff conceptualize the nature of the problem presented for each client presented, provide feedback about the medical/behavioral strategies used, describe alternative treatment approaches that are grounded in evidence-based therapies, and consider a process to implement, monitor, report, analyze, and interpret the results of the recommendations. Each case presented is discussed in subsequent meetings until the treatment package achieves the desired outcomes and the staff becomes more competent and independent with treatment implementation (see Box 8.1).

The PACT model was the only known consultative approach for agencies working with complex, high needs, high costs individuals with an ASD. This innovative approach could be a model for other high needs, high costs populations served by mental and behavioral health care settings. This model uses the current knowledge base of known evidence-based treatments for the adult ASD population, and reduces the research to practice gap from over a decade to within one year by partnering with local universities conducting research in these areas and with the clinical expertise to provide the consultation. Additionally, this approach is holistic in both its use of multiple disciplines and its therapeutic recommendations.

Interdisciplinary consultation approaches, such as the one described here, are vital to the ongoing care of adults on the autism spectrum. Mental, physical, and behavioral health providers are seeing staggering numbers of adults on the spectrum and have limited knowledge and capacity to navigate the complex situations, comorbid disorders, care coordination, and familial stressors that result in difficult-to-treat cases. Experts in behavioral psychology and applied behavior analysis, in particular, nursing, addiction, and psychiatry must work in coordination, and with these provider agencies to ensure that these complex cases, receive comprehensive and integrated treatment plans. The cost to the person and society will, in time, force more effective use of services that rely on expert use of evidence-based practices in integrated care plans.

Conclusion

The family and the individual must be part of any integrated care plan. Many of the adults with an ASD are indeed sitting at home on their parent's couches, with little contact with the social environment, postsecondary education, employment, or community integration. As a result, these individuals experience more health care concerns including obesity, obesity-related illnesses, depression, anxiety resulting in pharmacological intervention, and polypharmacy. The result of poorly developed and integrated services is a significant concern, which has a cruel effect on the individual and his or her family, and an enormous financial burden to the taxpayer. The need for new, testable and innovative models of interdisciplinary care is imperative. Models like PACT offer one alternative to be explored and tested, and if successful, scaled to other localities where university support, clinical expertise, and agency need are identified. Finally, the individual and the parents/caregivers must be active members of the interdisciplinary team for any chance of long-term success and sustainability. The parents of individuals with an ASD have spent the last 50 years advocating for their children and making changes in policy and service. Parent advocacy groups need the support of clinicians and researchers to understand the complexity of the service delivery gap, so they can effectively rally, with our support, once again.

References

Anderson, K. A, Shattuck, P. T., Cooper, B. P., Roux, A. M., & Wagner, M. (2013). Prevalence and correlates of postsecondary residential status among young adults with an autism spectrum disorder. *Autism, 18*(5), 562–570.

Ariane, V. S., Buescher, M. S., Zuleyha, C., Knapp, M., & Mandell, D. S. (2014). Costs of autism spectrum disorders in the United Kingdom and the United States. *Pediatrics, 168*(8), 721–728.

Buck, T. R., Viskochil, J., Farley, M., Coon, H., McMahon, W. M., Morgan, J., & Bilder, D.A. (2014). Psychiatric comorbidity and medication use in adults with autism spectrum disorder. *Journal of Autism & Developmental Disorders, 44*(12), 3063–3071.

Bureau of Autism Services, Pennsylvania Department of Public Welfare. (2011). Pennsylvania Autism Needs Assessment: A survey of individuals and families living with autism: Family impact. Retrieved from http://www.paautism.org/resources/AllResources/ResourceDetails/tabid/142/language/en-US/Default.aspx?itemid=280

Caplan, G. (1970). *Theory and practice of mental health consultation.* New York: Basic Books.

Caplan, G., & Caplan, R. B. (1993). *Mental health consultation and collaboration.* San Francisco: Jossey-Bass.

Cassidy, S., Bradley, P., Robinson, J., Allison, C., McHugh, M., & Baron-Cohen, S. (2014). Suicidal ideation and suicide plans or attempts in adults with Asperger's syndrome attending a specialist diagnostic clinic: A clinical cohort study. *The Lancet Psychiatry, 1,* 142–147.

Connell, J. E. (2010). Applications of performance feedback: Consultation in the home. *International Journal of Behavioral & Consultation Therapy, 6*(1), 17–23.

Erchul, W., & Martens, B. (2002). *School consultation: Conceptual and empirical bases of practice* (2nd ed.). New York: Springer.

Gerhardt, P. F. (Ed.). (2009). *The current state of services for adults with autism: Advancing futures for adults with autism.* New York: Organization for Autism Research.

Howlin, P., & Moss, P. (2012), Adults with autism spectrum disorders. *The Canadian Journal of Psychiatry, 57*(5), 275–283.

Individuals with Disability Education Act 20 U.S.C. § 1400. (1997). Retrieved from http://idea.ed.gov/

Kerns, C. M., Kendall, P. C., Zickgraf, H., Franklin, M. E., Miller, J., & Herrington, J. (2015). Not to be overshadowed or overlooked: Functional impairments associated with comorbid anxiety disorders in youth with ASD. *Behavior Therapy, 46*(1), 29–39.

Kolko, D., Campo, J., Kilbourne, A., & Kelleher, K. (2012). Doctor-office collaborative care for pediatric behavioral problems: A preliminary clinical trial. *Pediatrics, 166*(3), 224–231.

Lawer, L. (2014). *Pennsylvania autism census: Final report.* Harrisburg, PA: Pennsylvania Department of Public Welfare, Bureau of Autism Services.

Lawer, L., & Mandell, D. S. (2009). *Pennsylvania autism census: Final report.* Harrisburg, PA: Pennsylvania Department of Public Welfare, Bureau of Autism Services.

Mattila, M. L., Hurtig, T., Haapsamo, H., Jussila, K., Kuusikko-Gauffin, S., Kielinen, M., & Moilanen, I. (2010). Comorbid psychiatric disorders associated with Asperger syndrome/high-functioning autism: A community- and clinic-based study. *Journal of Autism & Developmental Disorders, 40*(9), 1080–1093.

Mazurek, M. O., Kanne, S. M., & Wodka, E. L. (2013). Physical aggression in children and adolescents with autism spectrum disorders. *Research in Autism Spectrum Disorders, 7*(3), 455–465.

McPheeters, M. L., Warren, Z., Sathe, N., Bruzek, J. L., Krishnaswami, S., Jerome, R. N., & Veenstra-VanderWeele, J. (2011). A systematic review of medical treatments for children with autism spectrum disorders. *Pediatrics, 127*(5), E1312–E1321.

National Autism Center. (2009). *National standards report.* Randolph, MA: The National Autism Center.

Noell, G., Witt, J., Slider, N., Connell, J., Gatti, S., Williams, K., . . . Duhon, G. (2005). Treatment implementation following behavioral consultation in schools: A comparison of three follow-up strategies. *School Psychology Review, 34*(1), 87–106.

Pellecchia, M., Connell, J. E., Eisenhart, D., Kane, M., Schoener, C., Turkel, K., . . . Mandell, D. (2011). Group performance feedback: Consultation to increase classroom team data collection. *Journal of School Psychology, 49,* 411–431.

Shattuck, P. T., Roux, A. M., Hudson, L. E., Taylor, J. L., Maenner, M. J., & Trani, J. F. (2012). Services for adults with an autism spectrum disorder. *Canadian Journal of Psychiatry, 57*(5), 284–291.

Shattuck, P. T., Narendorf, S. C., Cooper, B. P., Sterzing, P. R., Wagner, M., & Taylor, J. L. (2012). Postsecondary education and employment among youth with an autism spectrum disorder. *Pediatrics, 129*(6), 1042–1049.

Shattuck, P. T., Orsmond, G. I., Wagner, M., & Cooper, B. P. (2011), Participation in social activities among adolescents with an autism spectrum disorder. *PLoS ONE, 6*(11), e27176.

Simonoff, E., Pickles, A., Charman, T., Chandler, S., Loucas, T., & Baird, G. (2008). Psychiatric disorders in children with autism spectrum disorders: Prevalence, comorbidity, and associated factors in a population-derived sample. *Journal of the American Academy of Child & Adolescent Psychiatry, 47*(8), 921–929.

Smith, G. R., Monson, R. A., & Ray, D. C. (1986). Psychiatric consultation in somatization disorder. *New England Journal of Medicine, 314*(22), 1406–1413.

Smith, G. R., Rost, K., & Kasher, M. (1995). A trial of the effect of standardized psychiatric consultation on health outcomes and costs in somatizing patients. *Archives of General Psychiatry, 52*(3), 238–243.

Solomon, B. G., Klein, S. A., & Politylo, B. C. (2012). The effect of performance feedback on teachers' treatment integrity: A meta-analysis of the single-case literature. *School Psychology Review, 41*(2), 160–175.

Storch, E. A., Sulkowski, M. L., & Jacob, M. L. (2013). Exposure and response prevention and habit reversal training: Commonalities, differential use, and combined applications. *Journal of Contemporary Psychotherapy, 43*(3), 179–185.

Wang, L., & Leslie, D. L. (2010). Health care expenditures for children with autism spectrum disorders in Medicaid. *Journal of the American Academy of Child & Adolescent Psychiatry, 49*(11), 1165–1171.

Chapter 9

ASSISTING PARENTS IN
ADAPTING AND MAKING DECISIONS
REGARDING TREATMENT OPTIONS

Jennifer Harrison Elder

Introduction

P arents of individuals with autism spectrum disorder (ASD) face a variety of challenges, and because most individuals with ASD have normal life expectancies, these challenges can persist over a lifetime. Clinical reports indicate that without proper intervention, parents and siblings often experience extreme stress that may translate into anxiety and chronic depression. Consequently, it is vital for healthcare providers and other interveners to understand the disorder, assist and support parents, and identify ways to guide decision-making. In particular, many parents struggle to obtain a conclusive diagnosis; discern, acquire, and implement credible interventions; and face the financial burden of paying for services (Ekas, Lickenbrock, & Whitman, 2010; Elder & D'Alessandro, 2009). Unlike other disorders first noted in childhood, ASD has components of both acute and chronic conditions.

This chapter is designed to provide healthcare providers with an overview of the challenges individuals with ASD and their parents face and offer practical guidance for helping parents accept and manage this complex disorder. Discussed are a number of popular interventions, separating those that are evidence-based from those that have less empirical support. This information is important for health care providers engaged in advising parents and developing the most efficacious treatment plans.

Understanding the Unique Needs of
Parents of Individuals with ASD

In describing her ethic of caring, Nodding (1984) stated that healthcare providers must apprehend the reality of the other as the first moral imperative to caring. To be effective, healthcare providers must develop empathy, which involves careful listening, reflection, and recognition that ASD is challenging and ever-present. Thus, parents need varying degrees and types of assistance throughout the stages of adjustment and over the lifetime of care.

Common Reactions Related to Receiving a Diagnosis of ASD

The first challenge that health care providers face when interacting with parents of children with ASD is helping them acquire and accept an ASD diagnosis. Often, parents may suspect that the child has ASD long before a diagnosis. Even with increased media attention related to ASD, parents may find it difficult to locate knowledgeable healthcare providers for an evaluation. Once a diagnosis is made, parents face the difficult challenge of mourning the loss of their "perfect child" (Elder & D'Alessandro 2009). At this stage, healthcare providers must understand the range of family reactions to intervene effectively with compassion and proper guidance. This understanding can help parents adjust and eventually accept the diagnosis (Ross & Kessler, 2007). However, at first, parent reactions may include denial, anger and blaming, searching for a cure, depression, and embarrassment. Recognizing these common reactions is important because they may complicate the process of establishing therapeutic rapport.

Denial

Healthcare providers should understand that parents may experience denial, which involves disbelieving that the diagnosis is correct. Denial may occur because the child's physical appearance is typically normal, and it may serve to buffer the immediate shock of a diagnosis, which represents a new, uncertain future (Ross & Kessler, 2007). Fathers, who are usually less involved in the daily caregiving of the child, may experience more denial than mothers, who often have more opportunities to observe behavioral differences with other children. In addition, some fathers of children with ASD may express the broader autism phenotype (BAP) (Ingersoll & Hamrick, 2011) and have difficulty recognizing the core features of autism, which include marked deficits in social and communication skills. Healthcare providers can help parents by presenting factual information and connecting them to experienced parents who offer support. To ensure a positive, reciprocal partnership, health care providers must be willing to adapt instruction, communication, and expectations, and give parents adequate time to adjust to the diagnosis.

Anger and Blaming

Once the diagnosis is accepted, health care providers can help parents progress through a phase characterized by anger. Anger is often fueled by preceding frustration related to difficulties getting the initial diagnosis and questions such as "Why us?" and "Why our family?" In this phase, parents may displace their anger onto healthcare providers, who may have presented inaccurate information or responded too slowly. In addition, parents may examine their genealogy to identify a family history of symptoms that imply a genetic predisposition, and blame one side of the family. Healthcare providers may need to explain that both genetics and environment have been implicated in the etiology of ASD (Miles, 2011; Berry, Crider, & Yeargin-Allsopp, 2013; Volk, Lurmann, Penfold, Hertz-Picciotto, & McConnel, 2013). Although healthcare providers may tactfully correct misperceptions about the causes of ASD, they can best serve parents by listening actively to their concerns, providing emotional support, and requesting additional testing such as chromosomal microarray analysis (see Chapter 10).

Searching for a Cure

Soon after a diagnosis is made, many parents begin to search for a cure. In this phase, they may directly ask the healthcare provider for advice, search for remedies on the world wide web, or seek further input from parent support networks. Parents are particularly vulnerable during this time to false claims of "cures" from a variety of treatment approaches. Healthcare providers must recognize this phase, communicate closely with parents, direct them to credible information sources, and correct inaccurate information. It is for this reason that a later section of this chapter reviews the most common, empirically sound treatment approaches.

Depression

Parents may report that they feel guilty because they "gave" the disorder to their child, resulting in feelings of responsibility that can lead to depression (Elder, 2013). In addition, parents report feeling overwhelmed and tired because parenting a child with ASD can be a daily struggle (Hastings et al., 2005). For example, many children with ASD have sleep disturbances, become active at night, and engage in potentially dangerous activities (Souders et al., 2009). This may cause sleep deprivation, which can worsen depression and feelings of helplessness. Similarly, parents may feel incompetent and embarrassed in public when their child with ASD engages in tantrums, which can be difficult to control. Healthcare providers can help alleviate depression by correcting misperceptions, offering emotional support, and directing parents to resources for respite, such as family support groups, when they are available.

Acceptance

Acceptance is the ultimate goal for parents who struggle with a diagnosis of ASD. When parents accept the diagnosis, they may be willing to begin comprehensive care, which includes treatments that target deficits in communication and social interaction. The most successful parents become strong, well-informed advocates for their own children as well as others in the ASD community (Cappe, Wolff, Bobet, & Adrien, 2011). Health care providers can assist parents by helping them network with other parents through parent support groups. Parents who have accepted the diagnosis have described an increase in spiritual strength and hope, which are vital to successful family adaptation (Hall, 2012).

Navigating the System

Another challenge faced by parents is learning to navigate the healthcare system. Recently, with funding from a "Pipeline to PCORI" pilot grant from the University of Florida's Clinical and Translation Science Institute, the author and team conducted four focus groups with parents (n=38) of children and adults with ASD to determine barriers to early diagnosis and treatment. Responses indicated a need for a "navigator" to assist parents from the time of diagnosis until the securement of appropriate healthcare services. One focus group member, a mother of a 16-year-old boy with ASD, described how she "went crazy" after the diagnosis, and due to a lack of professional guidance, depended on the world wide web for treatment options, most of which had no empirical support. The mother stated, "In looking back, I did so many stupid and expensive things that were not helpful. I am lucky that they were not harmful, but they could have been. It was a dangerous time for my son" (Personal Communication). Other members of the group told similar stories and stated that they greatly benefited from the informal support they received from other, more informed parents in the ASD community. Unfortunately, none of the parents reported easy access to a knowledgeable healthcare provider, and this was especially true for parents who lived in remote locations, which often lacked the diagnostic and treatment services found in urban medical centers. Thus, healthcare providers should pay special attention to parents in rural or underserved areas because appropriate services may not be locally available. If this is the case, then healthcare providers may need to act as navigators, and help connect parents with appropriate treatment services in larger, urban areas.

Identifying Sources of Stress and Ways to Manage

Parents of children with chronic illnesses experience stress that can be detrimental to their health and family functioning. In a recently conducted systematic review, Hayes and Watson (2013) found that parents of children with ASD reported significantly more stress than did parents of children with other disabilities or disorders. Sources of stress included significant financial burden, changes in the family unit, and insecurity about long-term caregiving (Fletcher, Markoulakis, & Bryden, 2012; Lecavalier, Leone, & Wiltz, 2006). In addition, parents may experience stress due to caring for a child who turns down affection, fails to make eye contact, and dislikes being held. While the effects of acute stress may be apparent, unrelieved, prolonged stress may be more harmful over time as well as more difficult to assess and treat.

Research on parental stress and ASD has focused on mothers because they are usually the primary caregivers. However, more recent studies indicate that fathers also experience a high level of stress, are less likely to seek assistance with stress management (Little, 2013). Indeed, in the author's and team's prior work, they found that caring for a child with ASD affected both parents, with mothers and fathers both scoring over the 90th percentile on the Parenting Stress Index (Bendixen et al., 2011). Furthermore, Davis and Carter (2008) noted that although mothers had a higher rate of stress and depression, fathers reported more difficulty interacting with the children and reacted more negatively to overt behaviors such as tantrums, aggression, and loud or peculiar vocalizations. These findings suggest that mothers and fathers manifest stress differently and healthcare providers may need to work closely with fathers to effectively intervene.

Another consideration highlighted by Brobst, Clopton, and Hendricks (2009) was the quality of the marital relationship. Because both fathers and mothers are affected by stress related to raising a child with ASD, care needs to be taken to minimize negative effects on the marriage (Brobst, Clopton, & Hendricks, 2009). These researchers found this to be especially true if the child exhibited severe behaviors such as tantrums and/or physical aggression. Thus, health care providers should encourage parents to participate in support groups that focus on the couple's relationship, rather than the child's problems or the parental role. Parents may also benefit from enlisting the aid of an extended family member to provide the couple "date nights" and other periods of respite from parenting.

Resiliency Factors: Empowering Parents in Caring for the Person with ASD

It is clear from clinical practice that some parents adapt more readily to having a child with a disability than other parents. The Resiliency Model of Family Stress, which includes a strength-based versus a deficit-based model for factors of family functioning, may elucidate adaptation in parents of individuals with ASD. Health care providers can use this model to guide the development of effective interventions to mitigate stress and potentially enhance resiliency (McCubbin, McCubbin, Thompson, Han, & Allen, 1997). Analysis of this model and the relevant literature revealed that multiple factors predict resiliency in parents, and these include: social support; family cohesion; development of an internal locus of control; engaging fathers as primary interveners; flexibility, adaptation, and willingness to try new things; optimism; and understanding and empowering typically developing siblings in family training. These factors are discussed below.

Social Support

Social support has a key role in reducing the negative effects on parents who are raising a child with ASD. Twoy and colleagues (2007) referred to "external family coping strategies," where parents rely on community, social, and spiritual support to modulate their coping. Similarly, there is evidence that "informal support" provided by friends and family may benefit parents the most (Ekas, Lickenbrock, & Whitman, 2010). Ingersoll & Hambrick (2011) stressed the importance of obtaining informal social support at the time of diagnosis, which may consist of support groups that are popular among parents in the ASD community. Mandell and Salzer (2007) surveyed 1005 caregivers of children with ASD and found that two-thirds had participated in support groups and more than half were participating at the time of the study. Clifford and Minnes (2013) found similar results in their study of 149 parents of children with ASD, in which 75% reported having attended parent support groups. Not surprisingly, parents who currently attended support groups, both in-person and online, reported more adaptive coping strategies than nonattenders, and were more likely to seek emotional and instrumental support. These findings suggested that healthcare providers should encourage family engagement in support groups to facilitate adaptation after a diagnosis of ASD.

Family Cohesion

Greeff and Van de Walt (2010) found that family collaboration in the care of the child with ASD improved parent adaptation as measured by the Family Attachment and Changeability Index (McCubbin, Thompson, & McCubbin, 1996). This finding was corroborated with a clinical vignette from the author's early career, in which the mother of a 10-year-old boy with ASD established a schedule by which all family members, including five typically developing siblings, participated in the day-to-day routine care of the affected child. With this "family activity" arrangement, the child with ASD benefited and other members enjoyed having a role consistent with their levels of ability. Similarly, other researchers, including the author and team, have observed that sibling involvement in the care and treatment of the child with ASD may improve TD siblings' self-esteem and feelings of achievement, which can positively affect the family as a whole (Powers, 2000; Howlin & Rutter, 1987; Smith & Elder, 2010). As a result of these findings, healthcare providers may recommend to parents that they involve the whole family in the care of the child with ASD as a way to achieve greater family adaptation and harmony. This type of family involvement may also be useful in preparing the child with ASD in advance for medical procedures.

Development of an Internal Locus of Control

First purported by Rotter in the 1950s as part of "personality psychology," locus of control refers to the extent to which individuals believe that they control what affects them. A person's "locus" is conceptualized as either internal (a person believes he/she can control his/her life) or external (a person believes that decisions and life are controlled by environmental factors that cannot be influenced or changed) (Rotter, 1966). Research consistently shows that an internal locus of control is empowering because it involves a belief that events in life result from personal action (Clifford & Minnes, 2013; Hayes & Watson, 2013). This concept was clearly illustrated by a father who told the author, "I can spend an hour in my yard and produce something beautiful that is admired by the neighbors; however, I can spend the same hour or even several hours with my son, and I have nothing to show for it." This father naturally desired to feel control over variables in his environment—in this case, his son—that negatively affected his mood and well-being. After this admission, the father started to participate in family training, experienced positive results with his son, and eventually assumed the role of family school liaison—a role that was previously only held by the mother.

Including Fathers as Primary Caregivers

As illustrated by this case report, fathers may not readily accept roles as primary caregivers even though there is evidence that father involvement may benefit the child with ASD (Elder et al, 2011). In a systematic review of father involvement in early ASD intervention, Flippin and Crasis (2011) indicated that while father involvement is underreported in the literature, there was evidence that fathers were uniquely suited to enhancing play skills. This can improve child language and social skills. In addition, greater father involvement may result in more coparenting, which can lessen the maternal workload and increase family cohesion (Shannon et al., 2002).

Flexibility, Adaptation, and Willingness to Try New Things

Parents who are most successful in adapting to a family member with ASD are creative, flexible, and willing to try new things (Greeff & Van de Walt, 2010). For example, the author encountered parents of an eight-year-old with ASD that were concerned about the child's gaze aversion and lack of direct eye contact with visitors. As a result, they asked the child to tell them the guest's eye color at the end of the visit, and the child received a highly valued object if the answer was correct. This creative strategy enabled the parents to help the child interact in a more socially acceptable way, and served to address the communication deficits that are key features of ASD. While this strategy would not be appropriate for all children with ASD, it illustrates the importance of creative engagement and keen observation of the child's unique needs and preferences by parents (Elder et al., 2011).

Optimism

Ekas, Lickenhrock, and Whitman (2010) stated that optimism and the maintenance of hope, which were influenced by the level of familial support, improved family adaptation to a diagnosis of ASD. Hall (2012) noted that the quality of family services was related directly to the parents' optimism and that early intervention facilitated a hopeful outlook. Healthcare providers can help maintain this hopeful outlook through a process known as "reframing," which entails the replacement of negative views with positive ones or constructive acts (Hall, 2012; Hastings et al., 2005). Additional factors that may contribute to optimism are effective and open communication, parent advocacy, family routines and togetherness, healthy marital and parental relationships, and the level of independence of the child with ASD. Information-seeking that enables parents to be proactive in helping the child is also important to the creation of a positive mindset.

Helping Parents Make Informed Choices

In 2008, the American Academy of Pediatrics' Council on Children with Disabilities stated that treatment goals for children with ASD should be to: (a) Maximize the child's ultimate functional independence and quality of life by minimizing the core features, (b) facilitate development and learning, (c) promote socialization, (d) reduce maladaptive behaviors, and (e) educate and support parents (Myers & Johnson, 2008). Despite the fact that the Academy did not recommend ways to achieve these goals, parents need to make informed decisions regarding treatment options for their children with ASD.

Recent evidence indicates that children benefit most from early, intensive treatment programs that include care continuity, multidisciplinary education, and strong family support and education. Tonge and colleagues (2014) asserted, "Current early intervention models focus on parent involvement, teaching play and behavior skills, and improving social and communication skills" (p. 163). Just as importantly, Sherer and Schreibman (2005) noted that because of the "differential responsiveness to intervention programs" (p. 525), there is no single treatment approach for children with ASD. Instead, a variety of approaches are recommended depending on the child characteristics, autism severity, and functional level as well as service availability and family resources. Intervention approaches that have the most empirical support can be categorized as the following: Behavioral, educational and communication focused, social, and pharmacological (Elder, 2002). In each of these categories, health care providers can identify valid interventions that have undergone rigorous clinical trials and been endorsed by credible organizations such as Autism Speaks, Autism Society of America, Interagency Autism Coordinating Committee, and ASCEND.

Behavioral Interventions

In the 1970s, Lovaas and colleagues provided empirical evidence that trained therapists and parents could use behavioral interventions to help treat ASD (Lovaas, 1978; Lovaas, 1987). Lovaas's approaches are often referred to as discrete trail (DT), intensive behavior intervention (IBI), early intensive behavior intervention (EIBI), and applied behavior analysis (ABA), which focus on enhancing attention, imitation, receptive/expressive language, and preacademic and self-help skills. ABA typically uses a one-to-one therapist-child ratio and the "antecedent-behavior-consequence" (ABC) trials. Each trial or task has (a) an antecedent, which is a directive or request for the child to perform an action; (b) a behavior, or response from the child, which may be deemed successful, noncompliant, or nonresponsive; and (c) a consequence, defined as the reaction from the therapist, which can range from strong positive reinforcement to a strong negative response (Lovaas, 1987). Parents who are interested in ABA should consider the expense and intensity of the intervention, which are caused by the need for a therapist to engage the child 20–40 hours/week, often in the child's home. Although this arrangement is often helpful to the child, the extended presence of therapists in the home can further strain a stressed family system (Grindle, Kovshoff, Hastings, & Remington, 2009).

Another well-known approach is the Early Start Denver Model, which is less intensive, combines a variety of approaches, and is considered more developmentally appropriate for younger children (Dawson et al., 2010). Although there is currently more evidence supporting Lovaas' work, studies of both approaches indicate gains in communication, social interactions, and cognitive skills (Dawson & Burner, 2011; Vismara & Rogers, 2010; Warren et al., 2011). Researchers are also interested in integrated interventions, which combine two or more approaches and use interveners from various disciplines (e.g., special education, speech, and occupational therapy) who collaborate as a team (Mukherjee et al., 2014).

Pivotal response training (PRT) is another popular behavioral intervention that has some empirical support (Suhrheinrich et al., 2013). PRT is described as a "naturalistic intervention" based on principles of applied behavior analysis that facilitates generalization, increases spontaneity and motivation, and reduces prompt dependency. Some of these behaviors include response to multiple cues, self-management, and the initiation of social interactions (Koegel & Koegel, 2006). Parents may find this approach easier to implement because it seems more natural and less intense than the more traditional Lovaas approaches.

Educational and Communication-Focused Interventions

Healthcare providers can inform parents about several educational and communication-focused interventions that have empirical support. Project TEACCH (Treatment and Education of Autistic and Related Communication-Handicapped Children) also known as "structured teaching," is an educational intervention that focuses on visual learning and tries to accommodate the individual's ASD rather than overcome it (Mesibov & Shea, 2010). The Picture Exchange Communication System (PECS) (Bondy & Frost, 1994; Boesch, Wendt, Subramanian, & Hsu, 2012; Ganz, Davis, Lund, Goodwyn, & Simpson, 2012) focuses on teaching functional communication skills through progressive phases. Studies show that PECS successfully improves functional communication skills and decreases aberrant, frustration-produced behaviors that result from the child not being able to communicate effectively with adults (Yoder & Stone, 2006; Charlop-Christy, Carpenter, LeBlance, & Kellet, 2002). *DIR®/Floortime* is a child-directed approach designed to help the parent connect with the child, usually in the context of informal play that the child enjoys (Greenspan, 1992). The ultimate goal of the program is to increase turn-taking interaction and communication between the child and adult. Noting that most recipients of parent training are mothers, Elder et al. (2011) developed and tested the Father-Directed In-Home Training (FDIT) through a series of NIH funded studies. Like Greenspan's approach, the FDIT is play-based and incorporates four specific components (e.g., following the child's lead, imitation with animation, commenting on the child, and waiting expectantly for a child response). The primary goal of these interventions is to produce gains in the child's social and communications skills.

Social Interventions

Healthcare providers must prioritize social deficits, which are a hallmark of ASD, as they develop an integrated treatment program that targets the needs of the child with ASD and the family. It is particularly important that healthcare providers address joint attention, appropriate responses to questions, and understanding nonverbal communication to convey meaning and understanding.

While there is clear overlap among educational, communication, and social interventions, social interventions target the acquisition of social skills in individuals with ASD who are higher functioning. In this class of interventions, Gray's (1995) "social scripts" or "social stories" are popular and aim to help children with ASD understand social rules and the reciprocity of language. In this approach, the practitioner creates play scenarios or scripts that follow the child's lead, which differs markedly from traditional structured language therapies that direct the child to a story's conclusion. Evidence indicates that this method promotes language acquisition as well as play skills (Gray, 1995). Further, healthcare providers may use social stories to prepare both high-functioning children and adults with ASD for diagnostic and medical procedures.

Pharmacological Interventions

Parents of children with ASD often seek pharmacotherapeutics to help manage behavioral problems, such as head-banging, aggression, obsessive-compulsive behaviors and/or extreme hyperactivity. As a result, healthcare providers need to inform parents that many psychopharmaotherapeutics have not been empirically tested and validated for use in children with ASD.

In addition, healthcare providers need to clarify that medications do not cure autism; they only alleviate the most troublesome behaviors that impair or distress the child and interfere with other treatment (Malone, Gratz, Delaney, & Hyman, 2005; Tuchman & Rapin, 2002; West & Waldrop, 2006). If parents still express interest in pharmacotherapeutics, then healthcare providers may consider antidepressants, atypical antipsychotics, stimulants, α-adrenergic agonists, and anticonvulsants, which are commonly prescribed for children with ASD (Stachnik & Nunn-Thompson, 2007). These medications should be initiated carefully at low doses, and then gradually increased to control symptoms and minimize side effects (Correll, 2008; Bostic & King, 2008). It is important for healthcare providers to be aware of issues related to polypharmacy and the need to exercise due diligence when multiple untested treatments are employed.

Complementary and Alternative Therapies (CAT)

Researchers estimate that 32–92% of parents use one or more complementary and alternative treatments for their children with ASD (Matson et al., 2013). The most popular complementary and alternative therapies are sensory integration; the gluten-free, casein free diet; vitamins and nutritional supplements; hyperbaric oxygen chamber; and chelation therapy. Parents who are interested in these approaches should find a qualified practitioner and use them only as part of a larger, comprehensive, evidence-based treatment program. Similarly, healthcare providers should understand the basic science behind these interventions and be prepared to address parents' questions regarding these therapies. Some of them are briefly defined below.

Sensory Integration

Interventions that involve sensory integration help address common sensory processing problems and the modulation of responses (Case-Smith & Arbesman, 2008; Parham et al., 2007). They can be categorized as sensory-based (e.g., massage, brushing) or auditory (Dawson & Watling, 2000). Preliminary evidence demonstrated that therapeutic touch may also be effective. However, findings related to auditory integration interventions were inconclusive (Case-Smith & Arbesman, 2008) and more research is currently underway.

Gluten-free, Casein-free (GFCF) Diet

A commonly used CAT therapy is the gluten-free, casein-free (GFCF) diet, which includes the elimination of wheat (which contains gluten) and milk (which has casein) from the diets of children with ASD. It is based on the hypothesis that behavioral abnormalities of ASD may be a result of opioid peptides formed from the incomplete breakdown of gluten and casein (Elder, 2008; Christison & Ivany, 2006); however, to date, studies of the GFCF diet have revealed inconsistent findings (Whiteley et al., 2013). Indeed, studies have been limited by challenges related to dietary compliance, sufficient sample sizes, and experimental blinding in naturalistic, day-to-day settings and interactions. Despite these challenges, other researchers stated that individuals who respond positively may benefit from the GFCF diet (Herbert & Buckley, 2013; Whiteley et al., 2013) and that adopting the diet should be decided on an individual basis.

Vitamins and Nutritional Supplements

Many vitamins and nutritional supplements have been purported to be effective in treating symptoms of ASD. For example, B vitamins may positively affect the nervous system and Vitamins C and D may help avoid deficiency. Similarly, Super Nu-Ther® is popular because it contains high doses of B6 and magnesium and is available in pill, powder, or liquid form (Hamilton, 2000). Omega 3 fatty acids, another common supplement, may improve neurological health as well as mood, attention, and activity level, but studies have not shown that they are effective in improving symptoms (Lofthouse, Henndren, Hurt, Arnold, & Butter, 2012). In general, parents should be wary of the claims made by vitamin manufacturers, and ignore any suggestions that supplements should replace evidence-based treatments.

PROBIOTICS. GI problems (e.g., bowel patterns, stool inconsistency, and varying degrees of abdominal pain) are common among patients with ASD (Coury et al., 2012). Probiotics are microorganisms about which preliminary evidence is available. They may improve digestion and immune function as well as remove toxins (Adams, Audhya, & McDonough-Means, 2011; Lofthouse et al., 2012). While the literature currently lacks solid empirical evidence for these claims, there is mounting testimonial evidence suggesting that probiotics may improve gut flora and decrease self-stimulation, stereotypies, aggression, and hyperactivity, resulting in better socialization. Clearly, more research is needed, but probiotics are safe to use in individuals with ASD who have GI symptoms (Lofthouse et al., 2012).

Hyperbaric Treatment

Hyperbaric treatment assumes that the flow of oxygen to the brain is reduced in ASD; thus, advocates assert that exposure to high levels of oxygen will improve the symptoms of individuals with ASD. In 2009, the US

ABC News Network broadcasted a story, "The Search for a Cure," describing preliminary results from a trial by Dr. Daniel A. Rossignol, a father of two children with autism (Rossignol, 2009). He and his colleagues evaluated hyperbaric treatment in 56 children and reported that 30 percent who received the treatment had increased functioning (Brownstein, 2009). Those considering this treatment should know that while these results seem promising, this treatment lacks adequate empirical support, and is expensive (e.g., $100–$900 per treatment) because it is not covered by insurance.

Chelation

Chelation therapy aims to "cure" autism by removing heavy metals from the blood that has become toxic due to mercury overexposure. Despite this claim, to date, there is no proven link between mercury exposure and ASD (Schultz, 2010; Parker, Schwartz, Todd, & Pickering, 2004 Verstraeten et al., 2003), and the Institute of Medicine warns of possible risks and significant side-effects of chelation therapy (Lofthouse et al., 2012) such as potentially deadly liver and kidney damage.

The Health Care Provider's Role in Helping Parents

Parents of children with ASD need direction and support from knowledgeable health care providers from the time they first suspect ASD throughout the lifespan of the individual with ASD. Little (2013) noted that family-centered pediatric nurse practitioners, in particular, are positioned strategically to respond to the needs of parents and facilitate short and long-term adaptation. Caregiver burden must also be assessed, and the stress of mothers, fathers, and siblings equally considered. Mothers with limited education may need more guidance coping with the stress of raising a child with ASD and securing the necessary services (Little, 2013). Healthcare providers must take time to listen to parents in order to assess individual needs and provide practical guidance. This process should occur not only during childhood, but also during the challenging transition to adulthood and throughout the ASD individual's lifetime.

Finally, there is real promise for advancing science related to ASD in ways that are most meaningful and translatable into everyday life. Patient-Centered Outcomes Research Initiatives (PCORI) allow parents and other stakeholders from the ASD community (including high-functioning individuals with ASD) to determine the most relevant research questions and partner with scientists to address them in the most useful ways. Nurses and other health care providers are well positioned on the front line of care to lead these advances and improve the quality of life for those with ASD and their parents.

References

Adams, J., Audhya, T., & McDonough-Means, S. (2011). Effect of a vitamin/mineral supplement on children and adults with autism. *BMC Pediatrics, 11,* 111.

Berry, R. J., Crider, K. S., & Yeargin-Allsopp, M. (2013). Periconceptional folic acid and risk of autism spectrum disorders. *JAMA, 309*(6), 611–613.

Bendixen, R., Elder, J., Donaldson, S., Kairella, J., Valcante, G., & Ferdig, R. E. (2011). Effects of a father-based in-home intervention on perceived stress and family dynamics in parents of children with autism. *American Journal of Occupational Therapy, 65*(6), 679–687.

Boesch, M. C., Wendt, O., Subramanian, A., & Hsu, N. (2013). Comparative efficacy of the Picture Exchange Communication System (PECS) versus a speech-generating device: Effects on requesting skills. *Research in Autism Spectrum Disorders, 7*(3), 480–493.

Bondy, A., & Frost, L. (1994). The Picture Exchange Communication System. *Focus on Autistic Behavior, 9*(3), 1–19.

Bostic, J. Q., & King, B. H. (2008). Autism spectrum disorders: Emerging pharmacotherapy. *American Journal of Occupational Therapy, 62*(4), 416–29.

Brobst, J. L., Clopton, J. R., & Hendrick, S. S. (2009). Parenting children with autism spectrum disorders: The couple's relationship. *Focus on Autism and Other Developmental Disabilities, 24,* 38–49.

Brownstein, J. (2009, March 13). Hyperbaric autism treatment shows possible promise. *ABC News.* Retrieved from http://abcnews.go.com/Health/Autism News/story?id=7070353&page=1;%20retrieved%208-2-12

Cappe, E., Wolff, M., Bobet, R., & Adrien, J. (2011). Quality of life: A key variable to consider in the evaluation of adjustment in parents of children with autism spectrum disorders and in the development of relevant support and assistance programs. *Quality Life Research, 20,* 1279–1294.

Case-Smith, J., & Arbesman, M. (2008). Evidence-based review of interventions for autism used in or of relevance to occupational therapy. *American Journal of Occupational Therapy, 62*(4), 416–429.

Charlop-Christy, M., Carpenter, M., Le, L., LeBlanc, L., & Kellet, K. (2002). Using the Picture Exchange Communication System (PECS) with children with autism: Assessment of PECS acquisition, speech, social-communication behavior, and problem behavior. *Journal of Applied Behavior Analysis, 35*(3), 213–231.

Christison, G. W., & Ivany, K. (2006). Elimination diets in autism spectrum disorders: Any wheat amidst the chaff? *Journal of Developmental & Behavioral Pediatrics, 27,* S162–S171.

Clifford, T., & Minnes, P. (2013). Who participates in support groups for parents of children with autism spectrum disorders? The role of beliefs and coping style. *Journal of Autism & Developmental Disorders, 43,* 179–187.

Correll, C. U. (2008). Antipsychotic use in children and adolescents: Minimizing adverse effects to maximize outcomes. *FOCUS: The Journal of Lifelong Learning in Psychiatry, 6*(3), 368–378.

Coury, D. L., Ashwood, P., Fasano, A., Fuchs, G., Geraghty, M., Kaul, A., . . . Jones, N. E. (2012). Gastrointestinal conditions in children with autism spectrum disorder: Developing a research agenda. *Pediatrics, 130*(2), 160–168.

Davis, N. O., & Carter, A. S. (2008). Parenting stress in mothers and fathers of toddlers with autism spectrum disorders: Associations with child characteristics. *Journal of Autism & Developmental Disorders, 38*(7), 1278–1291.

Dawson, G., & Watling, R. (2000). Interventions to facilitate auditory, visual, and motor integration in autism: A review of the evidence. *Journal of Autism & Developmental Disorders, 30*(5), 415–421.

Dawson, G., Rogers, S., Munson, J., Smith, M., Winter, J., & Greenson, J. (2010). Randomized, controlled trial of an intervention for toddlers with autism: The Early Start Denver Model. *Pediatrics, 125*(1), e17–e23.

Dawson, G., & Burner, K. (2011). Behavioral interventions in children and adolescents with autism spectrum disorder: A review of recent findings. *Current Opinion in Pediatrics, 23*(6), 616–620.

Ekas, N. V., Lickenbrock, D. M., & Whitman, T. L. (2010). Optimism, social support, and well-being in mothers of children with autism spectrum disorder. *Journal of Autism & Developmental Disorders, 40*(10), 1274–1284.

Elder, J. H. (2002). Current treatments in autism: Examining the scientific evidence and clinical implications. *Journal of Neuroscience Nursing, 34,* 67–73.

Elder, J. H. (2008). The gluten-free, casein-free diet in autism: An overview with clinical implications. *Nutrition in Clinical Practice, 23*(6), 583–588.

Elder, J. H., & D'Alessandro, T. (2009). Supporting parents of children with autism spectrum disorders: Questions parent ask and what nurses need to know. *Pediatric Nursing, 35*(4), 240–250.

Elder, J. H., Donaldson, S. O., Kairalla, J., Valcante, G., Bendixen, R., Ferdig, R., . . . Serrano, M. (2011). In-home training for fathers of children with autism: A follow up study and evaluation of four individual training components. *Journal of Child and Family Studies, 20*(3), 263–271.

Elder, J. H. (2013). Empowering parents in the treatment of autism. In M. Fitzgerald (Ed.). *Autism: Book I.* Rijeka: Intech.

Fletcher, P. C., Markoulakis, R., & Bryden, P. J. (2012). The costs of caring for a child with an autism spectrum disorder. *Issues in Comprehensive Pediatric Nursing, 35*(1), 45–69.

Flippin, M., & Crais, E. R. (2011). The need for more effective father involvement in early autism intervention: A systematic review and recommendations. *Journal of Early Intervention, 33*(1), 24–50.

Ganz, J. B., Davis, J. L., Lund, E. M., Goodwyn, F. D., & Simpson, R. L. (2012). Meta-analysis of PECS with individuals with ASD: Investigation of targeted versus non-targeted outcomes, participant characteristics, and implementation phase. *Research in Developmental Disabilities, 33*(2), 406–418.

Gray, C. (1995). Teaching children with autism to "read" social situations. In K. Quill (Ed.), *Teaching children with autism: Strategies to enhance communication and socialization* (pp. 219–242). Stamford, CT: Cengage.

Greeff, A., & van der Walt, K-J. (2010). Resilience in parents with an autistic child. *Education and Training in Autism and Developing Disability, 45*(3), 347–355.

Greenspan, S. I. (1992). Reconsidering the diagnosis and treatment of very young children with autism spectrum or pervasive developmental disorder. *Zero to Three, 13,* 1–9.

Grindle, C. F., Kovshoff, H., Hastings, R. P., & Remington, B. (2009). Parents' experiences of home-based applied behavior analysis programs for young children with autism. *Journal of Autism & Developmental Disorders, 39,* 42–56.

Hall, H. R. (2012). Parents of children with autism: Behaviors of children, community support and coping. *Issues in Comprehensive Pediatric Nursing, 35*(2), 111–132.

Hamilton, L. M. (2000). *Facing autism: Giving parents reasons for hope and guidance for help.* Colorado: WaterBrook Press.

Hastings, R. P., Kovshoff, H., Ward, N. J., Espinosa, F., Brown, T. & Remington. (2005). Systems analysis of stress and positive perceptions in mothers and fathers of pre-school children with autism. *Journal of Autism & Developmental Disorders, 35,* 635–644.

Hayes, S. A., & Watson, S. L. (2013). The impact of parenting stress: A meta-analysis of studies comparing the experience of parenting stress in parents of children with and without autism spectrum disorder. *Journal of Autism & Developmental Disorders, 43*(3), 629–642.

Herbert, M., & Buckley, J. (2013). Autism and dietary therapy: Case report and review of the literature. *Journal of Child Neurology, 28*(8), 975–982.

Howlin, P., & Rutter, M. (1987). *Treatment of autistic children.* Hobeken, NJ: Wiley.

Ingersoll, B., & Hambrick, D. Z. (2011). The relationship between the broader autism phenotype, child severity, and stress and depression in parents of children with autism spectrum disorders. *Research in Autism Spectrum Disorders, 5*(1), 337–344.

Koegel, R. L., & Koegel, K. L. (2006). *Pivotal response treatments for Autism: Communication, social, and academic development.* Baltimore, MD: Brookes Publishing Company.

Lecavalier, L., Leone, S., & Wiltz, J. (2006). The impact of behaviour problems on caregiver stress in young people with autism spectrum disorders. *Journal of Intellectual Disability Research, 50*(3), 172–183.

Little, L. (2013). Differences in stress and coping for mothers and fathers of children with Asperger's syndrome and nonverbal learning disorders. *Pediatric Nursing, 28*(6), 565–570.

Lofthouse, N., Hendren, R., Hurt, E., Arnold, L. E., & Butter, E. (2012). A review of complementary and alternative treatments for autism spectrum disorders. *Autism Research and Treatment, 2012,* 1–21.

Lovaas, O. (1978). Parents as therapists. In E. Schopler & M. Rutter (Eds.), *Autism: A reappraisal of concepts and treatment* (pp. 369–377). New York: Plenum.

Lovaas, O. (1987). Behavioral treatment and normal educational and intellectual functioning in young autistic children. *Journal of Consulting and Clinical Psychology, 55,* 3–9.

Malone, R. P., Gratz, S. S., Delaney, M. A., & Hyman, S. B. (2005). Advances in drug treatments for children and adolescents with autism and other pervasive developmental disorders. *CNS drugs, 19*(11), 923–934.

Mandell, D. S., & Salzer, M. S. (2007). Who joins support groups among parents of children with autism? *Autism, 11*(2), 111–122.

Matson, J. L., Adams, H. L., Williams, L. W., & Rieske, R. D. (2013). Why are there so many unsubstantiated treatments in autism? *Research in Autism Spectrum Disorders, 7*, 466–474.

McCubbin, H. I., McCubbin, M. A., Thompson, A. I., Han, S. V., & Allen, C. T. (1997). Parents under stress: What makes them resilient? *Journal of Family and Consumer Sciences, 89*, 2–11.

McCubbin, H. L., Thompson, A. L., & McCubbin, M. (1996). *Family assessment, resiliency, coping and adaptation–inventories for research and practice.* Madison, WI: University of Wisconsin System.

Mesibov, G. B., & Shea, V. (2010). The TEACCH program in the era of evidence-based practice. *Journal of Autism & Developmental Disorders, 40*(5), 570–579.

Miles, J. H. (2011). Autism spectrum disorders: A genetics review. *Genetics in Medicine, 13*(4), 278–294.

Mukherjee, S., Rupani, K., Dave, M., Subramanyam, A., Shah, H., & Kamath, R. (2014). Evaluation of effectiveness of integrated intervention in autistic children. *The Indian Journal of Pediatrics, 81*(4), 339–345.

Nodding, N. (1984). *Caring, A feminine approach to ethics & moral education.* Berkeley, CA: University of California Press.

Parham, L. D., Cohn, E. S., Spitzer, S., Koomar, J. A., Miller, L. J., Burke, J. P., . . . Summers, C. A. (2007). Fidelity in sensory integration intervention research. *American Journal of Occupational Therapy, 61*(2), 216–227.

Parker, S. K., Schwartz, B., Todd, J., & Pickering, L. K. (2004). Thimerosal-containing vaccines and autistic spectrum disorder: A critical review of published original data. *Pediatrics, 114*(3), 793–804.

Powers, M. D. (2000). Children with autism and their parents. In M. D. Powers (Ed.), *Children with autism: A parents' guide* (2nd ed.). Bethesda, MD: Woodbine House.

Reichow, B., & Volkmar, F. R. (2010). Social skills interventions for individuals with autism: Evaluation for evidence-based practices within a best evidence synthesis framework. *Journal of Autism & Developmental Disorders, 40*(2), 149–166.

Ross, E. K-R., & Kessler, D. (2007). *Finding the meaning of grief through the five stages of loss.* New York: Scribner.

Rossignol, D. A., Rossignol, L. W., Smith, S., Schneider, C., Logerquist, S., Usman, A. . . . Mumper, E. A. (2009). Hyperbaric treatment for children with autism: A multicenter, randomized, double-blind, controlled trial. *BMC Pediatrics, 9*(1), 21.

Rotter, J. B. (1966). Generalized expectancies for internal versus external control of reinforcement. *Psychological Monographs: General & Applied, 80*(1), 1–28.

Shannon, J. D., Tamis-LeMonda, C. S., London, K., & Cabrera, N. (2002). Beyond rough and tumble: Low-income fathers' interactions and children's cognitive development at 24 months. *Parenting: Science and Practice, 2*, 77–104.

Sherer, M. R., & Schreibman, L. (2005). Individual behavioral profiles and predictors of treatment effectiveness for children with autism. *Journal of Consulting and Clinical Psychology, 73*(3), 525–538.

Smith, L. O., & Elder, J. H. (2010). Siblings and family environments of persons with autism spectrum disorder: A review of the literature. *Journal of Child and Adolescent Psychiatric Nursing, 23,* 189–195.

Souders, M. C., Mason, T. B., Valladares, O., Bucan, M., Levy, S. E., Mandell, D. S., . . . Pinto-Martin, J. (2009). Sleep behaviors and sleep quality in children with autism spectrum disorders. *Sleep, 32*(12), 1566–1578.

Stachnik, J. M., & Nunn-Thompson, C. (2007). Use of atypical antipsychotics in the treatment of autistic disorder. *Annals of Pharmacotherapy, 41*(4), 626–634.

Suhrheinrich, J., Stahmer, A. C., Reed, S., Schreibman, L., Rcisinger, E., & Mandell, D. (2013). Implementation challenges in translating pivotal response training into community settings. *Journal of Autism & Developmental Disorders, 43,* 2970–2976.

Tonge, B. J., Bull, K., Brereton, A., & Wilson, R. (2014). A review of evidence-based early intervention for behavioral problems in children with autism spectrum disorder: The core components of effective programs, child-focused interventions and comprehensive treatment models. *Current Opinion in Psychiatry, 27*(2), 158–165.

Tuchman, R., & Rapin, I. (2002). Epilepsy in autism. *The Lancet Neurology, 1*(6), 352–358.

Twoy, R., Connolly, P. M., & Novak, J. M. (2007). Coping strategies used by parents of children with autism. *Journal of the American Academy of Nurse Practitioners, 19*(5), 251–260.

Verstraeten, T., Davis, R. L., DeStefano, F., Lieu, T. A., Rhodes, P. H., Black, S. B., . . . Chen, R. T. (2003). Safety of thimerosal-containing vaccines: A two-phased study of computerized health maintenance organization databases. *Pediatrics, 112*(5), 1039–1048.

Vismara, L. A., & Rogers, S. J. (2010). Behavioral treatments in autism spectrum disorder: What do we know? *Annual Review of Clinical Psychology, 6,* 447–468.

Volk, H. E., Lurmann, F., Penfold, B., Hertz-Picciotto, I., & McConnell, R. (2013). Traffic-related air pollution, particulate matter, and autism. *JAMA Psychiatry, 70*(1), 71–77.

Warren, Z., McPheeters, M. L., Sathe, N., Foss-Feig, J. H., Glasser, A., & Veenstra-VanderWeele, J. (2011). A systematic review of early intensive intervention for autism spectrum disorders. *Pediatrics, 127*(5), e1303–e1311.

West, L., & Waldrop, J. (2006). Risperiodone use in the treatment of behavioral symptoms in children with autism. *Pediatric Nursing, 32*(6), 545–549.

Whiteley, P., Shattuck, P., Knivsberge, A., Seim, A., Reichelt, K. & Todd, L. (2013). Gluten- and casein-free dietary intervention for autism spectrum conditions. *Frontiers in Human Neuroscience, 6,* 1–8.

Yoder, P. J., & Stone, W. L. (2006). A randomized comparison of the effect of two prelinguistic communication interventions on the acquisition of spoken communication in preschoolers with ASD. *Journal of Speech, Language, and Hearing Research, 49,* 698–711.

Chapter 10

INTEGRATING GENETIC TESTING INTO HEALTH CARE

MARIAN REIFF AND SURABHI MULCHANDANI

Introduction

Advances in genetics have increased the ability to detect genetic changes associated with autism spectrum disorder (ASD). It is important to clarify that the diagnosis of ASD is based on developmental and behavioral assessments, and that clinical genetic testing is not used to diagnose ASD, but rather to determine the etiology of ASD after it is clinically diagnosed. A genetic etiology may lead to improved care and management for the patient, and to more informed risk-recurrence estimates for the family (Schaefer & Mendelsohn, 2013). Most genetic variants associated with ASD are also associated with intellectual disability, epilepsy, and psychiatric conditions, which suggests the possibility of shared biologic pathways (Carter & Scherer, 2013). Given the high prevalence of ASD (almost 1% of children in the United States), and the increasing use of genetic testing, healthcare professionals will need to integrate genetic information regarding ASD into their clinical practice. Healthcare providers will, therefore, need to be familiar with the relevant genetic information and to liaise with genetics professionals in order to facilitate optimal patient-centered care for ASD populations. Integration of genetics into the health care of individuals and families with ASD can help patients and healthcare providers to make informed decisions, thereby improving the quality of health care services (Agency for Healthcare Research and Quality [AHRQ], 2014).

This chapter presents current trends in genetic and genomic testing for ASD, beginning with an overview of recent advances in genetic testing for ASD and guidelines for use of genetic testing in pediatric clinical practice.

This is followed by a description of a standard genetics evaluation for individuals diagnosed with ASD. Some important psychosocial and ethical implications of genomic testing are considered, and several studies investigating the implications of genomic testing for healthcare providers and for families are presented, followed by recommendations to facilitate the integration of genetics and genomics into healthcare for people with ASD.

Chromosomal microarray analysis (CMA) is used as an example in this chapter to explore issues related to all larger-scale genetic and genomic testing including whole genome and whole exome sequencing. The challenges related to CMA, namely identification of novel variations, uncertainty in interpretation, and discovery of secondary are representative of all new larger-scale genomic tests. The lessons learned in the context of array-based testing can assist in preparing for the clinical integration of novel genome-wide sequencing methodologies.

Genetic Etiology of Autism Spectrum Disorder

Autism spectrum disorders (ASDs) is comprised of a group of heterogeneous conditions that share common features of impairment in social interaction and communication, and repetitive or stereotypic behavior (American Psychiatric Association, 2013). Based on high heritability, and comorbidity of ASD with epilepsy and intellectual disability, this neurobehavioral disorder is considered genetically influenced (Carter & Scherer, 2013). Given the heterogeneity of the condition, it is no surprise that various genetic, epigenetic, and environmental factors contribute to the etiology (Persico & Bourgeron, 2006).

Approximately 20% of autism cases can be explained by single genetic abnormalities (Schaefer & Mendelsohn, 2013). These include mutations in a single gene as seen in fragile X syndrome or submicroscopic copy number alterations such as 16p11.2 deletion syndrome. The percentage of individuals with ASD found to have a genetic abnormality has increased dramatically due to the use of genomic testing technologies such as CMA and next generation sequencing (Veenstra-VanderWeele, Christian, & Cook, 2004).

Genetic Testing in the Diagnostic Protocol

Genetic testing leading to an etiological diagnosis may provide benefits for patients and families, including providing recurrence-risk-based counseling, improving access to needed support or services, refining treatment options, providing prognosis, early detection of comorbid conditions, and avoiding unnecessary diagnostic tests (Manning & Hudgins, 2010; D. T. Miller et al., 2010). A recent literature review has pointed to a need for stud-

---

Box 10.1. Reasons for Recommending Genetic Testing in Autism Spectrum Disorder

- Limits the need for future diagnostic evaluations
- Provides prognostic information
- Provides anticipatory guidance to tailor treatments for comorbid conditions and associated features
- Provides information to tailor recommendations for early intervention services
- Contributes to the accuracy of recurrence risk estimates

---

ies to assess clinical utility by directly comparing health outcomes for use versus no use of genetic tests in order to assess clinical utility (AHRQ, 2014). Although randomized controlled studies have as yet not been conducted, several studies (Dawson et al., 2010; Eriksson et al., 2013; Hayward, Eikeseth, Gale, & Morgan, 2009; Heil & Schaaf, 2013; Lintas & Persico, 2009; Narcisa et al., 2012; Shen et al., 2010; Warren et al., 2011) [Coulter 2011] have delineated benefits of identifying genetic causation for ASD. These are listed in Box 10.1.

In a retrospective study involving patients with developmental delay, ASD and multiple congenital anomalies who had undergone CMA testing, Coulter et al. (2011) documented a substantial change in medical management based on the CMA results. The rate of recommendation for clinical action was 54% in individuals with pathogenic results and 34% for variations of unknown significance (VUS) results, and included referral to another specialty, specific imaging and targeted laboratory tests (Coulter et al., 2011). Even though genetic testing is not considered a diagnostic test for ASD, identification of all the factors that contribute to causation is important for counseling about prognosis and recurrence risk in the family, tailoring the care of affected individuals, and ending the parents' diagnostic odyssey.

Clinical Genetics Evaluation and Genetic Testing

Professional organizations, including the American Academy of Pediatrics, American Academy of Neurology, the National Society of Genetic Counselors, and the American College of Medical Genetics, recommend a clinical genetics evaluation for children with ASD in order to clarify etiology. A clinical genetics evaluation comprises a detailed review of medical and family history, physical examination to identify dysmorphic features, and determination of a differential diagnosis. This is followed by the genetic testing recommendation.

The family history review is focused on identifying others in the family with subclinical symptoms associated with the broader autism phenotype, neuropsychiatric and/or neurobehavioral conditions. Such findings are observed in up to 35% of ASD families (Miles, 2011). The physical examination includes height, weight, and head circumference to identify microcephaly or macrocephaly. The presence of microcephaly suggests specific monogenic or chromosomal etiology, whereas macrocephaly, which is seen in 35% of individuals with ASD, steers the evaluation towards other genetic causes such as *PTEN* gene mutation, fragile X syndrome or tuberous sclerosis. An in-depth dysmorphology exam further helps in the identification of features known to be related to genetic conditions such as Rett syndrome, thereby informing appropriate genetic testing (Miles, McCathren, Stichter, & Shinawi, 1993 updated 2010). Box 10.2 lists the genetic syndromes commonly associated with autism.

The clinical genetics evaluation helps in distinguishing essential or isolated autism from syndromic or complex autism. Essential autism is seen in 75% of all ASD cases. Syndromic autism is characterized by the presence of other comorbid conditions such as seizures, and clinically recognizable dysmorphic features and microcephaly (Miles, 2011; Schaefer & Mendelsohn, 2013).

Box 10.2. Genetic Syndromes Commonly Associated with Autism Spectrum Disorder

- Monogenic disorders
  - Fragile X syndrome
  - Mutations in PTEN gene
  - Rett syndrome
  - Tuberous sclerosis
- Sex chromosome abnormalities
  - Klinefelter syndrome (47,XXY) and 47,XYY
- Copy number alterations:
  - 22q11.2 deletion syndrome,
  - 16p11.2
  - 16p13.11
  - 15q13.3 deletion syndrome

A clinical genetics evaluation results in one of the three following outcomes:

1. Syndromic autism with a suspected genetic etiology,
2. Syndromic autism without a suspected genetic etiology, and
3. Essential autism.

The algorithm for clinical genetic evaluation is illustrated in Figure 10.1 showing the possible outcomes of a clinical genetics evaluation for ASD, and the testing options for each outcome (confirmatory genetic testing or CMA). If, after the clinical genetics evaluation, a syndromic form of ASD with a specific genetic etiology is suspected, confirmatory testing should be recommended. For example for an individual with ASD, seizures, and skin findings specific to tuberous sclerosis (TSC) syndrome; testing for TSC1 and TSC2 genes should be offered.

Chromosomal microarray analysis (CMA) is used in etiologic evaluation in all ASD subgroups, and in the case of essential autism, only CMA is recommended.

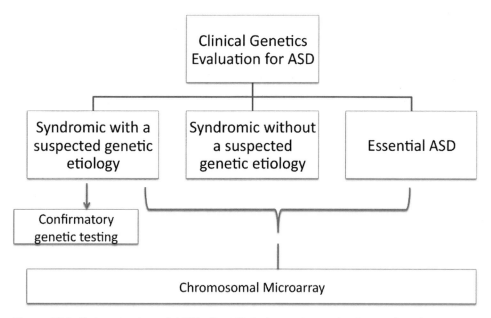

Figure 10.1. Categorization of ASD after clinical genetics evaluation and testing recommendation showing the possible outcomes of a clinical genetics evaluation for ASD, and testing options for each outcome.

First-Line Genetic Testing

CMA is the first line of testing for individuals with suspected ASD, as well as for developmental delay and multiple congenital abnormalities (D. T. Miller et al., 2010), and is increasingly used to obtain a genetic diagnosis for patients with autism spectrum disorder (ASD) (Manning & Hudgins, 2010; F. A. Miller, Hayeems, & Bytautas, 2010; Shen et al., 2010).

CMA is a DNA-based analysis used for identification of copy number variations (CNV). The normal copy number for most of chromosomes is two, since all human cells contain two sets of 23 chromosomes. The alterations identified by the CMA primarily include missing regions (known as deletions) and extra regions (duplications) of the chromosomes. Many deletions or duplications result in various clinical conditions.

Historically, chromosomal alterations (large deletions, duplications, or other structural changes) were identified under the microscope using karyotype analysis, and these alterations had to be at least 5 to 10 megabases (5 to 10 x 10^6 basepairs) in size to be detectable (the entire genome contains 3 billion or 3 x 10^9 basepairs). The resolution of CMA is 20–200 times higher than traditional karyotype analysis. CMA is used to identify copy number variations (CNVs) of 50 kilobases (50 x 10^3 basepairs) and larger, and can detect even smaller CNVs.

Interpretation of the clinical significance of the CNVs is based upon the gene content and absence of the CNV in the normal population. It is known that deletions and/or duplication of some parts of the genome are tolerated and do not result in a clinical abnormality. These benign CNVs are frequently found in healthy individuals and are considered to be polymorphisms of the genome (Pinto, Marshall, Feuk, & Scherer, 2007). In approximately 10% of clinically tested patients, the clinical significance of the CNV remains unknown based on the available data, leading to uncertainty in the interpretation of test results (Kohane, Masys, & Altman, 2006; Redon et al., 2006).

Results of CMA testing fall into three broad categories:

1. Positive or pathogenic or abnormal: Identification of a genetic alteration clearly known to cause pathology;
2. Negative or normal: Absence of a known pathogenic alteration; and
3. Ambiguous, variant of unknown significance (VUS): A genetic alteration that has not been described previously, has not been seen in controls so far studied, and for which there is incomplete data on the genes in the region.

Parental testing is recommended for cases with VUS results to determine whether the variant is inherited or *de novo* (i.e., when neither parent carries the variant). If one of the parents carries the variant and is phenotypically normal, the variant is more likely to be benign. However, the possibility exists that a parent carrying the variant has some minor anomaly or health problem that may or may not be associated with the variant. When the variant is either inherited from a similarly affected parent or is *de novo,* the variant is more likely to be associated with the phenotype. A similar pattern of inheritance needs to be observed in multiple families before assigning the status of benign or causative to a variant. In addition, there are several variants that have been identified with widely variable expressivity, which clouds the significance of findings in children whose normal parents also carry these variants (Mefford et al., 2008). There is, therefore, potential for considerable uncertainty in the interpretation of results, and in the implications of results for the children tested and for their parents (Ali-Khan, Daar, Shuman, Ray, & Scherer, 2009; Darilek et al., 2008; Tabor & Cho, 2007). Interpretational uncertainty decreases as information on VUS variants accumulates over time. Large datasets of CNVs in affected and unaffected populations are available to aid in clarifying the significance of VUS alterations, and information technologies can help clinicians to keep abreast of evolving knowledge (Aronson et al., 2012).

SECONDARY OR INCIDENTAL FINDINGS (IFs). The higher resolution genomic technologies also identify a higher rate of secondary or incidental findings (IFs), such as clinically relevant genetic variants unrelated to the reason for testing. In our experience, IFs were detected in1% of individuals undergoing CMA testing (Mulchandani, Conlin, Thiel, & Spinner, 2012). These findings included predisposition to later onset conditions, alterations in disease genes not related to the patient's current reason for study, or unexpected familial relationships. With the advent of higher resolution next generation sequencing technologies such as panels that include tens to hundreds of genes or exome sequencing, there is a greater attention on detection of IFs.

Guidelines developed for use in pediatric genomic research recommend that parents provide informed consent for disclosure of IFs based on specific criteria. One case might be when urgent clinical significance and potential benefit outweigh the risks of psychosocial harms (Abdul-Karim et al., 2013). The American College of Medical Genetics and Genomics (ACMG) recommendations for reporting of IFs in clinical exome and genome sequencing note that although predictive genetic testing for adult-onset diseases is generally not recommended for minors, IFs from genomic testing of a child that are relevant to some adult diseases have clinical implications for parents or other family members, and should, therefore, be disclosed to families undergoing genomic testing (Green et al., 2013). The ACMG has disseminated a list of conditions with proven clinical management that minimizes the risk of future adverse outcomes (Green et al., 2013). A presidential committee on bioethics has issued a report urging clinicians, diagnostics laboratories, and researchers to educate and prepare patients and research participants regarding the possibility of secondary findings in genomic tests like CMA or whole exome/genome sequencing (Gutmann et al., 2013).

Potential Psychosocial and Ethical Implications of Genomic Testing

The unanticipated and uncertain information generated by genomic technologies presents psychosocial and ethical challenges, particularly for testing in pediatric populations. An etiological diagnosis can provide psychological benefits for individuals and families, including decreased levels of uncertainty and anxiety, improved coping and adaptation, an increased sense of control, and relief from guilt for being in some way responsible for their child's condition (Lenhard, Breitenbach, Ebert, Schindelhauer-Deutscher, & Henn, 2005; Lipinski, Lipinski, Biesecker, & Biesecker, 2006; Makela, Birch, Friedman, & Marra, 2009). However, knowledge of genetic causation may also contribute to parents' anxiety and perceived stigma by increasing the perceived seriousness of a disorder and the concern that other family members could develop the same problem (McMahon, Baty, & Botkin, 2006; Phelan, Cruz-Rojas, & Reiff, 2002).

If parents undergo testing themselves, knowledge about their own genetic characteristics may be perceived as useful for family planning, but may also increase their sense of guilt if they discover that they carry a genetic alteration that may be associated with their child's medical condition. For parents interested in determining their risk for having a second child on the autism spectrum, VUS results can be especially challenging.

Uncertainties surrounding diagnosis and prognosis can be confusing for families and can lead to adverse psychosocial outcomes (Biesecker & Erby, 2008; Tabor & Cho, 2007; Timmermans & Buchbinder, 2010; Tluczek, Orland, & Cavanagh, 2011). However, for some people, having an inconclusive (rather than a pathogenic) result may have positive psychological outcomes, such as allowing for hope to be maintained (Lenhard et al., 2005; Lipinski et al., 2006; Whitmarsh, Davis, Skinner, & Bailey, 2007). Additionally, cultural norms may differentially affect perceptions of ASD-related behaviors and attitudes toward genomic testing (Chen, Xu, Huang, & Dhar, 2013; Mandell & Novak, 2005; Norbury & Sparks, 2013; Pachter & Dworkin, 1997).

In light of the differing perspectives regarding the nature of autism itself, important questions have been raised about the ethical implications of genomic testing for ASD (Lintas & Persico, 2009; Scherer & Dawson, 2011; Silverman, 2011; Walsh, Elsabbagh, Bolton, & Singh, 2011; Yudell et al., 2013). While many believe that detection of genetic etiology is beneficial, some contend that genetic research and clinical genetic testing have not helped find treatments or a cure for ASD (Pellicano & Stears, 2011; Walsh et al., 2011). Concerns have also been expressed that genetic advances could lead to the elimination of autism in the future, through prenatal testing and selective pregnancy termination (Pellicano & Stears, 2011; Sinclair, 2013).

Underutilization of Genetic Services

In spite of professional recommendations, studies have found that only approximately 24–28% of parents whose children were diagnosed with ASD reported that their child had undergone genetic testing (Amiet, Couchon, Carr, Carayol, & Cohen, 2014; Chen et al., 2013; Selkirk, McCarthy Veach, Lian, Schimmenti, & Leroy, 2009). Factors affecting underutilization of genetic services for ASD may include lack of awareness of the availability and utility of genetic testing, and lack of provider recommendation and referral for a genetics evaluation (Wydeven, Kwan, Hardan, & Bernstein, 2012). Some discrepancies in uptake of genetics services based on race/ethnicity and culture have also been reported (Amiet et al., 2014; Shea, Newschaffer, Xie, Myers, & Mandell, 2014). More research is needed in order to understand the decision-making process of providers and families regarding uptake of testing, and to facilitate the appropriate utilization of genetics services for ASD.

Practice Implications of Genomic Testing

With the recommendation to include genomic testing as part of the standard diagnostic routine, clinicians ordering testing have an important role to play in preparing families for testing and communicating results. At the same time, providers are confronting new challenges interpreting and conveying the results of genomic testing, particularly regarding uncertain and incidental findings (Grody, 2003; Wade, Wilfond, & McBride, 2010; Wilfond & Ross, 2009). Additionally, parents and families will be expected to understand the meaning and practical use of genomic test results.

Consideration of Healthcare Providers' Perceptions and Perspectives

In a study investigating providers' perspectives, clinicians ordering CMA rated their comfort level explaining results as lower for VUS results, compared with abnormal and normal results (Reiff et al., 2013b). Additionally, providers noted the high proportion of VUS results in CMA as compared with previous types of genetic testing, identified uncertainties associated with pathogenic results for which prognostic information was limited, and emphasized the importance of preparing families for potential uncertainties prior to testing (Reiff et al., 2014b).

Knowledge of the significance of a VUS often evolves over time as more data become available, and it can be challenging for providers to keep abreast of new information. Novel or rare pathogenic findings may have no immediate impact on treatment options or prognosis. In many cases, the boundaries between clinical care and clinical research are unclear, necessitating thoughtful communication about the benefits and limitations of genetic testing both pre- and posttest. Parents may incorrectly assume that they will be informed of relevant new discoveries; however, it is not feasible for providers to recontact patients to update them on new information (Pyeritz, 2011). Follow-up visits are an essential mechanism for keeping both providers and families up to date with new information.

REPORTING SECONDARY/INCIDENTAL FINDINGS (IFs). Some clinicians may not consider it pertinent, prior to testing, to discuss the potential for CMA to reveal information concerning biological parentage or predisposition to late-onset disease (Reiff et al., 2013b). Providers' reluctance to discuss IFs pretest was due to the considerable time required to discuss the wide range of potential findings, which may be impractical or unnecessary given their infrequent occurrence. Health care providers expressed a sense of duty to disclose IFs; however, they were also concerned about potential psychosocial harms of disclosing presymptomatic findings (Reiff et al., 2014a). Some providers also expressed reluctance to disclose risk information before a child developed symptoms, and were concerned for the potential psychological burden on families (Reiff et al., 2014a).

The potential psychosocial harms of overvigilance need to be weighed against the benefits of psychological preparedness and early prevention (Kohane et al., 2006; Lerman, Croyle, Tercyak, & Hamann, 2002; Nelson et al., 2001). Most reports agree that IFs that are clinically important and actionable should be disclosed; however, caution is recommended out of respect for the patient's right not to know, and due to implications for family members, especially when testing involves children (Christenhusz, Devriendt, & Dierickx, 2013). Clinical guidelines recommending informed consent for genomic testing were published prior to and since these studies were conducted. Additional recommendations regarding the need for informed consent for clinical whole exome sequencing have been disseminated. Outlined in these guidelines are a set of recommendations to help patients understand risks, benefits, and limitations of the testing. This discussion should specifically address "expected outcomes of testing, the likelihood and type of incidental results that may be generated, and the types of results that will or will not be returned. Patients should know if and what type of incidental findings may be returned to their referring physician by the laboratory performing the test" (ACMG Board of Directors, 2013, p. 748).

Consideration of Parents' Perceptions and Perspectives

Clinicians are offering CMA testing to an increasing number of families, yet little research has been conducted on the social and psychological impact of the test results. Given the challenges presented by the complex and uncertain information that CAM can provide, there is value in understanding the impact of the perspectives of the patients tested and their families regarding the testing experience and the impact of the test results. In a study involving parents of children with ASD who had undergone CMA, Reiff and colleagues (2014b) found that more than half of the parents reported that the CMA result had been moderately, very, or extremely helpful for their child. The perceived overall benefit of the test result for the child was significantly related to parents' understandings of the result, and their perceptions that the results: (a) Provided a definite diagnosis; (b) informed future medical care; (c) helped access services; (d) explained etiology; and (e) helped connect with others with the same condition (Reiff, Mulchandani, Giarelli, & Bernhardt, 2014b). Many parents reported that the blood draw itself was stressful for the child, and some delayed testing until a blood test was required for another purpose. Several respondents reported that the CMA results provided "concrete" biological evidence of a problem, which they reported might be helpful in obtaining special educational services for the child. Others reported they believed the test results might be used to help them seek and obtain the most appropriate treatments according to adjusted expectations of the child's functional potential. This included the option to avoid futile interventions. Table 10.1 presents parents' reports of how they believed test results could be used to inform medical care and guide educational and behavioral treatment strategies.

CHALLENGES IN PARENT'S UNDERSTANDINGS OF GENOMIC INFORMATION. Understanding of genetic test results tends to be poor in the general public (Condit, 2010), and in individuals undergoing genetic testing to assess disease risk (Klitzman, 2010). CMA results that involve genomic variations with uncertain clinical courses are especially challenging to understand (Darilek et al., 2008; Makela et al., 2009). Additionally, parents' reproductive decisions are influenced by their perceptions of recurrence risk, and these perceptions are frequently inaccurate (Selkirk et al., 2009).

Table 10.1
PARENTS' PERCEPTIONS OF CHROMOSOMAL MICROARRAY ANALYSIS
RESULTS: SELECTED THEMES AND ILLUSTRATIVE STATEMENTS ON
THE POTENTIAL USE OF TEST RESULTS

Potential Use	*Supporive Statement*
Guide medical care	There are medications for kids with ADHD [attention deficit hyperactivity disorder] and autism . . . Well, kids with [this result] react different to the normal meds that everybody says to put them on. Some of the meds can kill them. And if you do not know, you can give your kid something that everybody suggests you give to autism kids that will kill yours. [Result: Pathogenic]
Inform educational or behavioral approach	We were struggling . . . you know, what do we do? Do we teach him how to clear the dishes from our table, or do we teach him how to read and write? ... It does inform us about what his expectations can be . . . it has informed our [educational] goals. [Result: Pathogenic]
Inform reproductive decisions	It was something that we needed to have in our determination to continue our family [Result: Negative (normal)]
Inform expectations	I was able to realize that this is a permanent part of his genetic makeup and something that we'll be dealing with over the long term, instead of trying to find a quick solution. [Result: Variant of unknown significance (VUS)]
Alleviate sense of guilt	It helped me because the other way I looked at it was that pre-maturity-wise I really thought it was something that I did, that his water broke. And then when I started to think about geneti-cally, the genetics could have caused his prematurity and that really started to relieve some of my anxiety. [Result: VUS]
Validate parents' perceptions	I'm so glad I'm using my mother's intuition. So, it just con-firmed it, so I felt happy that I wasn't crazy. And everybody else would say–oh, nothing is wrong with him, he's fine. [Result: VUS]
Promote hope	It's nice to know there's a reason why there's certain parts of him that are the way they are and that other people have these things and they are functioning and surviving and it gives me hope that his future is positive. [Result: Pathogenic]
Raise new questions	I would have liked to have a follow-up appointment . . . and really talked about what that meant and . . . what do we do next, where do we go from here? [Result: Negative]

In a study of parental understanding of CMA results, parents who reported experiencing difficulty with comprehension of results also reported that they had received results by telephone, had long waits to see a geneticist to discuss results, received inconsistent information from different professionals, and conducted internet searches based on inadequate and/or inaccurate information. Comprehension tended to improve after discussing results with healthcare professionals and with medically informed relatives, friends, or support groups (Reiff et al., 2012). Research in other medical genetics settings has demonstrated increased satisfaction when patients have an option of receiving results by telephone or in person (Baumanis, Evans, Callanan, & Susswein, 2009; Fanos et al., 2011). Several parents articulated the challenges involved in having to take their special needs child to the consultation when results were discussed, which was required for insurance coverage for the visit. Although accommodations were usually made at the clinic to provide some time for parents to talk with providers without the child in the same room, parents would have preferred not to have to take child along, and this was a barrier to in-person consultations for some parents.

Most parents sought information on the internet, yet many reported that internet searches had limited value, and sometimes increased confusion (Reiff et al., 2012). This suggests an unmet need for sufficient and accurate information. Parents reported that when they tried to connect with other families with similar results, they used the chromosomal band name for the copy number variant (CNV) to identify other individuals with the same CMA result (Reiff 2012). CMA results are generally named based on the chromosomal band and subband designation, and each band can contain multiple different CNVs that may have no or minimal overlap. For example, a schematic representation of chromosome 1 shows the p (short) and q (long) arms of the chromosome and the region called 1p21.1 and 1p21.2 (see Figure 10. 2). Often, parents are aware only of the number of the chromosome in which the CNV was identified, the deletion/duplication or other unexpected finding. They may not know that any one of the chromosomes may have thousands of CNVs. When searching the internet without sufficiently detailed information, there is a tendency to find information that is irrelevant, too complicated, inaccurate, or misleading. For example, an internet search using the terms "chromosome 1p deletion or 1p21 deletion" may reveal a CNV comprising very large deletions or insertions associated with an extremely severe, and entirely unrelated condition in contrast with the accurate result "chromosome 1p21.1 deletion." If health professionals explain to parents the importance of using the specific details of the test result in internet searches, this could spare them the needless distress that occurs when uncovering disturbing information that is not relevant. By reducing the

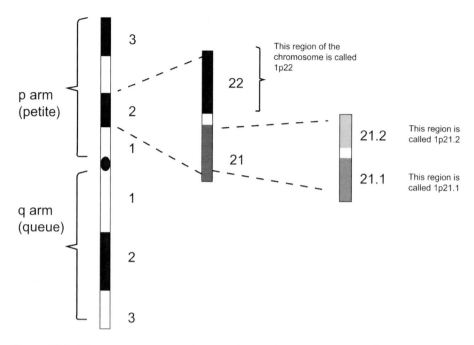

Figure 10.2. Chromosome nomenclature schema showing the p (short) and q (long) arms of chromosome 1 and the regions called 1p21.1 and 1p21.2.

negative outcomes associated with internet searches, the internet may become a valuable resource for information and/or support, as reported in several studies involving other types of genetic testing (Schaffer, Kuczynski, & Skinner, 2008).

Providing timely, in-person consultations to discuss results can help to reduce uncertainties associated with poor comprehension. However, uncertainties stemming from limitations in scientific knowledge can only be resolved by future discoveries. It can be helpful for families to differentiate between different types of uncertainties and identify those that can and cannot be reduced (Han, Klein, & Arora, 2011; Reiff et al., 2012). While scientific uncertainty will not be reduced by currently available information, it is possible to reduce other aspects of uncertainty and thereby improve understanding of the results. When uncertainties are differentiated, families' specific informational needs can be addressed more effectively. Scientific uncertainties that cannot be reduced at present may be addressed initially by acknowledging them clearly, and then by appropriate follow-up with health-care providers, and by participation in research studies, when available. This highlights the need for adequate follow-up care for patients with VUS and novel pathogenic findings. Healthcare professionals can also help families to interpret and find meaning in their results by clarifying uncertainties that can be reduced, and providing tailored information to address individual needs.

Recommendations

Several approaches have been suggested to facilitate the successful integration of genomic testing into health care for individuals with ASD. These may fall under categories of practice and policy recommendations.

Practice Recommendations

Clinical recommendations emphasize the importance of pretest counseling and informed consent to ensure that patients and families are prepared for the information and make an informed decision to receive it (Green et al., 2013; Gutmann et al., 2013; Kearney, Thorland, Brown, Quintero-Rivera, & South, 2011; Manning & Hudgins, 2010; D. T. Miller et al., 2010). This discussion should include the possibility of finding an etiologic explanation of ASD, the possibility of identifying a VUS, and the potential for secondary findings. Additionally, as for developmental disorders in general, the age of the individual tested should be considered in the decision to have genetic testing and the potential impact of genetic information. Varying information can be provided at different life stages in order to address the differing informational needs of individuals and families.

Delivery of results is crucial to understanding of the genetic information, which can be complex and involve multiple uncertainties. Results should, therefore, be provided by professionals with appropriate genetics expertise to accurately interpret and explain results, as articulated in professional guidelines (Kearney et al., 2011). For a variant of unknown significance (VUS), the guidelines recommend genetic consultation, genetic counseling, or both, and ongoing monitoring of the medical literature by the physician with an ongoing patient relationship (Kearney et al., 2011). As revealed by research on uncertainties in CMA testing, the type and level of uncertainty can be clarified by providers when results are communicated, and this clarification may facilitate patient understanding (Reiff et al., 2012). For example, it can be helpful to clarify whether uncertainties are at the level of patient comprehension, provider communication, or scientific limitations. Additionally, families should be provided with options for the mode of result delivery, either by telephone or in person.

Posttest genetic counseling should be available soon after results are delivered, in order to address the medical and psychosocial implications of CMA results for the child and other family members, and to inform families how to keep abreast of new relevant scientific information. Resources need to be developed to enable parents to access reliable information and connect with other families with the same CMA finding. It is imperative to provide details of the genetic test results to the patient's family, and to emphasize the importance of using the precise information in their searches, so that families can avoid focusing on misleading information, and can accurately identify other individuals with comparable genetic test results.

In order to make informed decisions about genomic testing, parents need adequate education and counseling about the potential benefits and limitations of genomic information, and healthcare providers need to convey the complexities and uncertainties of the information (Wilfond & Ross, 2009). Many nongenetics providers who order CMA may not have sufficient genetics knowledge to adequately explain the test and to interpret the results for patients. Genetics training for nongenetics specialists and primary healthcare providers can help them to provide appropriate support for families, and address the medical and psychosocial implications of test results. Additionally, the American Academy of Pediatrics AAP guidelines on genetic testing for ASD suggest collaboration with genetics professionals (Moeschler & Shevell, 2006; Nelson et al., 2001). Involving primary care practitioners is considered an effective means of providing integrated care to children with special health care needs (Rosenthal, 2008). The increasing use of genetics in health care will require continuing genetic education for primary care physicians, so they can provide care and guidance for families undergoing CMA and other types of genomic testing (Guttmacher, Porteous, & McInerney, 2007).

Policy Recommendations

The studies described above highlighted some of the benefits as well as the challenges posed by the increasing use of genomics for the providers and families of individuals with ASD, and suggest several provider-, family-, and system-level approaches that could facilitate the integration of genomics into healthcare (Reiff, Bernhardt, & Mulchandani, 2013a).

PROVIDER-LEVEL APPROACHES. Genetics expertise is crucial in communication of genomic test results to families, yet the medical genetics workforce is not sufficient to meet the demand for their services. More genetics professionals will be needed, and non-genetics health professionals will need training to improve their ability to interpret and convey genomic information (Greendale & Pyeritz, 2001). Additionally, providers may improve their comfort with interpreting genetic test results by appropriate liaison with genetic professionals. Providers will be in a position to help their patients to better understand the genetic information they impart by clearly identifying and categorizing uncertainties that can and cannot be reduced (Reiff et al., 2012). This can also help to improve provider-patient communication, promote clarity, and address informational needs of families.

FAMILY-LEVEL APPROACHES. Families need educational resources and support both before and after testing, as well as long-term, follow-up care, in order to be updated on scientific advances regarding uncertain and novel findings. Genetic literacy should be improved so that families can make informed medical decisions. Parents who have been through the testing experience could be a resource for new families having testing. Parent support groups and peer-to-peer counseling should be facilitated, and interested parents should be provided with training opportunities.

SYSTEM-LEVEL APPROACHES. The infrastructure for integrating genomics into health care could be improved by institutional policies encouraging compliance with best practice guidelines for ordering and explaining genetic testing. Access to genetics professionals is essential for pre- and posttest counseling and follow-up care. Collaboration among nongenetics providers and genetics professionals and testing laboratories should be facilitated. Insurance plans that do not allow for in-person consultations for parents to discuss results without the child present are problematic. Parents must either rely on the telephone to receive and discuss results, or discuss the results in the child's presence. Either scenario can lead to inadequate counseling and misunderstanding. Insurance coverage for a parents to consult with clinicians without the tested child present could help to improve understanding, and hence outcomes, of genomic testing of children.

Conclusions

Advances in genetic technologies have increased the ability to detect a genetic etiology for ASD, and clinical guidelines recommend that genetic testing should be discussed and offered for all patients and families with ASDs. A diagnosis of ASD should be made before a genetic consultation, and the primary care provider (PCP) should explain what a genetic consultation entails and the potential benefits and harms of testing. A clinical genetic evaluation includes a review of medical and family history, physical examination to identify dysmorphic features, and determination of a differential diagnosis, followed by when appropriate a genetic testing recommendation. A genetic evaluation can help in identifying and differentiating essential autism spectrum disorder from syndromic or complex autism. CMA is the first line of testing for individuals with ASD, developmental delay, and multiple congenital abnormalities and is increasingly used in the genetic evaluation of patients with ASDs. The complexities and uncertainties involved in

CMA and other types of genomic testing can create challenges for health-care providers and for individuals and families undergoing testing. Training and continuing education in genetics are essential for PCPs in order to integrate genetic information into their clinical practice. PCPs have an important role to play in informing families about genetic options, referring appropriately to genetics specialists, and following up on the information revealed by genetic testing. This includes helping families to understand and interpret the findings in ways that are meaningful not only to their medical situation but also to their life contexts, including the life stage of the individual tested and family members, and the potential impact of the specific genetic information on medical, educational, social, and reproductive options. In light of the rapid evolution of genetic technologies and identification of novel variants associated with ASD, follow-up genetic consultations should be considered periodically, in partnership with the medical team and the family.

References

Abdul-Karim, R., Berkman, B. E., Wendler, D., Rid, A., Khan, J., Badgett, T., & Hull, S. C. (2013). Disclosure of incidental findings from next-generation sequencing in pediatric genomic research. *Pediatrics, 131*(3), 564–571.

American College of Medical Genetics, Board of Directors. (2013). Points to consider for informed consent for genome/exome sequencing. *Genetics in Medicine, 15,* 748–749.

Agency for Healthcare Research and Quality (AHRQ). (2014). *Genetic testing for developmental disabilities, intellectual disability and autism spectrum disorders* (Technical Brief). Washington DC: AHRQ Agency for Healthcare Research and Quality, US Department of Health and Human Services.

Ali-Khan, S. E., Daar, A. S., Shuman, C., Ray, P. N., & Scherer, S. W. (2009). Whole genome scanning: Resolving clinical diagnosis and management amidst complex data. *Pediatric Research, 66*(4), 357–363.

American Psychiatric Association. (2013). *Diagnostic and statistical manual of mental disorders* (5th ed.). Washington, DC: American Psychiatric Association.

Amiet, C., Couchon, E., Carr, K., Carayol, J., & Cohen, D. (2014). Are there cultural differences in parental interest in early diagnosis and genetic risk assessment for autism spectrum disorder? *Frontiers in Pediatrics, 2*(32), 1–7.

Aronson, S. J., Clark, E. H., Varugheese, M., Baxter, S., Babb, L. J., & Rehm, H. L. (2012). Communicating new knowledge on previously reported genetic variants. *Genetics in Medicine, 14*(8), 713–719.

Baumanis, L., Evans, J. P., Callanan, N., & Susswein, L. R. (2009). Telephoned BRCA1/2 genetic test results: Prevalence, practice, and patient satisfaction. *Journal of Genetic Counseling, 18*(5), 447–463.

Biesecker, B. B., & Erby, L. (2008). Adaptation to living with a genetic condition or risk: A mini-review. *Clinical Genetics, 74*(5), 401–407.

Carter, M., & Scherer, S. (2013). Autism spectrum disorder in the genetics clinic: A review. *Clinical Genetics, 83*(5), 399–407.

Chen, L., Xu, L., Huang, T., & Dhar, S. U. (2013). Autism genetic testing: A qualitative study of awareness, attitudes, and experiences among parents of children with autism spectrum disorders. *Genetics in Medicine, 15*(4), 274–281.

Christenhusz, G. M., Devriendt, K., & Dierickx, K. (2013). To tell or not to tell? A systematic review of ethical reflections on incidental findings arising in genetics contexts. *European Journal of Human Genetics, 21,* 248–255.

Condit, C. (2010). Public understandings of genetics and health. *Clinical Genetics, 77*(1), 1–9.

Coulter, M. E., Miller, D. T., Harris, D. J., Hawley, P., Picker, J., Roberts, A. E., . . . Irons, M. (2011). Chromosomal microarray testing influences medical management. *Genetics in Medicine, 13*(9), 770–776.

Darilek, S., Ward, P., Pursley, A., Plunkett, K., Furman, P., Magoulas, P., . . . Eng, C. M. (2008). Pre-and postnatal genetic testing by array-comparative genomic hybridization: Genetic counseling perspectives. *Genetics in Medicine, 10*(1), 13–18.

Dawson, G., Rogers, S., Munson, J., Smith, M., Winter, J., Greenson, J., . . . Varley, J. (2010). Randomized, controlled trial of an intervention for toddlers with autism: The early start denver model. *Pediatrics, 125*(1), e17–e23.

Eriksson, M. A., Westerlund, J., Hedvall, Å., Åmark, P., Gillberg, C., & Fernell, E. (2013). Medical conditions affect the outcome of early intervention in preschool children with autism spectrum disorders. *European Child & Adolescent Psychiatry, 22*(1), 23–33.

Fanos, J. H., Gronka, S., Wuu, J., Stanislaw, C., Andersen, P. M., & Benatar, M. (2011). Impact of presymptomatic genetic testing for familial amyotrophic lateral sclerosis. *Genetics in Medicine, 13*(4), 342–348.

Green, R. C., Berg, J. S., Grody, W. W., Kalia, S. S., Korf, B. R., Martin, C. L., . . . Ormond, K. E. (2013). ACMG recommendations for reporting of incidental findings in clinical exome and genome sequencing. *Genetics in Medicine, 15,* 565–574.

Greendale, K., & Pyeritz, R. E. (2001). Empowering primary care health professionals in medical genetics: How soon? How fast? How far? *American Journal of Medical Genetics, 106*(3), 223–232.

Grody, W. W. (2003). Ethical issues raised by genetic testing with oligonucleotide microarrays. *Molecular Biotechnology, 23*(2), 127–138.

Gutmann, A., Wagner, J., Allen, A., Hauser, S., Arras, J., Kucherlapati, R., . . . Sulmasy, D. (2013). *Anticipate and communicate: Ethical management of incidental and secondary findings in the clinical, research and direct-to-consumer contexts.* Washington, DC: US: Presidential Commission for the Study of Bioethical Issues.

Guttmacher, A. E., Porteous, M. E., & McInerney, J. D. (2007). Educating health-care professionals about genetics and genomics. *Nature Reviews Genetics, 8*(2), 151–157.

Han, P. K. J., Klein, W. M. P., & Arora, N. K. (2011). Varieties of uncertainty in health care: A conceptual taxonomy. *Medical Decision Making, 31,* 828–838.

Hayward, D., Eikeseth, S., Gale, C., & Morgan, S. (2009). Assessing progress during treatment for young children with autism receiving intensive behavioural interventions. *Autism: The International Journal of Research and Practice, 13*(6), 613–633.

Heil, K. M., & Schaaf, C. P. (2013). The genetics of autism spectrum disorders—A guide for clinicians. *Current Psychiatry Reports, 15*(1), 1–8.

Kearney, H. M., Thorland, E. C., Brown, K. K., Quintero-Rivera, F., & South, S. T. (2011). American College of Medical Genetics standards and guidelines for interpretation and reporting of postnatal constitutional copy number variants. *Genetics in Medicine, 13*(7), 680–685.

Klitzman, R. L. (2010). Misunderstandings concerning genetics among patients confronting genetic disease. *Journal of Genetic Counseling, 19*(5), 430–446.

Kohane, I. S., Masys, D. R., & Altman, R. B. (2006). The incidentalome: A threat to genomic medicine. *Journal of the American Medical Association, 296*(2), 212–215.

Lenhard, W., Breitenbach, E., Ebert, H., Schindelhauer-Deutscher, H. J., & Henn, W. (2005). Psychological benefit of diagnostic certainty for mothers of children with disabilities: Lessons from Down syndrome. *American Journal of Medical Genetics, 133 A*(2), 170–175.

Lerman, C., Croyle, R. T., Tercyak, K. P., & Hamann, H. (2002). Genetic testing: Psychological aspects and implications. *Journal of Consulting and Clinical Psychology, 70*(3), 784–797.

Lintas, C., & Persico, A. M. (2009). Autistic phenotypes and genetic testing: State-of-the-art for the clinical geneticist. *Journal of Medical Genetics, 46*(1), 1–8.

Lipinski, S. E., Lipinski, M. J., Biesecker, L. G., & Biesecker, B. B. (2006). Uncertainty and perceived personal control among parents of children with rare chromosome conditions: The role of genetic counseling. *American Journal of Medical Genetics, Part C: Seminars in Medical Genetics, 142*(4), 232–240.

Makela, N. L., Birch, P. H., Friedman, J. M., & Marra, C. A. (2009). Parental perceived value of a diagnosis for intellectual disability (ID): A qualitative comparison of families with and without a diagnosis for their child's ID. *American Journal of Medical Genetics. Part A, 149A*(11), 2393–2402.

Mandell, D. S., & Novak, M. (2005). The role of culture in families' treatment decisions for children with autism spectrum disorders. *Mental Retardation and Developmental Disabilities Research Reviews, 11*(2), 110–115.

Manning, M., & Hudgins, L. (2010). Array-based technology and recommendations for utilization in medical genetics practice for detection of chromosomal abnormalities. *Genetics in Medicine, 12*(11), 742–745.

McMahon, W. M., Baty, B. J., & Botkin, J. R. (2006). Genetic counseling and ethical issues for autism. *American Journal of Medical Genetics—Seminars in Medical Genetics, 142 C*(1), 52–57.

Mefford, H., Sharp, A., Baker, C., Itsara, A., Jiang, Z., Buysse, K., . . . Eichler, E. (2008). Recurrent rearrangements of chromosome 1q21.1 and variable pediatric phenotypes. *New England Journal of Medicine, 359*(16), 1685–1699.

Miles, J. H. (2011). Autism spectrum disorders—a genetics review. *Genetics in Medicine, 13*(4), 278–294.

Miles, J. H., McCathren, R. B., Stichter, J., & Shinawi, M. (2010). Autism spectrum disorders. In R. A. Pagon, M. P. Adam, H. H. Ardinger, T. D. Bird, C. R. Dolan, C. T. Fong, . . . K. Stephens (Eds.), *GeneReviews*. Seattle, WA: University of Washington, Seattle.

Miller, D. T., Adam, M. P., Aradhya, S., Biesecker, L. G., Brothman, A. R., Carter, N. P., . . . Epstein, C. J. (2010). Consensus statement: Chromosomal microarray is a first-tier clinical diagnostic test for individuals with developmental disabilities or congenital anomalies. *The American Journal of Human Genetics, 86*(5), 749–764.

Miller, F. A., Hayeems, R. Z., & Bytautas, J. P. (2010). What is a meaningful result? Disclosing the results of genomic research in autism to research participants. *European Journal of Human Genetics, 18*(8), 867–871.

Moeschler, J. B., & Shevell, M. (2006). Clinical genetic evaluation of the child with mental retardation or developmental delays. *Pediatrics, 117*(6), 2304.

Mulchandani, S., Conlin, L. K., Thiel, B., & Spinner, N. B. (2012). Poster. Dealing with the unanticipated: Incidental findings from the lab's perspective. Presented at the: *International Standards on Cytogenetic Array Consortium*. Bethesda, MD. May 21–22.

Narcisa, V., Discenza, M., Vaccari, E., Rosen-Sheidley, B., Hardan, A. Y., & Couchon, E. (2012). Parental interest in a genetic risk assessment test for autism spectrum disorders. *Clinical Pediatrics, 52*(2), 139–146.

Nelson, R., Botkin, J. R., Kodish, E., Levetown, M., Truman, J., Wilfond, B., . . . Schwartz, P. (2001). Ethical issues with genetic testing in pediatrics. *Pediatrics, 107*(6), 1451–1455.

Norbury, C. F., & Sparks, A. (2013). Difference or disorder? Cultural issues in understanding neurodevelopmental disorders. *Developmental Psychology, 49*(1), 45–58.

Pachter, L. M., & Dworkin, P. H. (1997). Maternal expectations about normal child development in 4 cultural groups. *Archives of Pediatrics & Adolescent Medicine, 151*(11), 1144–1150.

Pellicano, E., & Stears, M. (2011). Bridging autism, science and society: Moving toward an ethically informed approach to autism research. *Autism Research, 4*(4), 271–282.

Persico, A. M., & Bourgeron, T. (2006). Searching for ways out of the autism maze: Genetic, epigenetic and environmental clues. *Trends in Neurosciences, 29*(7), 349–358.

Phelan, J. C., Cruz-Rojas, R., & Reiff, M. (2002). Genes and stigma: The connection between perceived genetic etiology and attitudes and beliefs about mental illness. *Psychiatric Rehabilitation Skills, 6*(5), 159–185.

Pinto, D., Marshall, C., Feuk, L., & Scherer, S. W. (2007). Copy-number variation in control population cohorts. *Human Molecular Genetics, 16 Spec No. 2*, R168–73.

Pyeritz, R. E. (2011). The coming explosion in genetic testing–is there a duty to recontact? *The New England Journal of Medicine, 365*(15), 1367–1369.

Redon, R., Ishikawa, S., Fitch, K. R., Feuk, L., Perry, G. H., Andrews, T. D., . . . Hurles, M. E. (2006). Global variation in copy number in the human genome. *Nature, 444*(7118), 444–454.

Reiff, M., Bernhardt, B. A., Mulchandani, S., Soucier, D., Cornell, D., Pyeritz, R. E., & Spinner, N. B. (2012). "What does it mean?": Uncertainties in understanding results of chromosomal microarray testing. *Genetics in Medicine, 14*(2), 250–258.

Reiff, M., Bernhardt, B. A., & Mulchandani, S. (2013a). Genomic variation: What does it mean? *LDI Issue Brief, 18*(4), 1–4.

Reiff, M., Mueller, R., Mulchandani, S., Spinner, N. B., Pyeritz, R. E., & Bernhardt, B. A. (2014a). A qualitative study of healthcare providers' perspectives on the implications of genome-wide testing in pediatric clinical practice. *Journal of Genetic Counseling, 23*(4), 474–488.

Reiff, M., Mulchandani, S., Giarelli, E., & Bernhardt, B. A. (2014b). Perceived value and use of genomic testing among parents of children with autism. *Abstracts, American College of Medical Genetics Annual Meeting,* Nashville, TN.

Reiff, M., Ross, K., Mulchandani, S., Propert, K. J., Pyeritz, R. E., Spinner, N. B., & Bernhardt, B. A. (2013b). Physicians' perspectives on the uncertainties and implications of chromosomal microarray testing of children and families. *Clinical Genetics, 83*(1), 23–30.

Rosenthal, T. C. (2008). The medical home: Growing evidence to support a new approach to primary care. *The Journal of the American Board of Family Medicine, 21*(5), 427–440.

Schaefer, G. B., & Mendelsohn, N. J. (2013). Clinical genetics evaluation in identifying the etiology of autism spectrum disorders: 2013 guideline revisions. *Genetics in Medicine, 15*(5), 399–407.

Schaffer, R., Kuczynski, K., & Skinner, D. (2008). Producing genetic knowledge and citizenship through the internet: Mothers, pediatric genetics, and cybermedicine. *Sociology of Health & Illness, 30*(1), 145–159.

Scherer, S. W., & Dawson, G. (2011). Risk factors for autism: Translating genomic discoveries into diagnostics. *Human Genetics, 130*(1), 123–148.

Selkirk, C. G., McCarthy Veach, P., Lian, F., Schimmenti, L., & Leroy, B. S. (2009). Parents' perceptions of autism spectrum disorder etiology and recurrence risk and effects of their perceptions on family planning: Recommendations for genetic counselors. *Journal of Genetic Counseling, 18*(5), 507–519.

Shea, L., Newschaffer, C. J., Xie, M., Myers, S. M., & Mandell, D. S. (2014). Genetic testing and genetic counseling among medicaid-enrolled children with autism spectrum disorder in 2001 and 2007. *Human Genetics, 133*(1), 111–116.

Shen, Y., Dies, K. A., Holm, I. A., Bridgemohan, C., Sobeih, M. M., Caronna, E. B., . . . Miller, D. T. (2010). Clinical genetic testing for patients with autism spectrum disorders. *Pediatrics, 125*(4), e727–e735.

Silverman, C. (2011). *Understanding autism: Parents, doctors, and the history of a disorder.* New Jersey: Princeton University Press.

Sinclair, J. (2013). Autism network international autreat 2013. Retrieved from http://www.autreat.com/intro.html

Tabor, H. K., & Cho, M. K. (2007). Ethical implications of array comparative genomic hybridization in complex phenotypes: Points to consider in research. *Genetics in Medicine, 9*(9), 626–631.

Timmermans, S., & Buchbinder, M. (2010). Patients-in-waiting: Living between sickness and health in the genomics era. *Journal of Health and Social Behavior, 51*(4), 408–423.

Tluczek, A., Orland, K. M., & Cavanagh, L. (2011). Psychosocial consequences of false-positive newborn screens for cystic fibrosis. *Qualitative Health Research, 21*(2), 174–186.

Veenstra_VanderWeele, J., Christian, S. L., & Cook, E. H. (2004). Autism as a paradigmatic complex genetic disorder. *Annual Review of Genomics and Human Genetics, 5,* 379–405.

Wade, C. H., Wilfond, B. S., & McBride, C. M. (2010). Effects of genetic risk information on children's psychosocial wellbeing: A systematic review of the literature. *Genetics in Medicine, 12*(6), 317–326.

Walsh, P., Elsabbagh, M., Bolton, P., & Singh, I. (2011). In search of biomarkers for autism: Scientific, social and ethical challenges. *Nature Reviews Neuroscience, 12*(10), 603–612.

Warren, Z., McPheeters, M. L., Sathe, N., Foss-Feig, J. H., Glasser, A., & Veenstra_VanderWeele, J. (2011). A systematic review of early intensive intervention for autism spectrum disorders. *Pediatrics, 127*(5), e1303–e1311.

Whitmarsh, I., Davis, A. M., Skinner, D., & Bailey, D. B., Jr. (2007). A place for genetic uncertainty: Parents valuing an unknown in the meaning of disease. *Social Science & Medicine (1982), 65*(6), 1082–1093.

Wilfond, B., & Ross, L. F. (2009). From genetics to genomics: Ethics, policy, and parental decision-making. *Journal of Pediatric Psychology, 34*(6), 639–647.

Wydeven, K. V., Kwan, A., Hardan, A. Y., & Bernstein, J. A. (2012). Underutilization of genetics services for autism: The importance of parental awareness and provider recommendation. *Journal of Genetic Counseling, 21*(6), 803–813.

Yudell, M., Tabor, H. K., Dawson, G., Rossi, J., Newschaffer, C. J., & Working Group in Autism Risk Communication and Ethics. (2013). Priorities for autism spectrum disorder risk communication and ethics. *Autism: The International Journal of Research and Practice, 17*(6), 701–722.

Section 3

ENVIRONMENTS, SERVICES, AND CONTEXT

Chapter 11

EDUCATING NURSES: FACULTY AND CURRICULAR ISSUES

MARCIA R. GARDNER AND MARIE FOLEY

Introduction

Creating improved healthcare experiences and more effective models of health care delivery for individuals on the autism spectrum is a significant, far-reaching, and important goal, but it is certainly one that is quite achievable. Modifications to a variety of healthcare processes and systems, including direct and indirect care, environmental, and regulatory processes and systems, will move us closer to the target. The healthcare provider-education system, as well, requires modification, so that new clinicians enter the healthcare delivery system well-prepared to use best practices in the care of people with autism, regardless of setting, level of care, or role in the health-care system. Various healthcare disciplines, including medicine and nursing, are beginning to explore ways to improve the preparation of clinicians for the care of people on the autism spectrum, their families, and their direct caregivers (Giarelli, Ruttenberg, & Segal, 2012; Major, Peacock, Ruben, Thomas, & Weitzman, 2013). Epidemiological data demonstrates that there is a larger-than-ever population of children on the autism spectrum, and the population continues to grow (Centers for Disease Control and Prevention (CDC), 2014).

Young children and teens will enter the pediatric autism "pipeline" and will be delivered thereafter into the adult health care delivery system. Nurses comprise the largest group of healthcare providers in the United States, and thus are highly likely to encounter, and need to design and implement, appropriate care for this population. This chapter will address preparation and education of nurses to care for people with autism, including issues related to practicing nurses, prelicensure and postlicensure programs of study, clinical experiences, and preparation of nursing faculty to teach their students about this important population.

Preparation of Nurses to Care for People with Autism

In order to ensure that the healthcare workforce is well-prepared for the care of people with autism, both prelicensure education and postlicensure education and continuing education must include content related to autism spectrum disorders (ASD) as well as clinical exposure to people with ASD across the lifespan. In the recent past, practicing nurses have reported less than adequate educational preparation and less than adequate comfort in caring for patients with a variety of developmental and other disabilities (Fisher, Frazer, Hasson, & Orkin, 2007; Singer, 2012; Smeltzer, Avery & Hayner, 2012), and little continuing education focused on people with developmental disabilities has been available for nurses. The nursing workforce must be knowledgeable about ASD and must have guided educational experiences to apply such knowledge and to develop skills to care for this diverse population of people. Unless ASD-related best practices are incorporated as standards in nursing curricula, patients on the autism spectrum may continue to be subject to difficult, unproductive, or distressing health encounters. Without effective preparation of nurses and nursing faculty in the care of people with autism and similar conditions, improved health care experiences and outcomes for this population will be much more difficult to achieve.

Components of Excellent Care across the Lifespan

Excellence in nursing care is related to the interaction of multiple factors including education for practice. The American Association of Colleges of Nursing's (AACN) Quality and Safety Education for Nurses (QSEN) enterprise outlines six components of high quality care: Patient-centered care, teamwork, evidence-based practice, quality improvement, safety, and informatics (AACN, n.d.). QSEN initiatives focus on helping students develop critical thinking and clinical decision-making skills in the context of these components of care, and encourage faculty development to support students' learning about these components (AACN, n.d.). People with ASD need nurses who understand how to tailor care to their individual needs; how to leverage the expertise of a variety of team members to support individualized care; how to understand, interpret, and apply evidence to their care; and how to use both technology and other tools to continually evaluate and improve the care environment and the quality of care.

Excellent nursing care delivery starts with the training of knowledgeable nurse educators. This leads to excellence in patient care across populations and along the lifespan, in primary care, acute, community, and long-term care settings. Nurse clinicians, educators, and administrators will need a deeper understanding of the population of children and *especially* adults on the autism spectrum. People with ASD are unique in their communication patterns, responses to behavioral and environmental stimuli, and social responsiveness. Nurses may find these differences difficult to understand and address. It is imperative that nurses develop the ability to incorporate knowledge of these differences when planning patient care (Fuentes, 2014; Gardner, 2012; Giarelli, Ruttenberg & Segal, 2012). This can begin when nursing faculty have skill in the care of this population along with the most updated information. Best practice care will expand when there is support for nursing faculty to improve their confidence and skills in caring for this population. Preparation of faculty and new nursing clinicians to care for individuals with autism across ages and setting are crucial components for improved quality of care.

There are few educational standards for preparation of nurses for the teaching role, and wide variation in their preparation for teaching. Regulations related to nursing faculty preparation vary by state and are specified by the respective nurse practice acts. Nursing faculty may have been educated as generalists, advanced/specialized clinicians (i.e., as nurse practitioners or clinical specialists), and/or specifically in the nurse educator role (Zungolo, 2004). Faculty in associate degree prelicensure programs may have baccalaureate or higher degrees, although many have masters degrees; faculty in baccalaureate and higher degree programs typically have master's or higher degrees, such as research doctorates (i.e., PhD) or doctor of nursing practice (DNP) credentials, although the advanced degrees vary by the type of academic institution and by rank and role (Roberts & Glod, 2013). Faculty teaching nursing students may or may not have had experiences with individuals on the autism spectrum and may or may not have a full knowledge base related to their care. No published data about nursing faculty preparation or advanced practice educational standards related to ASD were found. Supporting the development of nursing faculty expertise in care of this population will help to promote excellent nursing care.

Issues in Providing Health Care to People with ASD

There are several issues related to providing health care in general to people with ASD which have specific relevance for improving nursing care of this population: (a) Nurses' limited and variable experience with, and access to a patient population; (b) Needs for specialized training for faculty, and continuing education related to health needs of the population; and (c) providers' perceptions of the population. Studies have documented the difficulties that adults with developmental disabilities such as ASD and parents of children with ASD experience when trying to access care that meets their needs or those of their family members. Barriers to effective and appropriate health care in these populations include limited access to clinicians with best practice expertise related to the developmental conditions, poor communication among providers and patients/families, providers' difficulties understanding and managing behavioral challenges, misunderstandings of cultural preferences, lack of appropriate referrals for care, perceptions by clinicians of lower quality of life and negative attitudes toward individuals with disabilities (Carbone, Murphy, Norlin, Azor, Sheng, & Young, 2012; Hegge, 2009; Liptak et al., 2006; Minnes & Steiner, 2009; Smeltzer, Avery, & Hayner, 2012; Walsh et al., 2000; Will, Barnfather, & Leslie, 2013). Attention to the issues of experience with the population, education and continuing education, and perceptions of nurses about people with ASD should help to promote high quality, safe, effective nursing care.

Experiences with and Access to the Patient Population

Nurses will encounter people on the autism spectrum in settings that service broad populations of children and adults, such as primary care and medical specialty clinics or offices, emergency departments and hospital units, outpatient procedure units, nursing homes, and day care centers. Reliable statistics on the size of the adult population of people with ASD are not fully available. Considering that approximately 1% of the population is estimated to have an ASD (CDC, 2015), nurses will have intermittent exposures to patients with this diagnosis, despite its increased prevalence (CDC, 2014). People with ASD require the same health promotion, illness prevention, minor and major acute illness treatment, and support for daily life that are required by other population of patients (Melville, Cooper, Finlayson, Morrison, Allen, Robinson, et al., 2006), but the variability in the severity of their symptoms and related behavioral responses may mean that nurses have to spend more time planning and implementing plans of care for these clients. Their unique communication, behavioral, and environmental response patterns appear complicated and difficult to address, when their healthcare providers do not fully understand their needs.

Investigators have reported that nurses have had limited exposure to and preparation for assessment of health, management of challenging behaviors, interpreting and understanding needs, communicating effectively, supporting patients and their families, and implementing treatments in the population of people with developmental disabilities (Chenowith, Pryor, Jeong, & Hall-Puffin, 2004; Fisher et al., 2007; Melville et al., 2006; Melville et al., 2005; Singer, 2012; Smeltzer, Avery, & Hayner, 2012).

Specialized Training

Certification in developmental disabilities nursing is available, and a few autism-specific continuing education programs and certificates are now offered sporadically across US states. However, the majority of practicing nurses are not specialists in autism or developmental disabilities, nor do most clinicians practice in developmental disabilities settings. At this time, there are no data on the percent of nurses who have acquired advanced preparation in the care of this population.

However, McGonigle and colleagues (2014) discussed the critical need to train certain cohorts of professions such as emergency department staff, including first responders, paramedics, nurses, and others, about ASD and related emergency care. They advocated for the need to address delivery of services in this high-intensity environments involving urgent care, by a variety of providers, both professional and nonprofessional and the speed at which interventions are delivered. They emphasized the uneven access to continuing education about autism, despite availability of a limited amount of emergency-specific training materials from the Autism Society of America.

Providers' Perceptions of the Population

When patients are viewed as difficult to care for, such as when they manifest difficult to understand or disruptive behaviors, overall quality of care and patient safety can be affected; additional nursing time might also be needed to address patient needs (K. Addison & S. Luparell, 2014; Drake, Johnson, Stonez, Martinez, & Massey, 2012). In addition, some research suggests that exposure to individuals perceived to have unpleasant behaviors or attitudes may influence empathy toward patients (Bodner et al., 2015). Thus it is important to understand how nurses and nursing faculty view their interactions with people on the autism spectrum. Studies have documented that nurses and other healthcare providers do perceive caring for individuals with behavioral, communication, cognitive, and social challenges as difficult (Werner, 2011). The extent to which these perceptions influence the delivery of care in the population of people with autism is not known. However, education about the condition and exposure to the population can promote more positive perceptions and perhaps decrease nurses' concerns about the challenges involved in the care of people with ASD. Educational interventions, including clinical education, can help nurses to more effectively communicate with patients with ASD, to understand the wide range of behavioral manifestations associated with sensory processing dysfunction and anxieties in individuals with autism, and to respond more effectively to their health care needs.

A recent study of advanced practice nurses (pediatric and adult nurse practitioners) found self-reported competency in caring for individuals with ASD to be lower than for other chronic conditions; lack of provider education was listed as a significant barrier to effective care (Will, Barnfather, & Lesley, 2013). Strunk's (2009) study of school nurses' knowledge related to ASD demonstrated lower knowledge of the behavioral, communication, and safety components of ASD care than of medication-related and community resource components. In addition, negative attitudes of nurses toward people with the disruptive behaviors and communication deficits that can be associated with ASD, have been reported (Fisher, Frazer, Hasson, & Orkin, 2007; Walsh, 2000). Such attitudes may be due to misunderstanding, lack of knowledge and experiences, or both and may be barriers to the delivery of effective care.

Nursing Education

Considering the issues described above, attention needs to turn toward integration of best practices in ASD care into nursing curricula. There is a clear need to ensure that graduates of nursing education programs at all levels have exposure to the newest information about autism and have experiences with patients with autism across the lifespan.

Nurse Training in ASD

Surveys of nurses in practice have found that they recall having had limited information and minimal clinical contact with individuals with intellectual and developmental disabilities during their nursing education (Walsh, Hammerman, Josephson, & Krupka, 2000). A recent national survey was conducted with nursing faculty who were teaching primarily in associate and baccalaureate degree nursing programs (Gardner, Suplee & Jerome-D'Emilia, 2016). In this survey, a large majority of the 295 nursing faculty who responded to the survey recalled having less than two hours of prelicensure or postlicensure formal curricular content on ASDs. The vast majority had not had any clinical experiences with individuals on the autism spectrum in prelicensure or post-licensure formal education, and more than 70% reported having had no continuing education units or hours specific to ASDs in the past five years. The faculty reported low knowledge about ASD and about healthcare management issues related to ASD, and low confidence in their abilities to manage patients or clients with ASD, regardless of their clinical specialties or levels of education. Subjects reported three common and problematic deficits, in the nursing education programs in which they were currently teaching. *First,* ASD-specific content was addressed in the context of children, but rarely adults. *Second,* there were few to no planned clinical experiences with individuals or groups on the autism spectrum. *Third,* for the faculty who were aware of ASD content in their program curricula, ASD content in the entire curriculum accounted for approximately two hours or less (Gardner et al., 2016). These data reflect two likely scenarios. *First,* that nursing faculty are not well-versed in best-practices for the nursing care of people with autism. *Second,* that current nursing program curricula include limited information about and little clinical exposure to patients with autism. Recent graduates of nursing programs, regardless of level, are likely not adequately prepared to care for this population.

There is little other information in the literature about nursing faculty preparedness for teaching about autism. Smeltzer and colleagues (2005), however, demonstrated that faculty members' lack of comfort and expertise on the care of people with any kind of disability supports the need to increase and integrate such content in nursing curricula. It is likely that this phenomenon extends to ASDs, as well. Similar to other healthcare educators, nursing faculty need further training in the care of people with ASDs in order to develop appropriate knowledge and skills, use best practices, and feel comfortable and confident in the care of this population. Otherwise, how can they effectively support their students in developing these competencies?

Generalist Curriculum Issues

Considering the prevalence of ASD and its lifespan impact on individuals, families, and on society, it is crucial that ASD content and guided clinical experiences are appropriately incorporated into nursing curricula, and are not limited only to the pediatric context. Organizations including the American Association of Colleges of Nursing (AACN) have previously taken a leading role to ensure appropriate integration of selected specialized nursing content into nursing curricula and nursing practice, by drawing together experts across practice and education settings in specialized consortia (AACN, 2015). Integration of end-of-life care and care of older adults in nursing curricula are supported through the End of Life Nursing Education Consortium

(ELNEC) and Geriatric Nursing Education Consortium (GNEC) initiatives, which, in addition to communicating standards for practice, also provide curricular guidance related to the minimal competencies required for basic and advanced nursing practice, and help to support development of faculty expertise (AACN, 2015). Integration of genetics knowledge for nursing practice in nursing curricula has been addressed through development of *Essentials of Genetic and Genomic Nursing: Competencies, Curricula Guidelines and Outcome Indicators* (American Nurses Association, 2009). Such guidance regarding practice standards and related curricula for nursing care of people on the autism spectrum, at the generalist, specialist, and advanced practice nursing levels, are not yet available. We challenge our colleagues to join us to establish an autism education consortium along the lines of ELNEC and GNEC. Such an initiative would establish a framework for the preparation of clinicians with the requisite knowledge and skills to care for and teach about this population. However, some general guidance regarding the minimal competencies for care of individuals with ASD to be incorporated into prelicensure and advanced nursing education can be extrapolated from the literature.

Cervasio (2014) suggested a developmental disabilities pediatric curriculum for undergraduate education. She recommended incorporating 11 core competencies (see Box 11.1). These competencies can provide a foundation for understanding and teaching about developmental disabilities (DD) in general, in the context of pediatrics. These competencies may be revised and adapted to develop curricula specific to the care of children and adults with ASD. Pharmacotherapy, genetics/genomics, and family dynamics related to care of people on the autism spectrum are other areas of concern to be addressed in nursing curricula both at the undergraduate and graduate levels.

More generally, Willis (2011) identified in the Aspirational Standards of Developmental Disabilities Nursing Practice, eleven essential components of specialty practice in DD nursing, not restricted to setting or age. They are intended for specialty practice. These standards identify the domains for competencies in care of people with developmental disabilities but are applicable to teaching care of people with ASD. Table 11.1 illustrates how these competencies can be translated in the context of the ASD population (see Table 11.1).

Masterson, Dimitriou, Turko, and McPartland (2014) suggested that all undergraduates who are training to work directly with individuals with ASD as teachers or therapists should be prepared using a standardized, uniform curriculum. They argued that, regardless of the college setting, all graduates should develop a similar knowledge base and set of competencies for practice with individuals on the autism spectrum. While their recommendations

---

Box 11.1. Core Competencies to Incorporate with and Guide Autism-Specific Curricula for Undergraduate Nursing Education

- Communication
- Critical thinking
- Mobility skills
- Activities of daily living
- Sensory integration
- Behavior recognition and management
- Safety and cultural awareness
- Education and collaboration with other healthcare providers and staff
- Community resources
- Interpersonal skills
- Competency evaluation

Source: Cervasio, K. (2014). Inclusion of developmental disability nursing content into undergraduate nursing education: A renewed call for pediatric curricula reform. *International Journal of Nursing in Intellectual and Developmental Disabilities, 6*(1). http://ddna.org/vol6_issue1_article01

---

are focused on specialists' education, not on preparing health professionals, the argument that professionals who are likely to interface with individuals on the autism spectrum should develop a standardized knowledge base and set of competencies is important and valid. General curriculum standards for the incorporation of important concepts into nursing curricula are presented in Box 11.2.

Curricular Recommendations

The role of the nurse (i.e., generalist versus specialty practice, basic versus advanced practice, primary versus acute care) and the related standards of practice should determine the specific content, as well as the level of and expectations for clinical experiences for students. The curricular structure of the educational program would determine how the standards would be incorporated into courses and clinical experiences. Content and guided clinical experiences, along with the development of faculty expertise to support students are, however, both assumed and considered essential for effective preparation of new clinicians. Clinical experiences may be particularly im-

Table 11.1
ELEVEN ESSENTIAL COMPONENTS OF SPECIALTY PRACTICE*

Competency	Translation to Curriculum Element in Nursing of ASD
Therapeutic relationship establishment	Establish effective nurse-patient-family relationships in the context of individual patient communication dynamics
Interdisciplinary team collaboration	Collaborate with the interdisciplinary ASD care team
	Use effective interprofessional communication
Data collection	Collect relevant data for individualized care planning based on understanding of common manifestations of ASD
Identification of health care needs	Appraise health needs and environmental modification needs
Planning	Plan care to meet general and autism-specific health care needs
Implementation	Implement an individualized plan of care based on uniqueness of each patient with ASD
Evaluation	Evaluate care, integrating perspectives of patient, family, and caregivers
Quality assurance	Measure quality and safety indicators in the context of ASD
Advocate role	Advocate to meet unique needs of individuals with ASD in clinical settings and community
Educator role	Educate care providers, community members, and school staff, and professional colleagues about best practices
	Use best practices to educate patients with ASD, family members, and their caregivers
Continued competency	Maintain current knowledge of autism and related best nursing care practices

*Refer to Willis (2011) for additional information

Box 11.2. Proposed ASD-Specific Curriculum Standards for Nursing Education: Generalist and Advanced Practice

- Epidemiology and genetics of autism spectrum disorder (ASD)
- Definitions and diagnostic criteria, core features, and implications for health care
- Interdisciplinary team collaboration and nursing roles in multiple settings
- Family and cultural considerations and concerns
- Screening and diagnostic processes in children and adults
- Communication
- Sensory dysregulation
- Manifestations, interpretation, and management in health, school, and home settings
- Environmental implications and modifications
- Pharmacological therapy
- Health promotion and health surveillance in adults and children with ASD
- Common health problems in adults and children with ASD
- Treatments: evidence-based versus unproven
- Transitions from pediatric to adult models of health care
- Community supports and social integration
- Aging adults with ASD
- Ethical, regulatory, and legal considerations
- Required/guided pediatric clinical experiences
- Required/guided adult clinical experiences

---

portant because exposure to individuals with developmental disabilities has been associated with more positive attitudes about this population (Barr & Brachitta, 2008; Tracy & Iacona, 2008). It is also important to note that issues, contents, and clinical experiences related to adults with ASD, and especially aging adults with ASD, must also be part of the plan that addresses health needs across the lifespan.

In general, prelicensure and advanced practice nursing education about the care of individuals with autism can be improved. Gaps clearly exist in the knowledge and clinical expertise of nurses in current practice, reflected in the research on experiences of patients with autism, and parents of children with autism. In addition, despite significantly increased research attention to the prevalence, incidence, and causation of ASDs, screening and diagnostic methods and growing attention to intervention over the past decade or more, preparation of nurses to care for this population is still not adequate. In order to address this gap at the level of nursing education, regardless of the level of the educational program, nursing faculty will also need additional education, training, and clinical resources to best support their students' learning. Guidelines from other specialties, including geriatrics, genetics, and developmental disabilities provide some general direction for the targeted integration of autism content into prelicensure and graduate nursing education.

School Nurses

Of the estimated 1 in 68 children in the United States who were eight years old in 2010 are on the autism spectrum (Centers for Disease Control and Prevention, 2014), approximately 94% are enrolled in a public school setting (U.S. Department of Education, National Center for Education Statistics, 2013). Thus, the school nurse is the healthcare provider who will have the most daily interaction with children diagnosed with ASD from preschool (3–4 years) through age 21 and their families. School nurses are involved in assessment, consultation, planning, and collaboration with school staff and families to provide interventions and assist with providing a team approach when educating and ensuring a healthy school environment for children diagnosed with ASD. Furthermore, the school nurse is involved in health assessment and screening and may be the first person to identify subtle physiologic changes needing referral for further evaluation and/or change in treatment regime.

Management of children with ASD can present specific challenges for school nurses particularly related to communication, sensory dysfunction, behavior, safety and health concerns. Many children diagnosed with ASD have co-occurring conditions including learning disabilities, psychiatric disorders, and epilepsy (Klaiman, Fernandez-Carriba, Hall, & Saulnier, 2014), which also require management by school nurses in the school setting. Since some children with ASD may experience problems with language and communication, as well as hypersensitivity to sensory stimuli (American Psychiatric Association, 2013), it can be especially challenging for a school nurse to assess a child for an impending illness, change in behavior, or other healthcare concern. Referring to a set of best practices for assessment of a student with ASD will facilitate this procedure.

In a busy nurse's office, there may be a flurry of activities, lights, and noise which could be problematic for students who are hypersensitive to sensory stimuli. School nurses need to be cognizant of these issues when assessing and caring for the student with ASD and attend to decreasing environmental stimuli, speaking in a slow and soothing tone, and limiting the number of individuals in the health office. Being familiar with individual students, their sensitivities, normal behaviors, and triggers will assist the school nurse with screening, assessment, and provision of care for the student with ASD. Parents/guardians are usually the most familiar with the special needs of the child and the best able to distinguish "typical" behavior (i.e., normal for their child) from abnormal behavior that is precipitated by physical or emotional distress (Solodiuk, 2013)

The Individuals with Disabilities Education Improvement Act (2004) mandates that students with disabilities, including those with ASD, be educated without additional cost in a public school, in the least restrictive environment. The school nurse, as a key member of the interprofessional education team, can support parents as they negotiate the educational system to ensure an appropriate education for their child. The school nurse can provide information and access to resources including developmental and educational assessment and support parental collaboration in creating appropriate multidisciplinary interventions. To best serve their student population, school nurses need to be knowledgeable about ASD including screening, diagnosis, treatment, and intervention strategies which are helpful to the student, staff, and family.

Siblings and Families of Children with ASD

School nurses care for the child with ASD and also interact with and care for siblings who may be in the school system. Furthermore, the school nurse is the individual in the school setting parents often seek for guidance related to health care and educational concerns for their children. Therefore, the school nurse has a pivotal role in caring for not only the child with ASD, but also to assess family coping of siblings and parental caregivers. The school nurse can assist with guiding family members to understand and implement coping mechanisms and provide resources and referrals for needed services for family functioning and management (Kenny & Corkin, 2011).

School Nurse Curricula

While school nurses report having an adequate understanding of the disorder, including symptoms and medication management, they have reported inadequate knowledge related to communication, behavioral management, and safety in the school setting (Strunk, 2009). Therefore, it is imperative that school nursing curricula include topics related to content areas to assist school nurses to provide care to and assist the student with ASD to succeed in school and in future academic and social development.

In the US, school nursing services are state-regulated; therefore, educational preparation of school nurses varies by state. Many states have specific certification educational requirements such as specific content beyond licensure related to the role, scope, and practice of the school nurse, and specific state and federal laws governing school nursing practice. Some US states require courses either at the bachelor's or master's level which incorporate content in physical assessment of the school-age child including screening and health promotion, content in health education along with a supervised teaching experience, courses in special education including learning disabilities; while other states have no requirements beyond licensure.

Likewise, educational requirements for school nurses vary from state to state. For example, in Alabama, Arkansas, and Florida, licensure as a nurse either as a licensed practical nurse or a registered nurse is sufficient. In Illinois, New Jersey, and California, an RN with a bachelor's degree (not necessarily in nursing) is required plus additional courses beyond the bachelor's degree (Baccalaureate- or Master's-level courses) are required. In Massachusetts, Colorado, Delaware, and Pennsylvania, a BSN plus additional credits are required. Many states require a supervised practicum in school nursing and others do not. For a list of school nurse requirements by state, please see the following website: http://www.nasbe.org/healthy_schools/hs/bytopics.php?topicid=2130, or refer to individual state school nurse consultants.

Since school nursing is defined as a specialized practice (American Nurses Association [ANA] & National Association of School Nurses [NASN], 2011), it is the position of NASN (2012) that every child deserves a school nurse who has a baccalaureate degree in nursing from an accredited college or university and is licensed as a registered nurse through the State Board of Nursing. These requirements constitute minimal preparation needed to practice at the entry level of school nursing (American Nurses Association & National Association of School Nurses, 2011). Additionally, NASN supports state and national school nurse certification. Therefore, one should expect that certification requirements include specialty courses related to school nursing practice including a clinical practicum with exposure to students with special needs. Specific content related to the care and support of students with chronic conditions, including ASD, should be included in all school nurse certification programs. This content should not only include information related to prevalence, etiology, screening, diagnoses, and treatment of ASD, but it should also include content related to the role of the school nurse in the management of the student with ASD in the school setting.

CONTENT AREAS MOST USEFUL FOR NURSING CARE OF ASD. Content must focus on the understanding that each child presents differently and can be located anywhere on the spectrum of the disorder. Therefore, the need for a comprehensive evaluation of the student's symptoms and their severity, strengths, weaknesses as well as co-occurring conditions is important (Close, Lee, Kaufmann, & Zimmerman, 2012). As each student exhibits individual behaviors and symptoms, no single treatment for ASD is effective for all students. Content should stress that interventions must be individualized using multiple modalities and including all necessary members of the educational and healthcare team is important. The team may comprise some or all of the professions including teacher, nurse, occupational therapist, physical therapist, psychologist, social worker, special education teacher, pharmacist, speech therapist, and neurologist. A nurse might be the ideal case manager for the child's comprehensive care team.

Introduction of principles of applied behavioral analysis (ABA) (Warren et al., 2011) into school nurse education will provide the nurse with useful tools to manage behavior in the school setting. ABA can be effectively used in preparation for anticipated assessments and treatments to minimize or control behaviors that might become barriers to care.

In addition, content related to medication management is important for school nurse education. Students with ASD are often prescribed psychotropic medications both alone and in combination. These medications are not only a combination of conventional medications, but can include alternative medications as well. Students with co-occurring conditions such as epilepsy, bipolar disorder, and/or ADHD (Spencer et al., 2013) as well as those who exhibit challenging behaviors such as aggression, inattention, hyperactivity, and irritability (Granich, 2014) are typically those on multiple medications. Therefore, school nurses need course content related to types of medications, both conventional and alternative that students may be taking as well as possible interactions and side effects of these medications. The need to monitor students for medication effectiveness and to educate parents, school staff, and members of the interdisciplinary team about changes in behavior or side effects is necessary. To provide optimal care for students with ASD related to polypharmacy, the school nurse must serve as the case manager for the student's care and keep all members of the team including the student's primary care provider aware of any side effects or behavior changes.

Some side effects of the psychotropic medications include anorexia and/or gastric upset. Therefore, school nurses also need content on the importance of nutritional assessment and management. Medication side effects related to anorexia, as well as sensory processing dysfunction which can result in aversion to specific textures, can lead to the need for nutritional referrals and interventions. School nurse education related to safety concerns associated with visual or auditory impairment as well as the well-publicized concern with wandering outside of the school environment is necessary. Some students with ASD may exhibit self-mutilating behaviors; therefore, inclusion of evidence-based activities to assist the student to refrain from self-injury is important.

The school nurse in the high school can be a resource to students as they transition out of the public school setting, especially for those who are higher functioning. This period can be very difficult for the student and family as they struggle with the overlapping issues of emerging adulthood, changing social expectations, and the core characteristics of ASD. Providing support is imperative. Encouraging school nurses to be aware of local and national resources available to families and how to access those resources will be appreciated by students and their families.

PRACTICAL EXPERIENCE. It is recommended by the authors that a practicum experience be included in all school nurse certification programs. It would be helpful for school nurse students to have some time during their practicum in a special school for students with ASD as well as other behavioral and cognitive difficulties. While most students are not educated in these types of environments, experience observing how school nurses manage students with ASD would be helpful to the school nurse student.

As with all nursing practice, encouraging school nurses to be lifelong learners and stay abreast of the most current evidence-based information related to the care and support of students and families with ASD is the most important concept to be incorporated into school nursing education. As the population of students with ASD continues to grow, opportunities to better educate school nurses to care for students with ASD will improve educational, social, and behavioral outcomes for students.

Educational Effectiveness and Innovation

Limited information is available for critical review about the general value of specialized training on nursing care of patients with ASD. Moreover, little is known about how effectively such increased knowledge about and clinical practice with patients with ASD translates into improved outcomes for this population (Cervasio, 2014; Gardner, 2012). We have some evidence that knowledge leads to changes in practice, and it is reasonable to assume that improving knowledge of best practices will lead to better care for the population.

Swanson and colleagues (2014) reported that training of a small group of primary care pediatricians regarding screening for ASD resulted in an 85% increase in children identified as at-risk. Giarelli, Ruttenberg, and Segal (2012) reported that a continuing education program for nurses resulted in sharing of information about ASD with colleagues and employers, and in incorporation into their practice in a large majority of the participants. A modular, case-based educational model to train pediatric residents resulted in significantly improved knowledge of ASD and significant increase in self-reported competence to manage patients with ASD. Virtual (computer-based) training for care of people with developmental disabilities in general has been effective in improving attitudes toward disabled individuals and increasing knowledge of developmental disabilities and related health problems (Boyd et al., 2008; Sanders, Kleinert, Free, Slusher, Clevenger, & Boyd, 2007; Sanders, Kleinert, Free, King, Slusher, & Boyd, 2008).

The increasing availability of high fidelity simulation and standardized patient (human) simulation may offer additional opportunities for clinicians, nursing faculty, and students to use knowledge and develop improved clinical and interpersonal skills for the care of individuals with ASD and their families. Simulation scenarios which require application of knowledge and skills related to ASD can be easily developed and offered across the curriculum. Standardized patient-care scenarios can portray individuals on the autism spectrum and offers learners opportunities to practice, make mistakes, and correct them prior to caring for patients. Students might screen the standardized patients for ASD, to interact with individuals on the autism spectrum in primary and acute care settings, to address family concerns, to participate in interdisciplinary team discussions, all in the safe educational environment of the simulation laboratory. The advantages of simulation training, compared to other learning modalities, include opportunities for interaction and use of clinical judgment, reviewing recorded scenarios and critiquing self and others, debriefing and guided reflection, some of which may not be available in the "real world" clinical experience (Ebersold & Tschannen, 2013).

Conclusion

The large and growing population of individuals with ASD creates challenges for nurses and other healthcare providers. ASD is a lifelong condition with a unique set of core features which affect interaction and responses to care including impaired communication, impaired socialization, restricted/repetitive behavioral repertoire, and sensory processing difficulties. In the past, families of children with developmental disabilities such as autism have had less than optimal healthcare experiences for their children. Adults with developmental disabilities have overall poorer health, have less access to appropriate health care, and receive fewer illness prevention and health promotion interventions than others (Havercamp, Scandlin, & Roth, 2004; Liptak et al., 2005; Melvill et al., 2005; Minnes & Steiner, 2009). Much more research into healthcare experiences and outcomes in adult population of people with ASD is needed, but it is clear that health care of people of all ages on the autism spectrum can be improved on many fronts.

Nurses, regardless of level of practice and roles, will encounter people with autism in all healthcare settings across the lifespan and will be challenged to innovate with their individual patients, to create and test new models of care, and to use the best evidence-based practices currently available for care of individuals with ASD. Therefore, new clinicians need to be prepared to care for this population, and should be exposed to epidemiological, genetic, family, pharmacological, sensory, environmental, communication, and behavioral concepts related to ASD, to screening and management, to the interdisciplinary team approach, and to ethical, legal, and regulatory issues related to the care of people with ASD during their educational preparation. If available, nurses should seek continuing education and certification in the nursing care of ASD. One such program is offered at Drexel University for nurses who have obtained their baccalaureate degree (Post-Baccalaureate Certificate in Nursing of ASD, 2015).

Students should explore community and other resources available to individuals on the autism spectrum and their families and will benefit from clinical experiences with people of all ages who have ASD, guided by faculty with expertise in the care of this population. Innovative educational modalities such as case-based and simulation-based scenarios will help students translate knowledge to clinical practice. These components of care apply to nurses being prepared at the generalist, prelicensure, as well as at the specialist, advanced practice levels. Special attention to the preparation of school nurses as both care providers and as consultants to school staff is extremely important, as school nurses are the healthcare providers who are most likely to interact with, and care for, children and teens with ASD on an ongoing basis.

References

Addison, K., & Luparell, S. (2014). Rural nurses' perception of disruptive behaviors and clinical outcomes. *Online Journal of Rural Nursing and Health Care, 14*(1), 66–82. Retrieved from http://eds.b.ebscohost.com/eds/pdfviewer/pdfviewer ?sid=7dfcfe17-ea51-4810-81eb-5cd0cf0a9b94%40sessionmgr114&vid=5&hid=10

American Association of Colleges of Nursing. (2015). *End of life nursing education consortium.* Retrieved from http://www.aacn.nche.edu/elnec

American Association of Colleges of Nursing. (2015). *GNEC project.* Retrieved from http://www.aacn.nche.edu/geriatric-nursing/gnec

American Association of Colleges of Nursing (n.d). *Quality and Safety Education for Nurses.* Retrieved from http://www.aacn.nche.edu/qsen/home

American Nurses Association (ANA) and National Association of School Nurses (NASN). (2011). *School nursing: Scope and standards of practice* (2nd ed.). Silver Spring, MD: Nursebooks.org.

American Psychiatric Association. (2013). *Diagnostic and statistical manual of mental disorders* (5th ed.): DSM-5. Arlington, VA: American Psychiatric Association.

Bodner, E., Cohen-Fridel, S., Mashiah, M., Segal, M., Grinshpoon, A., Fischel, T., & Iancu, I. (2015). The attitudes of psychiatric hospital staff toward hospitalization and treatment of patients with borderline personality disorder. *BMC Psychiatry, 15*(2). Retrieved from http://www.biomedcentral.com/1471-244X/15/2

Boyd, S. E., Sanders, C. L., Kleinert, S. L., Huff, M. B., Lock, S., Johnson, S., . . . Clark, T. L. (2008). Virtual patient training to improve reproductive health care for women with intellectual disabilities. *Journal of Midwifery and Women's Health, 53*(5), 453–460.

Carbone, P. S., Murphy, N. A., Norlin, C., Azmor, V., Sheng, X., & Young, P. C. (2013). Parent and pediatrician perspectives regarding the primary care of children with autism spectrum disorder. *Journal of Autism & Developmental Disorders, 43,* 964–972.

Centers for Disease Control. (2015). *Autism spectrum disorders: Data & statistics.* Retrieved from http://www.cdc.gov/ncbddd/autism/data.html

Centers for Disease Control and Prevention. (2014). Prevalence of autism spectrum disorders–Autism and Developmental Disabilities Monitoring Network, 11 sites, United States, 2010. *MMWR Surveillance Summary, 63*(2), 1–22.

Cervasio, K. (2014). Inclusion of developmental disability nursing content into undergraduate nursing education: A renewed call for pediatric curricula reform. *International Journal of Nursing in Intellectual and Developmental Disabilities, 6*(1). Retrieved from http://ddna.org/vol6_issue1_article01

Chenowith, L., Pryor, J., Jeong, Y., & Hall-Puffin, L. (2004). Disability specific preparation programme plays an important role in shaping students' attitudes toward disablement and patients with disabilities. *Learning in Health and Social Care, 3*(2), 83–91.

Close, H. A., Lee, L. Kaurmann, C., & Zimmerman, A. (2012). Co-occurring conditions and change in diagnosis in autism spectrum disorders. *Pediatrics, 129*(2), e305–e316.

Drake, J., Johnson, N., Stonek, A. V., Martinez, D. M., & Massey, M. (2012). Evaluation of a coping kit for children with challenging behaviors in a pediatric hospital. *Pediatric Nursing, 38*(4), 215–221.

Ebersold, M., & Tschannen, D. (2013). Simulation in nursing practice: The impact on patient care. *Online Journal of Issues in Nursing, 18*(2). Retrieved from http: //nurs-

ingworld.org/MainMenuCategories/ANAMarketplace/ANAPeriodicals/OJIN
/TableofContents/Vol-18-2013/No2-May-2013/Simulation-in-Nursing-
Practice.html

Fisher, K., Frazer, C., Hasson, C., & Orkin, F. (2007). A qualitative study of emergency room nurses' perceptions and experiences of caring for individuals with
intellectual disabilities in the United States. *International Journal of Nursing in
Intellectual and Developmental Disabilities.* Retrieved from http://ddna.org
/publications/journal/vol-3-issue-1-article-1/

Fuentes, J. (2014). Ten tips to support me. *Journal of the American Academy of Child and
Adolescent Psychiatry, 53*(11), 1145–1146.

Gardner, M. R. (2012). Preparing nurses to care for people with developmental disabilities: Perspectives on integrating developmental disabilities concepts and
experiences into nursing education. *Nursing Clinics of North America, 47*(4),
517–527.

Gardner, M. R., Suplee, P., & Jerome-D'Emilia, B. (2016). Survey of nursing faculty
preparation for teaching about autism spectrum disorders. *Nurse Educator, 41*(4).

Giarelli, E., Ruttenberg, J., & Segal, A. (2012). Continuing education for nurses in the
clinical management of autism spectrum disorders: Results of a pilot evaluation.
Journal of Continuing Education in Nursing, 43(4), 169–176.

Granich, J., Hunt, A., Ravine, D., Wray, J., & Whitehouse, A. J. O. Complementary
and alternative medication among children with autism is not associated with
the severity of core symptoms. *Journal of Autism, 1*(4). Retrieved from http:
//www.hoajonline.com/journals/pdf/2054-992X-1-4.pdf

Havercamp, S. M., Scandlin, D., & Roth, M. (2004). Health disparities among adults
with developmental disabilities, adults with other disabilities and adults not
reporting disability in North Carolina. *Public Health Reports, 119,* 419–426.

Klaiman, C., Fernandez-Carriba, S., Hall, C., & Saulnier, C. (2014). Assessment of
autism across the lifespan: A way forward. *Current Developmental Disorders
Reports, 1*–9.

Kenny, J., & Corkin, D. (2011). The challenges of caring for an exceptional child.
Learning Disability Practice, 14(9), 14–18.

Liptak, G. S., Orlando, M., Yingling, J. T., Thereur-Kaufman, K. L., Malay, D. P.,
Tomkins, L. A., & Flynn, J. R. (2006). Satisfaction with primary health care
received by families of children with developmental disabilities. *Journal of
Pediatric Health Care, 20*(4), 245–252.

Major, N. E., Peacock, G., Ruben, W., Thomas, J., & Weitzman, C. C. (2013). Autism
training in pediatric residency: Evaluation of a case-based curriculum. *Journal of
Autism and Developmental Disorders, 43,* 1171–1177.

Melville, C., Cooper, S. A., Morrison, J., Finlayson, J., Allen, L., Robinson, N.,
Burns, E., & Martin, G. (2006). The outcomes of an intervention study to reduce
the barriers experienced by people with intellectual disabilities accessing primary health care services. *Journal of Intellectual Disability Research, 50,* 11–17.

Melville, C. Finlayson, J., Cooper, S. A., Allen, L., Robinson, N., Burns, E., Martin,
G., & Morrison, J. (2005). Enhancing primary care health services for adults with
intellectual disabilities. *Journal of Intellectual Disabilities Research, 49,* 190–198.

Minnes, P., & Steiner, K., (2009). Parent views on enhancing the quality of healthcare for their children with fragile X syndrome, autism or Down syndrome. *Child Healthcare and Development, 35*(2), 250–256.

National Association of School Nurses. (2012). *Position statement: Education, licensure, and certification of school nurses.* Retrieved from http://www.nasn.org/Policy Advocacy/PositionPapersandReports.

Post-Baccalaureate Certificate in Nursing of ASD. (2015). *Integrated nursing care of autism spectrum disorder.* Retrieved from http://www.drexel.edu/cnhp/academics /post-baccalaureate/Certificate-PB-Integrated-Nursing-Care-of-Autism-Spectrum -Disorder/

Roberts, S. J., & Glod, C. (2013). Faculty roles: Dilemmas for the future of nursing education. *Nursing Forum, 48*(2), 99–105.

Sanders, C. L., Kleinert, H. L., Free, T., King, P., Slusher, I., & Boyd, S. (2008). Developmental disabilities: Improving competence in care using virtual patients. *Journal of Nursing Education, 47*(2), 66–73.

Sanders, C. L., Kleinert, H. L., Free, T., Slusher, I., Clevenger, K., & Boyd, S. (2007). Caring for children with intellectual and developmental disabilities: Virtual patient instruction improves students' knowledge and comfort level. *Journal of Pediatric Nursing, 22*(6), 457–465

Singer, B. (2012). Perceptions of school nurses in the care of students with disabilities. *Journal of School Nursing, 29*(5), 329–336.

Smeltzer, S. C., Avery, C., & Haynor, P. (2012). Interactions of people with disabilities and nursing staff during hospitalization. *American Journal of Nursing, 112*(4), 30–37.

Soloduik, J. C. (2013). Parent described pain response in nonverbal children with intellectual disability. *International Journal of Nursing Studies, 50*(8), 1033–1044.

Spencer, D., Marshall, J., Post, B., Kulakodlu, M., Newschaffer, C., Dennen, T., Azocar, F., & Jain, A. (2013). Psychotropic medication use and polypharmacy in children with autism spectrum disorders. *Pediatrics, 132*(5), 833–840.

Strunk, J. A. (2009). School nurses' knowledge of autism spectrum disorders. *Journal of School Nursing, 25*(6), 445–452.

Swanson, A. R., Warren, Z. E., Stone, W. L., Vehorn, A. C., Dohrman, E., & Humberd, Q. (2014). The diagnosis of autism in community pediatric settings: Does advanced training facilitate practice change? *Autism, 18*(5), 561–565.

U.S. Department of Education, National Center for Education Statistics. (2013). *Digest of Education Statistics, 2012 (NCES 2014-015), 6*(4), 333–342.

Warren, Z., McPheeters, M. L., Sathe, N., Foss-Feig, J., Glasser, A., & Veenstra-VanderWeele, J. (2011). A systematic review of early intensive intervention for autism spectrum disorders. *Pediatrics, 127*(5), e1303–e1311.

Walsh, K. K., Hammerman, S., Josephson, F., & Krupka, P. (2000). Caring for people with developmental disabilities: Survey of nurses about their education and experience. *Mental Retardation, 38*(1), 33–41.

Will, D., Barnfather, J., & Lesley, M. (2013). Self- perceived autism competency of primary care nurse practitioners. *Journal for Nurse Practitioners, 9*(6), 350–355.

Willis, M.A. (2011). *Aspirational standards of developmental disabilities nursing practice.* Texas: Developmental Disabilities Nursing Association.

Zungolo, E. (2004). Faculty preparation: Is clinical specialization a benefit or a deterrent to quality nursing education? *Journal of Continuing Education in Nursing, 35*(1), 19–23.

Chapter 12

EMERGENCY MEDICINE
AND IMPROVING SERVICES

ROMY NOCERA

Introduction

People with autism spectrum disorder (ASD) use emergency medicine services significantly more often than their neurotypical counterparts. Given the core characteristics and sensory adversities inherent to ASD, the chaotic emergency department (ED) environment may prove difficult for these patients, their caregivers, and medical professionals, resulting in fear, frustration, and substandard care. The purposes of this chapter are to present the experiences of ASD patients in the ED, describe the influence of ASD-related traits in this context, examine ways of improving emergency care to these individuals, and discuss approaches to conducting research concerning this issue.

Medical Needs Precipitating ED Use by Persons with ASD

Adults with ASD report over twice the odds of using the ED in a given year compared with adults who are neurotypical (Nicolaidis et al., 2013), and children with ASD seek emergency care with far greater frequency than children not on the spectrum (Gurney, McPheeters, & Davis, 2006). Typical treatments given to these individuals can result in adverse events that need prompt medical attention (Venkat, Jauch, Russell, Crist, & Farrell, 2012), and numerous other causes and conditions leading to ED use have been identified.

Psychiatric Conditions Treated in the ED

Urban EDs have a high percentage of patients admitted with psychiatric emergencies. Psychiatric conditions are highly prevalent in ASD. Anxiety and mood disorders are common, along with attention deficit disorder/ attention deficit hyperactivity disorder (ADD/ADHD), psychotic symptoms, depression, behavioral and conduct problems, obsessive-compulsive disorder, and oppositional defiant disorder (Gurney, McPheeters, & Davis, 2006; Hofvander et al., 2009; Levy, Mandell, & Schultz, 2009). Suicidality has been identified in 10–50% of samples studied (Segers & Rawana, 2014), and people with autistic traits are more likely to engage in substance misuse, including alcohol, cannabis, and nicotine (de Alwis et al., 2014).

Psychiatric problems are often the impetus for ED visits. Seventy percent of children aged 10–14 years with ASD were reported to have at least one comorbid psychiatric disorder; and the likelihood of a psychiatric ED visit was increased nine-fold and more likely due to psychotic disorders or externalizing (behavioral) problems (Simonoff, Pickles, Charman, Chandler, Loucas, & Baird, 2008). An extensive database review found 13% of ED visits by children with ASD were due to a psychiatric problem, compared with 2% of visits made by neurotypical children (Kalb, Stuart, Freedman, Zablotsky, & Vasa, 2012). Over a two-year period, 24 children and adults with ASD had a combined total of 39 visits to the ED, 30 of which were for psychiatric or behavioral crises (Tint, Robinson, & Lunsky, 2011). Over half (54%) resulted from the patient's physical or verbal aggression; 13% were due to self-harm and/or suicidal behavior.

ED usage for psychiatric problems is somewhat driven by families and caregivers turning to the ED in times of crisis, partly due to deficiency of community mental healthcare professionals who offer ASD-specialized services. Use of emergency services sometimes seems the only option for assistance, if mainstream mental health services and specified resources are inaccessible or scarce, or families lack the resources needed to manage psychiatric situations (Bradley & Lofchy, 2005; Kalb, Stuart, Freedman, Zablotsky, & Vasa, 2012; Lunsky, Gracey, & Gelfand, 2008). Family members of children and adults with ASD have reported heightened stress levels, often increasing risk for crises. A common response to this crisis is the use of emergency services, especially among parents of high-school age children (White, McMorris, Weiss, & Lunsky, 2012).

Medical Comorbidities Treated in the ED

Most people with ASD have one or more concurrent disorders, which are at times severe enough to warrant emergency care. Kohane et al. (2012)

identified numerous overrepresented conditions in persons with ASD under age 35 years, all of which are commonly treated as emergencies. These individuals had significantly higher rates of epilepsy, CNS/cranial anomalies, Type I diabetes, muscular dystrophy, sleep disorders, inflammatory bowel disease and gastric syndromes, and numerous additional disorders. Gastrointestinal disorders, predominantly chronic diarrhea and constipation, have an estimated prevalence of 24–42% (Molloy & Manning-Courtney, 2003; Wang, Tancredi, & Thomas, 2011). Respiratory, food, and skin allergies are commonplace in children with ASD (Gurney, McPheeters, & Davis, 2006), and adults show high rates of hypertension (Tyler, Schramm, Karafa, Tang, & Jain, 2011).

Epilepsy and seizure disorders are of particular concern, with an estimated prevalence of 20–35% in adults (Minshew, Sweency, & Bauman, 1997). Average prevalence in children has been reported as approximately 12%, reaching 26% by adolescence (Viscidi et al., 2014). Undoubtedly many people seek emergency care at the onset of the first seizure episode and when the seizure disorder is not pharmacologically controlled.

Injuries

Children with autism are over twice as likely to incur an injury that necessitates emergency treatments (Lee, Harrington, Chang, & Connors, 2008). Injuries are also more severe and have a higher likelihood of fatality (Cavalari & Romanczyk, 2012). Common injuries are open wounds, burns, and internal injuries, upper limb injuries and fractures, with incidence of head, face, and neck injuries especially elevated (McDermott, Zhou, & Mann, 2008).

Self-injurious behaviors (SIBs) are common, as an estimated 50% of persons with ASD engage in moderate to severe SIB at some time (Billstedt, Gillberg, & Gillberg, 2005). SIBs causing enough harm to require medical care include head banging/shaking, self-biting, excessive self-scratching or rubbing, self-choking, and hair pulling (Minshawi, Hurwitx, Fodstad, Biebl, Morriss, & McDougle, 2014). Self-inflicted injury and/or suicide attempts occurred 7.6 times more compared to children without disability. Additionally, McDermott et al. (2008) found that ED/hospital treatment for poisoning was 7.6 times more frequent among children with autism or PDD and concurrent intellectual disability (ID) or developmental disability/delay (DD).

ASD Patients and the Emergency Department

The ED experience for ASD patients, their caregivers, and healthcare providers (HCP) is multifaceted and complex, with many interactive components (see Figure 12.1). People with any type of DD face complications in

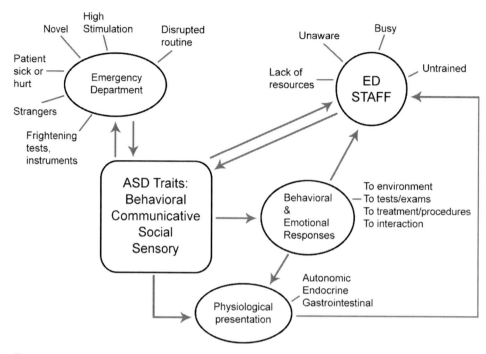

Figure 12.1. Representation of the interactive components of the visit to the emergency department for the patient with autism spectrum disorder. Each component may be complemented by a set of guidelines and used to develop a staff training program.

the ED, but having comorbid autism results in a more atypical presentation (Bradley & Lofchy, 2005). The combination of the presenting complaint and the complex traits and medical disorders associated with ASD can prove perplexing for ED practitioners. Most HCPs do not have ASD-specific education or experience in interacting with these patients. Some are conspicuously uncomfortable with or resistant to providing treatment (Tint, Robinson, & Lunsky, 2011). Across medical specialties, only 36% of physicians caring for adults with ASD reported receiving some specialized training; 67% stated that they would like or needed more (Bruder, Kerins, Mazzarella, Sims, & Stein, 2012).

The ED experience can also be difficult for family members and family caregivers, with compounded stressors of the emergency situation and daily life as a caretaker, especially if the patient displays aggressive or disruptive behaviors. Families may be frustrated by the staff's lack of training and understanding, or fear that misunderstanding typical ASD-related idiosyncrasies may lead to substandard treatment. Caregivers and parents have noted that HCPs lack of awareness of the complexities of ASD and awareness of the appropriate methods for assessing these patients. They emphasized the need for increased training (Venkat, Jauch, Russell, Crist, & Farrell, 2012; White, McMorris, Weiss, & Lunsky, 2012).

An ED visit is highly stressful for the ASD patient and can elicit fear, confusion, and overstimulation. Furthermore, the acute nature and novelty of the emergency situation and environment can intensify ASD-related traits or concurrent psychiatric symptoms (Kalb, Stuart, Freedman, Zablotsky, & Vasa, 2012) and negatively affect the outcomes of treatment.

Communication Disorders and ASD-related Traits

Many individuals with ASD have impaired communication skills (Owley, 2004) and have trouble following directions, understanding and using words. Speech is often repetitive, idiosyncratic, and/or echolalic. Many individuals demonstrate impairment in conversation. They misconstrue abstract aspects of language, and interpret figures of speech or "kidding around" quite literally, resulting in anger, confusion, or embarrassment (Owley, 2004, p. 188). Individuals with ASD may not comprehend another's perspective; fail to use and interpret social cues such as facial expressions, voice tone, and body postures/language; or refuse to make eye contact (Owley 2004; Thorne, 2007). They may utilize black-and-white or "concrete" thinking and struggle with abstract reasoning and thinking from multiple perspectives (Meyer & Minshew, 2002, p. 158). Skillful communication is essential to the delivery of appropriate and efficient care in the ED.

EFFECT OF ASD SYMPTOMS ON CARE. These traits frequently bring about unique challenges to care (Tint, Robinson, & Lunsky, 2011). Idiosyncrasies of speech plus lack of nonverbal gestures inhibit the patient from describing his/her symptoms, degree of pain, and other discomforts (Owley 2004; Tint, Robinson, & Lunsky, 2011). Symptoms may be expressed in such a manner that they are mistaken for a psychiatric disorder rather than a physical ailment (Bradley & Lofchy, 2005). Limited comprehension makes it hard for the patient to grasp information given by medical personnel, and cognitive deficits and impaired language processing may limit understanding of medical tests, procedures, interventions, and expectations in the ED (Kalb, Stuart, Freedman, Zablotsky, & Vasa, 2012; Lunsky, Gracey, & Gelfand, 2008; McGonigle, Venkat, Beresford, Campbell, & Gabriels, 2014a). Among physicians who treated adults with ASD, 54.7% stated that these patients could not understand and follow medical recommendations (Bruder, Kerins, Mazzarella, Sims, & Stein, 2012). That their attempts to communicate are not understood is often frustrating to the patient; indeed, adults with autism have reported lower satisfaction with patient-provider communication (Nicolaidis et al., 2013).

Many patients with ASD dislike and/or avoid physical contact and resist being touched by unknown ED personnel or medical instruments, which can be frightening or make them uncomfortable (Gurney, McPheeters, & Davis, 2006). Conversely, some are attracted to shiny objects and may grab for instruments (CARD, 2009). Doctors, nurses, and hospitals are associated with unpleasant or painful procedures, instigating a heightened level of anxiety. Persons with ASD often exhibit compulsive rituals or adhere to rigid routines. A medical emergency and trip to the ED are disruptions to the patient's schedule and often involve a long and unpredictable waiting period in a busy room; this is upsetting and can trigger anxiety, frustration, aggression, or withdrawal (CARD, 2009; Owley, 2004; Vaz, 2010).

Additionally, motor stereotypies such as teeth clenching, body rocking, self-biting, and head banging are escalated by anxiety and easily misconstrued as symptoms of an underlying disorder or injury. If unaware of the usual behavior of an ASD patient, the physician cannot determine if the stereotypic pattern has changed or increased due to an underlying pathology (Venkat, Jauch, Russell, Crist, & Farrell, 2012).

Under physiological stress, some ASD patients have inflated levels of lactate or ammonia (Manzi, Loizzo, Giana, & Curatolo, 2008); some also show autonomic abnormalities, manifest as higher baseline heart rate, diastolic pressure, and mean arterial pressure (Ming, Julu, Brimacombe, Connor, & Daniels, 2005). These situation-induced physiologic responses may subsequently lead to misinterpretation of vital sign measurements and unreliable laboratory test results.

Psychiatric Issues and Emergency Care

ASD patients reporting to the ED with psychiatric issues bring a host of challenges. Neurotypical individuals presenting with mental health problems can be disruptive and dangerous. For ASD patients, core traits or concurrent psychiatric symptoms are often exacerbated (Kalb, Stuart, Freedman, Zablotsky, & Vasa, 2012). Some become violent, at times to levels that are recurrent or severe enough to cause concern (Billstedt, Gillberg, & Gillberg, 2005). An unusually high likelihood of ED-diagnosed psychotic disorders among children with ASD has been reported, possibly because ED physicians confuse the complex psychiatric presentation, combined with the defining traits of ASD, with actual psychosis (Kalb, Stuart, Freedman, Zablotsky, & Vasa, 2012). Similarly, this report noted that lower rates of ED visits for mood and anxiety disorders are possibly due to overshadowing behavioral and psychotic issues, along with the ED staff's difficulty in identifying mood disorders in these children. Importantly, physicians should not dismiss symptoms as solely due to the patient's neuropsychiatric problems, as this poses a risk of not addressing the symptoms' primary etiology (Owley, 2004).

Sensory Stimulation

Sensory procession dysfunction is commonly found among patients with ASD, and is a critical source of adversity in the ED. Some individuals paradoxically show both over- and underreactivity to sensory stimuli (McGonigle, Venkat, Beresford, Campbell, & Gabriels, 2014a), or a combination of hypersensitivity and hyposensitivity to certain stimuli (Kern et al., 2006). Parents of toddlers with ASD reported greater tactile sensitivity, abnormal responses or heightened sensitivity to taste and smell, stimulation seeking, and auditory filtering compared to both typically developing children and children with other forms of DD (Rogers, Hepburn, & Wehner, 2003).

Research has shown that children with ASD may experience enhanced motion perception and weaker spatial suppression, seeing some movements twice as fast as neurotypically developing children (Foss-Feig, Tadin, Schauder, & Cascio, 2013). Auditory defensiveness (hyperacusis) is especially pronounced in environments with loud or multiple sources of noise (Kern, Miller, Cauller, Kendall, Mehta, & Dodd, 2001). Of great concern, many individuals have either an amplified or diminished threshold for, or a lowered response to, pain (Pellicano, 2013). One may anticipate that adults might experience the same problems.

Environment as Barrier. The ED is an environment in which overstimulation is the norm. Giarelli et al. (2014) found elevated levels of noise and light in numerous areas of a large urban ED. The waiting room was significantly brighter than other areas, and had the highest mean sound level and highest consistent but fluctuating noise levels, potentially triggering greater agitation and discomfort. Treatment rooms had among the widest ranges in light intensity, the least space, and the greatest degree of clutter, thus posing a high risk for inciting behavioral reactions and intensifying the patient's uneasiness. Fluorescent lights are almost ubiquitously used in the ED and are sources of great disturbance for those ASD patients with an enhanced capacity for sensing distressing flickers (Beaver, 2006). Buzzing sounds from these lights are upsetting and aggravating, and such lighting is reported to increase repetitive behaviors (Long, 2010). Importantly, 50% of surveyed ED staff were unaware that sensory overload in the ED can exacerbate behavioral problems in ASD (Vaz, 2010).

The ASD patient's hyper- and hyposensitivity to stimuli can greatly affect emergency medical care. The patient with sensory processing abnormalities may be highly reactive to lights, sounds, and odors (Gurney, McPheeters, & Davis, 2006). Fear, frustration, and distress may be displayed by behavioral outbursts or self-injurious actions (Owley, 2004; Pellicano, 2013). Sensory overload provokes anxiety (Vaz, 2010), and abnormal sensory reactivity has been associated with worsening of repetitive and restrictive actions, ultimately affecting the individual's adaptive behavior (Rogers, Hepburn, & Wehner, 2003) and becoming a barrier to effective assessment and treatment.

PHYSIOLOGICAL RESPONSE. High levels of stimulation also generate physiological effects that alter patient presentation and skew interpretation of symptoms. Loud noise arouses the autonomic and endocrine nervous systems (Lusk, Gillsepie, Hagerty, & Ziemba, 2004), elevates systolic and diastolic blood pressure and heart rate, and releases stress hormones (Babisch, 2005). Exposure to artificial bright lights can influence heart rate, elevate temperature, heighten alertness and mood (Küller, 2006), promote suppression of melatonin, and alter cortisol levels (Ruger, Gordijn, Beersma, de Vries, & Daan, 2006). Laboratory tests and vital signs measurements are thus doubly affected, by the high stimulation of the ED environment and the anxiety and agitation of the ASD patient.

Improving Emergency Care for the Patient with ASD

ED visits are undoubtedly stressful and potentially traumatizing events for individuals with ASD, but careful management can improve compliance and ultimate outcome (Owley, 2004), and the incorporation of environmental modifications and communication techniques can assist health care providers in treating ASD patients (Venkat, Jauch, Russell, Crist, & Farrell, 2012). Numerous strategies can lessen the emotional and behavioral impact of excessive sensory input and core traits of ASD, increase cooperation, and reduce anxiety. Many are geared toward general healthcare encounters, but may be applicable in the ED (see Box 12.1).

Environmental Modifications

For the benefit of the patient and all persons in the healthcare setting, several environmental alterations and effective accommodations have been described (CARD, 2009; Owley, 2004; Tint, Robinson, & Lunsky, 2011; Vaz, 2010; Venkat, Jauch, Russell, Crist, & Farrell, 2012). As waiting is extremely problematic for some persons with ASD, likely more so in the ED, the ASD patient should be triaged, registered, and seen by medical staff as quickly as possible (CARD, 2009; Owley, 2004; Vaz, 2010). If an extended waiting period is inevitable, moving the individual someplace quieter, away from high traffic and activity, or having the parent/caregiver wait with the patient outside of the medical environment altogether is advised.

Box 12.1. Modifying Patient-Staff Interactions and the Emergency Department Environment for Patients with Autism Spectrum Disorder*

Environmental Modifications
- Quiet waiting area
- Closed door
- Dimmed lights
- Less clutter in exam/ treatment rooms
- Nonfluorescent lights
- Cloth gowns and table covers
- Distracting toys/objects
- Means for nonverbal communication

Staff Behavioral Modifications
- Allow more time
- Engage parent/caregiver
- Approach patient slowly
- Speak directly to patient, as appropriate
- Speak slowly, in neutral voice tone
- Use short, direct phrases
- Speak in nonmedical terms as possible
- Explain procedures prior to beginning
- Limit physical contact
- Allow patient to see/touch instruments
- Demonstrate procedures on doll/stuffed animal
- Be prepared for behavioral/ emotional outbursts
- Give praise and positive reinforcement

Additional Modifications
- Alert staff of patient's ASD
- Decrease wait time
- Allow parent/caregiver to remain with patient during procedures and transport
- Limit number of personnel interacting with patient

*Adapted from Bradley & Lofchy, 2005; CARD, 2009; Owley, 2004; Scarpinato, Bradley, Kurbjun, Bateman, Holtzer, & Ely, 2010; Tint, Robinson, & Lunsky, 2011; Vaz, 2010; Venkat, Jauch, Russell, Crist, & Farrell, 2012.

THE EXAMINATION ROOM. Patients should be examined in a private, quiet room, with a door that shuts and lights that can be dimmed or blocked. To ease tactile sensitivity, cloth gowns and exam table coverings can replace paper. Unnecessary objects should be removed, and the room arranged so the parent/caregiver can remain. Allowing the patient sufficient personal space, having as few physicians and nurses as possible in the treatment room at one time, and limiting the number of staff involved and the amount of time they interact with the patient will decrease activity, help the patient understand what is happening, reduce anxiety, and improve behavior (CARD, 2009; Owley, 2004; Scarpinato et al., 2010; Vaz, 2010). One of the first "autism-friendly" EDs uses a sensory box, with toys and other objects of different textures the patient can use to self-soothe (Mulvaney, 2014).

Modifications in Physician and Staff Practices

Overall, healthcare workers must be sensitive to the unique qualities and needs of ASD patients; keeping in mind this is a greatly diversified group, heterogeneous in clinical presentation and in severity, type, and frequency of symptoms (Levy, Mandell, & Schultz, 2009). Although important to be aware of core symptomology, assumptions should not be made about the person's communicative, cognitive, or social capabilities. Persons on the spectrum display a wide range of intellectual ability, from severe disability to average or even above-average intelligence and therefore be intellectually capable despite impaired ability to interact socially or communicate with others (Charman, Pickles, Simonoff, Chandler, Loucas, & Baird, 2010; Thorne, 2007).

THERAPEUTIC RAPPORT. While interacting with ASD patients, personnel must adjust their activities and manner, first acknowledging that examining and treating someone with ASD will require more time (Bradley & Lofchy, 2005; Vaz, 2010). If urgent care is not needed, staff can first discuss with the caregiver the best way to approach and communicate with the patient (Thorne, 2007). When engaging the patient, eye contact should not be forced (Venkat, Jauch, Russell, Crist, & Farrell, 2012).

Speaking slowly in a neutral tone of voice, using simple nonmedical phrases, and explaining to the patient and caregiver all that the medical team is about to do are recommended (CARD, 2009). If the patient is completely nonverbal or prefers nonverbal communication, staff can use alternative modes, including paper and pencil, gestures and sign language, symbol and picture cards, or a communication device, such as iPads with autism-specific applications (CARD, 2009; Scarpinato, Bradley, Kurbjun, Batemen, Holtzer, & Ely, 2010; McGonigle, Venkat, Beresford, Campbell, & Gabriels, 2014a; Venkat, Jauch, Russell, Crist, & Farrell, 2012). A doll or stuffed animal can be used to demonstrate where the patient will be touched and how procedures will be performed, and when possible, the patient should see and handle any instruments and equipment that will be used (CARD, 2009; Olejnik, 2004; Thorne, 2007).

When obtaining medical history, Venkat et al. (2012) stressed addressing the patient directly; keeping questions short, direct, and simple; and assessing baseline behavior, communication, and social abilities along with dietary habits, sleep patterns, pharmacological therapy, etc. However, anomalies in comprehensive and language skills may necessitate input from the caregiver. Personnel should use positive reinforcement, including praise, encouragement and rewards for cooperation while ignoring unwanted or inappropriate behaviors (CARD, 2009; Scarpinato, Bradley, Kurbjun, Batemen, Holtzer, & Ely, 2010; Thorne, 2007; Vaz, 2010).

It is helpful to reduce exposure to tactile stimuli that the patient finds annoying or agitating, limit the amount of physical contact, and inform the patient before getting close or touching (CARD, 2009; Olejnik, 2004; Vaz, 2010). Auditory capacity should be gauged, as for those with hyperacusis, normal voice tones may be too loud or perceived as harsh; with hearing loss, speaking in normal tones can result in further communication failure. Similarly, the patient's pain threshold and tolerance should be assessed. At times medical staff are unsure if they are causing pain, or if the patient is displaying a heightened reaction to procedures or contact.

MEDICATIONS AND TREATMENTS. Medications must be administered carefully, as ASD commonly includes oral or textural aversions. Patients may chew pills that should not be chewed, or refuse to take medication unless crushed in food, potentially influencing choice of medication and dosing schedule in order to avoid drug interactions (Owley, 2004; Venkat, Jauch, Russell, Crist, & Farrell, 2012). Modified assessment strategies such as visual analog scales and careful observation of the patient's facial expressions are useful, and for injections or blood draws, the procedure should be carefully explained, and a lidocaine-based topical cream used when necessary (Scarpinato, Bradley, Kurbjun, Bateman, Holtzer, & Ely, 2010).

SAFETY AND CONTROL. Staff must also be prepared for a fight-or-flight response or aggressive or resistant behavior, such as kicking, biting, or dropping to the floor (CARD, 2009). Management of aggression can be complicated, as the origin for this behavior may be unclear, possibly stemming from pain, overstimulation, or any number of sources. Although long-term therapeutic interventions are useful, acute action is needed in the ED. This includes physical restraint if the patient or others are in imminent danger (Sturmey, 2002) and pharmacological treatment, namely atypical antipsychotics (Levy, Mandell, & Schultz, 2009). The latter should be used with caution and only when necessary, as they may obscure the clinical picture and because people with ASD are heterogeneous in their response to psychoactive medications (Owley, 2004).

It is also crucial that caregivers be directly involved and engaged (Owley, 2004; Vaz, 2010; Venkat, Jauch, Russell, Crist, & Farrell, 2012). Parents understand the child's patterns and idiosyncracies of behavior, language, and general communication; comprehend and translate verbalizations; and help provide a soothing, safe environment (Owley, 2004). Cargivers are familiar with the patient's response to medical encounters, and can prepare, calm, and distract the individual, identify his/her specific sensitivities, give advice regarding strategies they use in stressful situations and to reduce anxiety (CARD, 2009; Scarpinato, Bradley, Kurbjun, Batemen, Holtzer, & Ely, 2010; Vaz, 2010), and alert staff to the stimuli that may increase or decrease agitation (McGonigle, Venkat, Beresford, Campbell, & Gabriels, 2014a). Such input helps practitioners identify symptoms that indicate pathology, rather than ASD-related traits. Importantly, physicians should not speak to the caregiver as if the patient are not there, nor assume he/she does not understand what is being said about his/her behavior, condition, or plans for treatment. Although he/she may have little expressive language ability, receptive language skills may be highly developed (Owley, 2004).

Training and Education for Emergency Care Practitioners

Possibly the most effective interventions in improving emergency care are education, training, and the provision of resources for staff. There are currently no widespread practical training curricula for emergency department personnel on the characteristics and comorbidities associated with ASD and their impact on emergency care (McGonigle et al., 2014b). Several educational programs and training tools are being developed for emergency care practitioners. Debbaudt and Brown (2006) described the concept of an autism response team, among first responders in times of medical emergency, comprised of highly trained and experienced volunteers from police, fire rescue, emergency medical, and hospital ED. McGonigle and colleagues (2014b) devised a training manual and DVD for time efficient presentation to EMS personnel and ED nurses, and eventually ED physicians, based on key information about the ASD community: Epidemiology and core characteristics, myths that need to be dispelled, medical comorbidities that might necessitate emergency care, and an approach to assessing, examining, and treating the ASD patient.

Similarly, the Assess Communicate Treat for Autism (ACT) training manual was developed by an ED physician and experts in ASD and special education, and is being promoted in hospitals across Pennsylvania with the goal of helping health systems and medical practitioners nationwide in treating patients with ASD (Autism Speaks, 2013). Such programs could easily be incorporated into school curricula and continuing education for ED physicians and nurses.

Educational material might be made accessible on a hospital intranet (Vaz, 2010). For access to rapid assistance, emergency psychiatric staff suggested developing a resource list of available services, available by website and 24-hour telephone line, noting that improved access to experts would alleviate stress involved in diagnosing and treating psychiatric crises in the ED (Lunsky, Gracey, & Gelfand, 2008). Gurney, McPheeters, and Davis (2006) suggested that healthcare systems employ a coordinated care or case management plan with a central contact person who is familiar with the ASD child's specific medical and psychological needs. A similar plan for the ED can involve consultants who are trained and on call as needed by emergency room personnel.

Conducting Emergency Medicine Research in ASD

Information regarding emergency treatment of ASD patients is largely from the perspectives of parents, caregivers, and medical staff. Disabled and persons with ASD have not often been included as partners in research, and research is not representative of their knowledge and experience (Kitchin, 2000; Nicolaidis et al., 2013). The importance of the patient's perspective is underscored by the findings of the limited existing research, as a survey of adults with and without ASD found those with ASD reported lower satisfaction with general health care and chronic condition self-efficacy and higher odds of unmet care needs (Nicolaidis et al., 2013).

Research Challenges and Improvement Strategies

People with ASD, or any developmental disability, are a vulnerable and potentially exploitable group (Dalton & McVilly, 2004). This raises various ethical concerns. The relationship between investigator and research participant is not perceived as one of equal power. Vulnerable subjects may question the agenda of social scientists and might believe themselves to be more "victims" of research rather than participants (Kitchin, 2000, p. 26). Robison (2004) stressed that medical researchers must maintain their ethical obligations to the autistic community, and that their ultimate responsibility is to the individual with ASD. An integral component of the assuring fair treatment of subjects is obtaining informed consent (Nind, 2008).

CONSENTING. The consent process should include information concerning why, how, and by whom the research is being conducted, all that it involves, possible risks and outcomes, how information will be kept and who might see it, and the patient's right to decline or withdraw participation without consequence (Dalton & McVilly, 2004). ASD-related disabilities can impair the capacity to provide informed consent. The International Association for the Scientific Study of Intellectual Disabilities (IASSID), has endorsed a position statement outlining guidelines for conducting research involving and affecting people with ID, their families, and community, making recommendations regarding ethical review processes, study designs and methodology, and consent processes (Dalton & McVilly, 2004). In determining the capacity to give consent, the investigator should consider if the person has previously participated in research, their decision-making capacity in daily situations, their demonstrated ability to say "no," and their ability to understand and explain the research protocol, risks, and their right to decline participation without consequences (Dalton & McVilly, 2004).

Cognitive, communicative, and social limitations can impact all phases of the research process and must be considered in study design and implementation. Flaws and necessary changes to research methods have been identified in the current literature regarding particular features of ASD. These include strategies for matching comparison groups in studies of cognitive abilities (Mottron, 2004), alternatives to matching designs in general autism research (Jarrold & Brock, 2004), and procedures for conducting language research (Tager-Flusberg, 2004). Investigators must act inclusively and responsibly to incorporate techniques for communicating abstract ideas and enabling subjects to discuss their views and experiences (Nind, 2008).

TECHNOLOGY. As with interactions in the ED, alternative methods of communication may be needed. For data collection, Nicolaidis and colleagues (2013) noted that computers and the Internet play an important role in the autistic community, as technology-assisted communication can overcome the problems of in-person communication.

Another useful method is the Interactive Autism Network (IAN), an online community within a research framework that provides a large database of information that has been voluntarily submitted by families and can reduce the challenges of recruiting subjects with ASD (Rosenberg, Law, Yenokyan, McGready, Kaufmann, & Law, 2009). This network connects researchers to people with ASD and their families, helps advance understanding of the value of research participation, and influences research direction. Within this network, those with ASD, their families, and caregivers could respond to surveys assessing their utilization and opinions of emergency care services.

Also employing an online survey, Nicolaidis et al. (2013) used a community-based participatory research (CBPR) approach to adapt validated health services questionnaires to more accurately assess the healthcare experiences of adults with ASD. Importantly, members of both academia and the community, the majority of whom are on the spectrum, are involved and are equitable partners throughout all stages of the research process. This method addresses several criticisms of disability research, by including persons with disability as investigators and ensuring that studies are designed with their best interests in mind, with the goal of improving some aspect of living with ASD.

Qualitative Research and ASD

Persons with developmental disabilities reported some wariness of structured questionnaires (Kitchin, 2000) and standardized instruments may not be fully applicable to this population. Therefore, qualitative methods may yield a rich set of data on the ASD patient's experiences in the ED. The value of conducting qualitative research lies in the natural-setting focus of these studies. Open interviews, observation, and audiovisual materials (Creswell, 2003; Nind, 2008) allow subjects more freedom and less restriction concerning the topic of interest. Qualitative research does not introduce treatments, manipulate variables, or impose operational definitions of variables. Rather, it aims to get a better understanding through firsthand experience, truthful reporting, and quotation of actual conversations, and to understand how participants derive meaning from their surroundings and how their meaning influences their behavior.

Audiovisual recording could be especially beneficial and robust in the ED, as it combines verbal and nonverbal data, encompasses the encounter in its entirety, and provides firsthand view of the environment. An accurate real-time depiction would be captured of the ASD patient in these highly-charged surroundings, providing an excellent record of patient and staff behavior and leading to effective protocols in examining, treating, and interacting with these individuals. However, there are limitations in what can appropriately and ethically be taped or recorded.

Conclusion

Emergency care of persons with ASD is a singular realm of medicine that has not received adequate attention and intervention. The special medical needs of this population, combined with the distinct characteristics and presentation associated with the autism spectrum require an approach to emergency care that is generally not implemented. The recommended environmental modifications, changes in practitioner behavior, and educational programs can greatly improve the emergency care experience for everyone involved. Future research is needed, with particular attention to the uniqueness of the person with ASD as a participating subject, in order to fully develop protocols of emergency care for these patients.

References

Autism Speaks. (2013). Training in autism friendly protocols help to improve ER care. Retrieved from http://www.autismspeaks.org/news/news-item/training -autism-friendly-protocols-help-improve-er-care

Babisch, W. (2005). Noise and health. *Environmental Health Perspectives, 113*(1), A14– A15.

Beaver, C. (2006). *Designing environments for children and adults with ASD.* Paper presented at the 2nd World Autism Congress & Exhibition, South Africa.

Billstedt, E., Gillberg, I. C., & Gillberg, C. (2005). Autism after adolescence: Population-based 13- to 22-year follow-up study of 120 individuals with autism diagnosed in childhood. *Journal of Autism & Developmental Disorders, 35*(3), 351– 360.

Bradley, E., & Lofchy, J. (2005). Learning disability in the accident and emergency department. *Advances in Psychiatric Treatment, 11*(1), 45–57.

Bruder, M. B., Kerins, G., Mazzarella, C., Sims, J., & Stein, N. (2012). Brief report: The medical care of adults with autism spectrum disorders: Identifying the needs. *Journal of Autism & Developmental Disorders, 42*(11), 2498–2504.

CARD–Center for Autism and Related Disorders. (2009). *Autism and the hospital emergency room.* University of South Florida (Ed.). Tampa: Florida Center for Inclusive Communities, University of South Florida.

Cavalari, R. N., & Romanczyk, R. G. (2012). Caregiver perspectives on unintentional injury risk in children with an autism spectrum disorder. *Journal of Pediatric Nursing, 27*(6), 632–641.

Charman, T., Pickles, A., Simonoff, E., Chandler, S., Loucas, T., & Baird, G. (2011). IQ in children with autism spectrum disorders: Data from the Special Needs and Autism Project (SNAP). *Psychological Medicine, 41*(3), 619–627.

Creswell, J. (2003). *Research design: Qualitative, quantitative, and mixed methods approaches.* Thousand Oaks, CA: Sage.

Dalton, A. M., & McVilly, K. R. (2004). Ethics guidelines for international, multi-center research involving people with intellectual disabilities. *Journal of Policy and Practice in Intellectual Disabilities, 1*(2), 57–70.

De Alwis D., Agrawal, A., Reiersen A. M., Constantino, J. N., Henders, A., Martin, N. G., & Lynskey, M. T. (2014). ADHD symptoms, autistic traits, and substance use and misuse in adult Australian twins. *Journal of Studies on Alcohol and Drugs, 75*(2), 211–221.

Debbaudt, D., & Brown, M. (2006). The autism response team: A concept whose time has come. *Autism Spectrum Quarterly, Spring,* 8–10. Retrieved from asert911 .com/wp-content/uploads/2014/02/Debbaudt_Brown_ASQ71.pdf

Foss-Feig, J. H., Tadin, D., Schauder, K. B., & Cascio, C. J. (2013). A substantial and unexpected enhancement of motion perception in autism. *Journal of Neuroscience, 33*(19), 8243–8249.

Giarelli, E., Nocera, R., Turchi, R., Hardie, T. L., Pagano, R., & Yuan, C. (2014). Sensory stimuli as obstacles to emergency care for children with autism spectrum disorder. *Advanced Emergency Nursing Journal, 36*(2), 145–163.

Gurney, J. G., McPheeters, M. L., & Davis, M. M. (2006). Parental report of health conditions and health care use among children with and without autism: National Survey of Children's Health. *Archives of Pediatrics & Adolescent Medicine, 160*(8), 825–830.

Hofvander, B., Delorme, R., Chaste, P., Nyden, A., Wentz, E., Stahlberg, O., & Leboyer, M. (2009). Psychiatric and psychosocial problems in adults with normal-intelligence autism spectrum disorders. *BioMedical Central Psychiatry, 9,* 35–43

Interactive Autism Network. (2014). Retrieved from http://www.iancommunity.org

Jarrold, C., & Brock, J. (2004). To match or not to match? Methodological issues in autism-related research. *Journal of Autism & Developmental Disorders, 34*(1), 81–86.

Kalb, L. G., Stuart, E. A., Freedman, B., Zablotsky, B., & Vasa, R. (2012). Psychiatric-related emergency department visits among children with an autism spectrum disorder. *Pediatric Emergency Care, 28*(12), 1269–1276.

Kern, J. K., Miller, V. S., Cauller, L . J., Kendall, R., Mehta, J., & Dodd, M. (2001). The effectiveness of N, N-Dimethylglycine in autism/PDD. *Journal of Child Neurology, 16*(3), 169–173.

Kern, J. K., Trivedi, M. H., Garver, C. R., Grannemann, B. D., Andrews, A. A., Savla, J. S., Johnson, D. G., Mehta, J. A., & Schroeder, J. L. (2006). The pattern of sensory processing abnormalities in autism. *Autism, 10*(5), 480–494.

Kitchin, R. (2000). The researched opinions on research: Disabled people and disability research. *Disability & Society, 15*(1), 25–47.

Kohane, I. S., McMurry, A., Weber, G., MacFadden, D., Rappaport, I., Kunkel, L., . . . Weber, G. M. (2012). The co-morbidity burden of children and young adults with autism spectrum disorders. *PLoS ONE, 7*(4), e33224.

Küller, R. (2006). The impact of light and colour on psychological mood: A cross-cultural study of indoor work environments. *Ergonomics, 49*(14), 1496–1507.

Lee, L. C., Harrington, R. A., Chang, J. J., & Connors, S. L. (2008). Increased risk of injury in children with developmental disabilities. *Research in Developmental Disabilities, 29*(3), 247–255.

Levy, S. E., Giarelli, E., Lee, L. C., Schieve, L. A., Kirby, R. S., Cunniff, C., Joyce, N., Reaven, J., & Rice, C. E. (2010). Autism spectrum disorder and co-occurring developmental, psychiatric, and medical conditions among children in multiple populations of the United States. *Journal of Developmental Behavioral Pediatrics, 31*(4), 267–275.

Levy, S. E., Mandell, D. S., & Schultz, R. T. (2009). Autism. *Lancet, 374*(9701), 1627–1638.

Long, E. A. (2010). Classroom lighting design for students with autism spectrum disorders. Report submitted for degree of Master of Science, Kansas State University, Manhattan, KS.

Lunsky, Y., Gracey, C., & Gelfand, S. (2008). Emergency psychiatric services for individuals with intellectual disabilities: Perspectives of hospital staff. *Intellectual and Developmental Disabilities, 46*(6), 446–455.

Lusk, S. L., Gillespie, B., Hagerty, B. M., & Ziemba, R. A. (2004). Acute effects of noise on blood pressure and heart rate. *Archives of Environmental Health, 59*(8), 392–399.

Manzi B., Loizzo, A. L., Giana, G., & Curatolo, P. (2008). Autism and metabolic diseases. *Journal of Child Neurology, 23*(3), 307–314.

Masterson, T. L., Dimitriou, F., Turko, K., & McPartland, J. (2014). Developing undergraduate coursework in autism spectrum disorders. *Journal of Autism and Developmental Disorders, 44*(10), 2646–2649.

McDermott, S., Zhou, L., & Mann, J. (2008). Injury treatment among children with autism or pervasive developmental disorder. *Journal of Autism & Developmental Disorders, 38*(4), 626–633.

McGonigle, J. J., Venkat, A., Beresford, C., Campbell, T. P., & Gabriels, R. L. (2014a). Management of agitation in individuals with autism spectrum disorders in the emergency department. *Child and Adolescent Psychiatric Clinics of North America, 23*(1), 83–95.

McGonigle, J. J, Migyanka, J. M., Glor-Scheib, S. J., Cramer, R., Fratangeli, J. J., Jegde, G. G., Shang, J., & Venkat, A. (2014b). Development and evaluation of educational materials for pre-hospital and emergency department personnel on the care of patients with autism spectrum disorder. *Journal of Autism & Developmental Disorders, 44,* 1252–1259.

Meyer, J. M., & Minshew, N. J. (2002). An update on neurocognitive profiles in Asperger syndrome and high-functioning autism. *Focus on Autism and Other Developmental Disabilities, 17*(3), 152–160.

Ming, X., Julu, P. O., Brimacombe, M., Connor, S., & Daniels, M. L. (2005). Reduced cardiac parasympathetic activity in children with autism. *Brain Development, 27*(7), 509–516.

Minshawi, N. F., Hurwitz, S., Fodstad, J. D., Biebl, S., Morriss, D. H. & McDougle, C. J. (2014). The association between self-injurious behaviors and autism spectrum disorders. *Psychology Research and Behavior Management, 7,* 125–136.

Minshew, N., Sweeney, J.A., & Bauman, M.I. (1997). Neurologic aspects of autism. In D. V. Cohen, FR. (Ed.), *Handbook of autism and pervasive developmental disorders* (2nd ed., pp. 344–369). New York: Wiley.

Molloy, C. A., & Manning-Courtney, P. (2003). Prevalence of chronic gastrointestinal symptoms in children with autism and autistic spectrum disorders. *Autism, 7*(2), 165–171.

Mottron, L. (2004). Matching strategies in cognitive research with individuals with high-functioning autism: Current practices, instrument biases, and recommendations. *Journal of Autism & Developmental Disorders, 34*(1), 19–27.

Mulvaney, N. (2014, October 14). Capital Health-Hopewell opens 1st 'autism-friendly' pediatric emergency department in N.J. Times of Trenton. Retrieved from http://www.nj.com/mercer/index.ssf/2014/10/capital_health_-_hopewell_to _launch_first _autism-friendly_pediatric_emergency_department_in_nj.html

Nicolaidis, C., Raymaker, D., McDonald, K., Dern, S., Boisclair, W. C., Ashkenazy, E., & Baggs, A. (2013). Comparison of healthcare experiences in autistic and non-autistic adults: A cross-sectional online survey facilitated by an academic-community partnership. *Journal of General Internal Medicine, 28*(6), 761–769.

Nind, M. (2008). Conducting qualitative research with people with learning, communication and other disabilities: Methodological challenges. *Economic & Social Research Council, National Centre for Research Methods review paper.* 1–24. Southampton, UK: University of Southampton.

Olejnik, L. (2004). Understanding autism. How to appropriately & safely approach, assess & manage autistic patients. *Journal of Emergency Medical Services, 29*(6), 56–61, 64.

Owley, T. (2004). Treatment of individuals with autism spectrum disorders in the emergency department: Special considerations. *Clinical Pediatric Emergency Medicine, 5,* 187–192.

Pellicano, E. (2013). Sensory symptoms in autism: A blooming, buzzing confusion? *Child Development Perspectives, 7*(3), 143–148.

Robison, J. E. (2011). *Ethical issues in autism research.* Retrieved from https://iacc .hhs.gov/non-iacc-events/2011/slides_elsi_john_robison_092611.pdf

Rogers, S. J., Hepburn, S., & Wehner, E. (2003). Parent reports of sensory symptoms in toddlers with autism and those with other developmental disorders. *Journal of Autism & Developmental Disorders, 33*(6), 631–642.

Rosenberg, R. E., Law, J. K., Yenokyan, G., McGready, J., Kaufmann, W. E., & Law, P. A. (2009). Characteristics and concordance of autism spectrum disorders among 277 twin pairs. *Archives of Pediatrics & Adolescent Medicine, 163*(10), 907–914.

Ruger, M., Gordijn, M. C., Beersma, D. G., de Vries, B., & Daan, S. (2006). Time-of-day-dependent effects of bright light exposure on human psychophysiology: Comparison of daytime and nighttime exposure. *American Journal of Physiology: Regulatory, Integrative and Comparative Physiology, 290*(5), R1413–R1420.

Scarpinato, N., Bradley, J., Kurbjun, K., Bateman, X., Holtzer, B., & Ely, B. (2010). Caring for the child with an autism spectrum disorder in the acute care setting. *Journal of Specialized Pediatric Nursing, 15*(3), 244–254.

Segers, M., & Rawana, J. (2014). What do we know about suicidality in autism spectrum disorders? A systematic review. *Autism Research, 7*(4), 507–521.

Simonoff, E., Pickles, A., Charman, T., Chandler, S., Loucas, T., & Baird, G. (2008). Psychiatric disorders in children with autism spectrum disorders: Prevalence, comorbidity, and associated factors in a population-derived sample. *Journal of the American Academy of Child and Adolescent Psychiatry, 47*(8), 921–929.

Sturmey, P. (2002). Treatment interventions for people with aggressive behavior and intellectual disability. In G. B. Holt& N. Bouras (Eds.), *Autism and related disor-*

ders: The basic handbook for mental health, primary care, and other professionals.* Great Britain: Henry Lang LTD.

Tager-Flusberg, H. (2004). Strategies for conducting research on language in autism. *Journal of Autism & Developmental Disorders, 34*(1), 75–80.

Thorne, A. (2007). Are you ready to give care to a child with autism? *Nursing, 37*(5), 59–61.

Tint, A. R., Robinson, S., & Lunsky, Y. (2011). Brief report: Emergency department assessment and outcomes in individuals with autism spectrum disorder. *Journal on Developmental Disabilities, 17*(2), 56–59.

Tyler, C. V., Schramm, S. C., Karafa, M., Tang, A. S., & Jain, A. K. (2011). Chronic disease risks in young adults with autism spectrum disorder: Forewarned is fore-armed. *American Journal of Intellectual & Developmental Disabilities, 116*(5), 371–380.

Vaz, I. (2010). Improving the management of children with learning disability and autism spectrum disorder when they attend hospital. *Child: Care, Health and Development, 36*(6), 753–755.

Venkat, A., Jauch, E., Russell, W. S., Crist, C. R., & Farrell, R. (2012). Care of the patient with an autism spectrum disorder by the general physician. *Postgraduate Medical Journal, 88*(1042), 472–481.

Viscidi, E. W., Triche, E. W., Pescosolido, M. F., McLean, R. L., Joseph, R. M., Spence. S. H., & Morrow, E. M. (2013). Clinical characteristics of children with autism spectrum disorder and co-occurring epilepsy. *PLoS One, 8*(7), e67797.

Wang, L. W., Tancredi, D. J., & Thomas, D. W. (2011). The prevalence of gastro-intestinal problems in children across the United States with autism spectrum disorders from families with multiple affected members. *Journal of Developmental Behavioral Pediatrics, 32*(5), 351–360.

White, S. M., McMorris, C., Weiss, J. A., & Lunsky, Y. (2012). The experience of crisis in families of individuals with autism spectrum disorder across the lifespan. *Journal of Child and Family Studies, 21,* 457–465.

Chapter 13

PHYSICAL THERAPY TO PROMOTE HEALTH, FUNCTION, AND COMMUNITY PARTICIPATION

MARGARET E. O'NEIL AND MARIA FRAGALA-PINKHAM

Overview of Physical Therapy Services

Physical therapy (PT) is a health profession that uses evidenced-informed practice to restore, maintain, and promote optimal physical function (American Physical Therapy Association (APTA) Guide to Physical Therapy Practice, 2014). Physical therapists provide services to help individuals achieve goals of improved function, mobility, activity, and participation in activities of daily living. The APTA has adopted the International Classification of Functioning, Health and Disability (ICF) Model as a framework to describe patient/client health and function and to guide management (see Figure 13.1, The ICF Model) (World Health Organization (WHO), 2002). The ICF Model provides a common language for health professionals (APTA, Board of Directors (BOD Guidelines, 2014; WHO, 2002; Steiner, Ryser, Huber, Uebelhart, Aeschlimann et al., 2002).

PT services are provided for individuals of all ages across the lifespan to prevent, eliminate, or reduce body function and structure impairments, activity limitations, or participation restrictions. Individuals with ASD receive PT services because of the abnormal motor function and motor impairments often associated with this diagnosis that often leads to decreased activity and participation. Motor impairments found in individuals with ASD include hypotonia, motor apraxia, toe-walking, and gross motor delay. See Figure 13.1 for an illustration of the International Classification of Functioning, Health and Disability (ICF) Model.

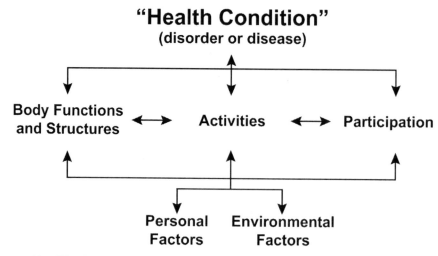

Figure 13.1. The International Classification of Functioning, Health and Disability ICF Model© (World Health Organization, 2007) was created by the World Health Organization and has been adopted by the APTA to identify and describe patient health and function and to guide patient management (WHO, 2002). Reprinted with permission from the World Health Organization.

Family-centered or patient/client-centered approaches are used in PT to ensure that goals, needs, and preferences of child and adult patients/clients and their families/caregivers are included in the plan of care (Barry & Edgman-Levitan, 2012). Family-centered care is based on the tenets that parents and families are experts and constants in their children's lives (O'Neil & Palisano, 2000). Similarly, in patient/client-centered care, the adult patient/client and caregivers are partners in care. PT must be meaningful to patient/client and family/caregiver routines (Reuben & Tinetti, 2012).

Historically, interdisciplinary models of care are used in rehabilitation services and special education to address the needs of the patient/client. Physical therapists are members of the interdisciplinary team and provide expertise in the management of motor function and performance (Steiner, Ryser, Huber, Uebelhart, Aeschlimann, & Stucki, 2002). Physical therapists are trained in care coordination, communication, and documentation to ensure effective, efficient, and collaborative patient services to optimize patient outcomes (APTA, Guide to Physical Therapy Practice, 2014).

The APTA advocates use the Patient/Client Management Model in patient/client care (APTA Guide to Physical Therapy Practice, 2014). The six elements of this model are: (1) examination, (2) evaluation, (3) PT diagnosis, (4) prognosis, (5) intervention, and (6) outcomes. The APTA has created a list of recommended outcome measures for a number of different patient/client populations (APTA Guide to Physical Therapy Practice, 2014). Intervention strategies and measures that may be appropriate for individuals with ASD are discussed in this chapter.

Physical Therapists' Roles to Promote Function and Participation

Although the Patient/Client Management Model is recommended by the APTA, the Bronfenbrenner's Social Ecological Model (1993) provides a complimentary framework to highlight areas beyond the clinic that may be important to promote carry-over of functional goals (Bronfenbrenner, 1993; O'Neil, Fragala-Pinkham, Ideishi, & Ideishi, 2012) (see Figure 13.2 The Social Ecological Model). The Social Ecological Model includes five levels: (1) individual, (2) interpersonal, (3) organizational, (4) community, and (5) public policy. Engaging in public policy and advocacy may not be considered part of the physical therapist's traditional role, but it is an important component of patients/client management (Sullivan, Wallace, O'Neil, Musolina, Mandich, & Bottomly, 2011).

Physical Therapy for Individuals with ASD

The American Psychiatric Association's Diagnostic and Statistical Manual, Fifth Edition (DSM-5) provides updated standardized criteria for autism spectrum disorders (ASDs) (American Psychiatric Association, 2013). The criteria include persistent deficits in social communication and social interaction and restricted, repetitive patterns of behavior, interests, or activities with symptoms present in early development. Symptoms do not include intellectual disability or global developmental delay; however, intellectual disability and ASD often co-occur (Wing, Gold, & Gillberg, 2011).

Three severity levels of ASD are identified in the DSM-5 and each level is described by two categories (social communication and restricted, repetitive behavior). Individuals with ASD level one require support, those at ASD level two require substantial support, and those at ASD level three require very substantial support. Although DSM-5 has been recently adopted, individuals with a DSM-IV autism diagnosis, Asperger's disorder, or pervasive developmental disorder not otherwise specified should be given the diagnosis of ASD (Wing, Gold, & Gillberg, 2011).

Motor Function in Individuals with ASD

It is critical for physical therapists to understand motor function and motor activity in individuals with ASD (Downey & Rapport, 2012). Brain development in individuals with ASD is different from individuals with typical

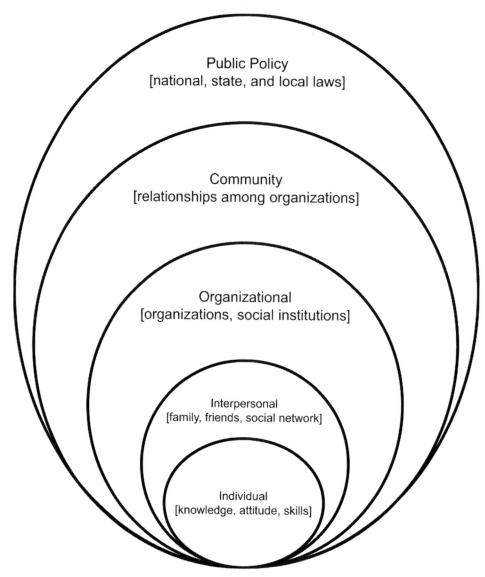

Figure 13.2. The Social Ecological Model. This material is copyrighted and any further reproduction and distribution requires written permission from the journal editors. Source: M. E. O'Neil, M. Fragala-Pinkham, R. I. Ideishi, & S. K. Ideishi. (2012). Community-based programs for children and youth: Our experiences in design, implementation and evaluation. *Physical & Occupational Therapy in Pediatrics, 32*(2), 111–119.

development and is a contributing factor to the motor impairments in this patient population. For individuals with ASD, brain development usually occurs in three stages with overgrowth in early years (infants and toddlers), slow growth and arrested development in late childhood, and a decline in growth with possible degeneration after preadolescence and adulthood (Bhat, Bubela, & Landa, 2015; Courchesne, Redcay, & Kennedy, 2004). Decreased long-range connectivity results in poor integration of sensorimotor, social communication, and cognitive function and may contribute to decreased coordination and motor control difficulties seen in children with ASD (Williams, Goldstein, & Minishew, 2006; Mostofsky, Powell, Simmonds, Goldberg, Caffo, & Pekar, 2009; Fournier, Hass, Naik, Loda, & Cauraugh, 2010). Also, youth with ASD may have mirror neural system impairments in the frontoparietal cortices making action production and action observations difficult and which may explain poor imitation skills and difficulties with social and motor learning (Cattaneo & Rizzolatti, 2009; Dapretto et al., 2006). Postural control mechanisms including the motor systems ability to respond to sensory perturbation (i.e., feedback system) or to anticipate sensory perturbation or challenges (i.e., feed-forward system) are present in individuals with ASD but at a lower level compared to peers with typical development (Minshew, Sung, Jones, & Furman, 2004; Fournier, Hass, Naik, Loda, & Cauraugh, 2010).

Some individuals with ASD have poor postural control or stability when visual or somatosensory input is removed, suggesting that postural responses rely on multimodal sensory integration, and may operate on feedback or feed-forward mechanisms (Schmitz, Martineau, Barthelemy, & Assinante, 2003).

Individuals with ASD exhibit gross and fine motor delay, limitations in acquisition of developmental motor skills, and decreased manual dexterity and development of reaching and grasping skills. Individuals with ASD often demonstrate motor stereotypes including repetitive motion and/or banging of objects which are a core feature of ASD. They may have decreased imitation skills and poor praxis (or decreased coordination and motor planning) (Bhat, Landa, & Galloway, 2011; Bhat, Bubela, & Landa, 2015).

The prevalence of specific motor impairments associated with ASD (i.e., hypotonia, motor apraxia, toe-walking, delayed gross motor milestones, and reduced ankle mobility) have been established in a cohort of 154 children and adolescents with hypotonia at highest prevalence (51%) followed by apraxia (34%), toe-walking (19%), gross motor delay (9%), and finally, reduced ankle mobility (2%) (Ming, Brimacombe, & Wagner, 2007). A comparison of motor function in youth with high functioning autism (HFA) or Asperger's syndrome compared to youth with typical development indicates that youth with HFA or Asperger's syndrome have balance deficits, slower speed on repetitive movements, increased motor dysrhythmia (awkward or improperly timed motor task performance), increased motor overflow (extraneous or involuntary movements), and abnormal gait characteristics compared to youth with typical development (Jansiewicz, Goldberg, Newschaffer, Denckla, Landa, & Mostofsky, 2006). Table 13.1 (Motor Limitations in Individuals with or at Risk for ASD) illustrates select motor impairments in individuals with ASD by age and motor skill development.

Sensory Modulation in Individuals with ASD

Children with ASD may have sensory modulation disorders (SMDs) which may affect motor performance. SMDs are deficits in regulation and organization of the type and intensity of behavioral responses to sensory input (e.g., tactile, olfactory, visual, auditory, vestibular, or proprioceptive). There are three categories of SMDs that have been observed in children: (1) "Underresponsive" children (i.e., slow to respond to verbal cues or pain); (2) "overresponsive" children have exaggerated or prolonged responses to sensory input (i.e., covers ears when noises are loud; covers eyes when lights are bright); and (3) "sensory seeking" children need sensory input and may use repetitive, stereotypic motor behaviors (i.e., rocking, hand flapping) (Bhat, Landa, & Galloway, 2011). Adults with ASD may have SMDs and will have similar motor responses and behaviors as those described for children (Bhat, Landa, & Galloway, 2011).

Physical Therapy Clinical Management of ASD

PT clinical management includes use of the three models discussed previously. The Social Ecological Model (Bronfenbrenner, 1993) provides a broad context to promote interdisciplinary services that translates from clinical care to community participation. Although participation in public policy may not be a traditional role for therapists, it may be important to promote optimal functional outcomes (O'Neil, Fragala-Pinkham, Ideishi, & Ideishi, 2012).

The ICF Model (WHO, 2002) provides structural organization in designing the PT plan of care and underscores the importance of a multipronged approach when developing plans of care. For example, the personal dimensions of the ICF Model encourage the therapist to consider the patient/client needs across body structure and function; activity and participation while including interventions that address environmental factors to optimize sustained function (Steiner, Ryser, Huber, Uebelhart, Aeschlimann, & Stucki, 2002). The therapist may provide interventions to the patient/client with ASD to promote strength and balance (body structure and function) while

Table 13.1
MOTOR LIMITATIONS IN INDIVIDUALS WITH OR AT RISK FOR ASD

Motor Limitations	*Infants and Young Children*	*Children and Adults*
Gross motor skills and coordination	Delays in movement in supine, prone and sitting; delayed walking skills; decreased balance and coordination with gross motor activities such as walking on stairs and uneven terrain outdoors or using playground equipment such as swings or slides	Difficulty initially with gross motor skills such as jumping jacks in physical education classes, problems learning to jump rope, swim, ride a bike; difficulty coordinating steering and cycling movements, throwing, catching, and kicking a ball
Fine motor skills	Decreased reaching and grasping; difficulty grabbing dangling toys, limited ability to clap or to point (to indicate wants); difficulty with self-feeding such as picking up small cut-up pieces of food or crackers or cereal	Limited fine motor coordination including manual dexterity tasks such as difficulty with buttons, shoe tying, hand writing, opening individual food packages at lunch, manipulating small toys or objects
Stereotypic motor behaviors	Repetitive banging of objects or unusual sensory exploration often emerges by two years of age	Motor stereotypes such as body rocking or hand movements may be observed in older children and adults
Posture and developmental movements	Delay in maintaining postural alignment and control in side-lying and transitions into and out of sitting; delay in floor mobility (rolling, crawling, creeping); delay in standing	Delays in postural control and balance reactions for both anticipatory (feed forward) and responsive (feedback) postural perturbations which impacts walking on uneven surfaces or sports skills requiring balance and agility such as soccer drills around cones, roller blading, ice skating or skiing
Imitation and motor planning	Limited ability to stack blocks or scribble or "bang" on high chair; limited ability to play with Duplos® or to connect blocks or to play with puzzles	Delays in postural, gestural, and oral imitation; deficits in completing complex movement sequences (dyspraxia) which impacts learning of new skills or sports

Adapted from: Bhat, A.N., Landa, R.J., & Galloway, J.C. (2011). Current perspectives on motor functioning in infants, children, and adults with autism spectrum disorders. *Physical Therapy, 91,* 1116–1129. .

providing recommendations to increase walking and physical activity (activity) and identifying community resources where the patient/client may engage in these new motor skills to practice and promote participation.

The Elements of Patient/Client Management Model (APTA Guide to Physical Therapy Practice, 2014) provides guidelines for the physical therapist to ensure that all six elements are addressed for comprehensive and complete patient/client care. A thorough examination and evaluation will lead to a clear PT diagnosis and prognosis and a clear, comprehensive plan of care that should address the patient/client goals and result in improved functional motor outcomes. For the individual with ASD, it is critical to have a clear understanding of motor function by observation, specific motor measures, and in-depth interview with the patient/client of caregiver to understand the focus of PT interventions.

Examination, Evaluation, Diagnosis, and Prognosis

Individuals with ASD receive PT services to improve functional mobility, activity, performance and/or participation. These services may be delivered in various environments depending on the patients'/clients' needs. The examination process includes interview and record review to identify patient/client and family goals and to document history and impact of the condition; systems review to identify critical body structures and function impairments and activity limitations that will be addressed in the intervention and plan of care; and tests and measures to document patient/client status and to readminister after the plan of care to examine outcome effectiveness (APTA, Guide to Practice, 2014). The therapist uses a lifespan approach to ensure the use of proper measures and development of functional goals and plans of care that are age appropriate for the individual with ASD.

The physical therapist should obtain information on patient/client medications when reviewing the medical chart or during the patient/client or caregiver interview. The therapist must know how the medications may affect motor skills and behaviors. Therapists should be aware of any potential side effects of medications and how they influence an exercise program. Common medications for ASD include neuroleptics, selective serotonin reuptake inhibitors, tricyclic antidepressants, lithium, mood stabilizers, and anxiolytics (American Academy of Child and Adolescent Psychiatry (AACAP), 1999; Chugani, 2005).

Physical therapists conduct a comprehensive fine and gross motor examination to identify motor control, planning, performance, and/or imitation skills and impairments. The physical therapist may administer special tests such as those identified in Table 13.2 (Examples of Tests and Measures in

Physical Therapy Examination for Individuals with ASD). In addition to history taking and tests and measures, a comprehensive examination usually consists of observation of play, physical activity, or functional mobility in natural environments for the individual with ASD.

Results of the examination will be considered in the therapist's evaluation of finding to determine an optimal plan of care to meet patients'/clients' goals and needs and address functional motor and mobility skills. Based on the examination and evaluation findings, the physical therapist determines the "physical therapy diagnosis and prognosis" and plan of care. The PT diagnosis and prognosis usually consists of the neuromuscular and musculoskeletal comorbid conditions associated with ASD. For example, the PT diagnosis may be "decreased participation in active play at recess due to decreased balance, motor coordination and motor planning." However, because motor delays have been identified in patients/clients with ASD at all cognitive levels, it is sometimes difficult to determine if poor motor performance is due to motor delay or cognitive and language challenges which may limit the individual's ability to understand the instructions or request during the examination (Bhat, Landa, & Galloway, 2011).

TESTS AND MEASURES. Table 13.2 provides examples of tests and measures in physical therapy examination for individuals with ASD, contains select tests and measures that are used to determine effectiveness of PT interventions. The table is formatted by patient age ranges including infants and toddlers, children and adolescents; and adults. The table also groups by categories (i.e., dimensions of the ICF Model, gross motor, imitation, and motor control). It is important to choose tests and measures that are age-appropriate and that will provide information on PT outcome effectiveness for specific functional goals and interventions.

Gross motor. Motor assessment tools are age and impairment specific. Multiple motor assessments are available to document motor skills and function. These motor assessments have been validated on youth with disabilities and provide information on motor skills, balance, agility, coordination, and motor development. Although these measures are used in individuals with ASD, not all measures have been validated for this patient population.

Developmental and functional mobility. The tests of developmental and functional mobility provide information on overall development (e.g., gross motor, fine motor, social/cognitive, communication), functional activities, mobility and adaptive behaviors. These tests and measures have been widely used to examine motor function and skills in individuals with ASD. Tests of functional mobility may be performance-based (i.e., the School Function Assessment) or judgment-based (i.e., The Pediatric Evaluation Disability Inventory–Computerized Adapted Testing (PEDI-CAT).

For adults with ASD, self-reported measures of functional ability include measures of communication, social reciprocity, repetitive behaviors, stereotyped interests, and maladaptive behaviors (Shattuck, Seltzer, Greenberg, Orsmond, Bolt, & Trani, 2007).

Physical activity. Evidence suggests that both self-report and objective physical activity measures should be used to document physical activity frequency and intensity in individuals with disabilities (Cervantes & Porretta, 2010; Trost & O'Neil, 2014). Accelerometers and pedometers are valid and reliable objective measures of physical activity in youth with typical development and disabilities (Trost, 2007; O'Neil, Fragala-Pinkham, Lennon, George, Forman et al., in press). Self-report measures help describe physical activity behaviors. Both types of measures may be important to document outcomes of interventions when the goal is increased physical activity for individuals with ASD.

Fitness. Total fitness is comprised of health-related fitness and skill-related fitness (American College of Sports Medicine, 2010). The fitness measures are mostly health-related measures that have been used with individuals with ASD.

Dole and Chafetz (2010) wrote a handbook for physical therapists referenced in this section of Table 13.2. This handbook provides useful information on normative values for fitness measures in typically developing youth which is useful when interpreting fitness outcomes for youth with ASD. The Brockport Test uses 27 items to assess fitness across four categories: Muscular strength/endurance and musculoskeletal function, body composition, aerobic function, and flexibility) (Winnick & Short, 1999). The 16 or 20 meter PACER (Progressive Aerobic Cardiovascular Run) or "beep test" is a field-based measure adapted from the Fitnessgram® which provides information on aerobic capacity for individuals with disabilities. Use of a heart rate monitor during a PACER test is recommended to determine exercise intensity and maximal heart rate (Winnick & Short, 1999). A self-reported rating scale of perceived exertion is used to determine exercise intensity during the PACER (Presidential Youth Fitness Program, 2013). Modified curl-ups, the isometric pushup, or the trunk lift can be used to measure muscular strength/endurance. The Fitnessgram® and Brockport tests use the sit-and-reach box to measure hamstring flexibility. Both tests also provide information on how to calculate BMI from height and weight to determine weight category (i.e., underweight, healthy weight, overweight, obese) as a marker for body composition (Presidential Youth Fitness Program, 2013).

Praxis and imitation batteries. Three age-specific praxis tests are included in Table 13.2. These tests describe the individual's motor imitation and motor planning abilities. These measures are used to document intervention outcomes (Bhat, Landa, & Galloway, 2011).

Participation. Measures of participation include parent and patient/client report and observation tools. Participation measures include self-report or structured interviews of individuals, parents, or caregivers. The Canadian Occupational Performance Measure (COPM) is a self-report measure used with adult and child patients. The COPM generates patient/client individualized goals and provides a rating scale for the individual or caregiver to rate importance, performance and satisfaction on these goals (Law, Baptiste, Carswell, McColl, Polatajko, & Pollock, 2005). The Child Assessment of Participation and Enjoyment (CAPE) questionnaire is a 55-item survey to identify activities in which youth participate after school (King et al., 2004) which has been validated for children with autism (Potvin, Snider, Kehavia, & Wood-Dauphinee, 2013). The CAPE provides information in several dimensions of participation (frequency, intensity, diversity, and enjoyment) and may provide information in change over time to examine intervention effectiveness when the goal is to increase participation by youth with ASD.

Contextual factors. The environment can be a facilitator or barrier to functional mobility, motor planning and control, physical activity and fitness. Although there are several questionnaires to identify social and physical environmental factors, there are none that are specific to individuals with ASD. Therefore, it is useful to conduct interviews with individuals with ASD, caregivers and teachers to identify environmental factors that promote health, function, and community participation and those that present as barriers. Information on contextual factors should be included in the plan of care to promote translation of clinical goals to community environments. Physical therapists can help individuals and families adapt the environment and find resources to promote function, health, and participation.

Interventions

PT interventions are designed to address patient/client and family/caregiver goals. Strategies must be appropriate for the individual's age, developmental level, and functional abilities.

INTERVENTION SETTINGS FOR CHILDREN WITH ASD. Early Intervention Services are available for individuals of different ages. This includes infants and toddlers with or at risk for ASD. These services are critical to promote mobility, exploration, and development of social skills and to reduce the risk for future functional delay (Bhat, Landa, & Galloway, 2011). Core signs that may indicate that an infant or young child may have or be at risk for ASD are: (1) Difficulty in social communication and interactions and (2) a ten-

Table 13.2
EXAMPLES OF TESTS AND MEASURES IN PHYSICAL THERAPY
EXAMINATIONS FOR INDIVIDUALS WITH ASD

Tests and measures	Infants & Toddlers	Children and Adolescents	Adults
Gross motor	Gross & Fine Motor Subtests of the Mullen Scale of Early Learning (Mullen, 1995)	Movement Assessment Battery for Children (MABC) (Croce, Horvak, & McCarthy, 2000)	Autism Diagnostic Interview–Revised (ADI-R) (Shattuck, et al., 2007)
	Alberta Infant Motor Scale (AIMS) (Piper, Darrah, 1994)	Bruininks-Oseretsky Test of Motor Proficiency (Bruininks & Bruininks, 2005)	Scales of Independent Behavior–Revised (SIB-R) (Shattuck et al., 2007)
	Autism Observational Schedule for Infants (Bryson et al., 2008)	Test of Gross Motor Development (TGMD2, 2000)	
	Peabody Developmental Motor Scales-2 (Folio & Fewell, 2000)		
Developmental & functional mobility	Parent Interview & Observations	Pediatric Evaluation Disability Inventory–Computerized Adapted Testing (PEDI-CAT) (Dumas & Fragala-Pinkham, 2012) (www.pedicat.com)	Autism Diagnostic Interview–Revised (ADI-R) (Shattuck et al., 2007)
	Mullens Scales of Early Learning (Mullen, 1995; Landa & Garret-Mayer, 2006)	PEDI-CAT Autism Module (in development) (Kramer, Coster, Kao, Snow, & Orsmond, 2013)	Scales of Independent Behavior–Revised (SIB-R) (Shattuck et al., 2007)
	Vineland II Scales of Adaptive Behavior (Sparrow, Ciccheti, & Barra, 2005)	School Function Assessment ~~(SFA, 1998)~~	
Physical activity	Accelerometers (Trost, 2007) Observation of Physical Activity and Play	Accelerometers (Trost, 2007) Pedometers (Tudor-Locke, 2004)	Accelerometers (Trost, 2007) Pedometers (Tudor-(Locke, 2004)

Table 13.2–*Continued*

		System for Observing Play and Leisure Activity in Youth (SOPLAY) (McKenzie, 2006)	Systematic Observation
		Physical Activity Log (Sallis, 1993)	Physical Activity Log (Sallis, 1993)
Fitness	Body Mass Index (BMI) (Krebs et al., 2007)	BMI, waist circumference, skin fold thickness (Krebs et al., 2007)	BMI, waist circumference, skin fold thickness (Krebs et al., 2007)
	Heart rate during activity (Dole & Chafetz, 2010)	Heart rate during PACER walk/run tests (FITNESSGRAM or Brockport) www.pyfp.org	Heart rate during walk/run tests (Fegan, 2009)
	Respiratory rate (Dole & Chafetz, 2010)	Respiratory rate and/or oxygen consumption during PACER walk/run tests (FITNESSGRAM or Brockport) (www.pyfp.org)	Respiratory rate and/or oxygen consumption during walk/run tests (Fegan, 2009)
		Functional Muscular Strength & Endurance Tests (sit-ups, push-ups, etc.) (FITNESSGRAM or Brockport) (www.pyfp.org)	Functional Muscular Strength & Endurance Tests (sit-ups, push-ups, etc.) (Fegan, 2009)
Praxis & imitation batteries	Autism Observational Scale for Infants (Bryson, Zwaigenbaum, & McDermott, 2008)	Sensory Integration and Praxis Test (Ayres, 1989)	Florida Apraxia Battery (Power, Code, Croot, & Sheard, 2010)
Participation	Parent-Child Interaction	Play-based Assessment	Environmental Assessment

continued

Table 13.2–*Continued*

		Canadian Occupational Performance Measure (COPM) ˋ(Law et al., 2005)	Canadian Occupational Performance Measure (COPM) (Law et al., 2005)
		Child Assessment of Participation and Enjoyment (CAPE, 2004) (Potvin, Snider, Prelock, Kehayia, & Wood-Dauphinee, 2013)	
Contextual factors	Parent interview on personal and environmental factors	Parent, child, teacher interview on personal and environmental factors	Patient or caregiver or employer interview on personal and environmental factors

Adapted from A. N. Bhat, R. J. Landa, & J. C. Galloway (2011). Current perspectives on motor functioning in infants, children, and adults with autism spectrum disorders. *Physical Therapy, 91,* 1116–1129; and S. M. Srinivasan, L. S. Pescatello, & A. N. Bhat (2014). Current perspectives on physical activity and exercise recommendations for children and adolescents with autism spectrum disorders. *Physical Therapy, 94,* 875–889.

dency for the child to engage in restricted, repetitive motor behavior patterns (Glumac et al., 2014).

Infants at risk for ASD may not have motor delays in the first year of life because some delays (such as onset of walking) do not manifest until the end of the first year (Bhat, Landa, & Galloway, 2011). Therefore, it is important that infants at risk be followed closely and that they have repeated motor development PT examinations in follow-up clinics or in early intervention settings (Bhat, Landa, & Galloway, 2011). In early intervention programs, it is important for the physical therapist to work closely with the family and the interdisciplinary team (i.e., educator, psychologist, speech and language pathologist, occupational therapist, nurse) to address the motor development issues associated with ASD such as strategies to promote exploratory play, redirect motor activities, and facilitate social, active play (O'Neil & Palisano, 2000).

School-aged children and adolescents (3–21 years old) may qualify for special education and related services including PT. These services may be delivered in the home, preschool, or day care settings for young children

(3–5 years old) and in school for older children (5–21 years old) (Kaminker, Chiarello, O'Neil, & Dichter, 2004). Some school-aged children and adolescents may also receive PT services in outpatient clinics (Kaminker, Chiarello, O'Neil, & Dichter C, 2004).

INTERVENTION SETTINGS FOR ADULTS. Adults may receive PT services to address specific functional mobility or motor needs. However, they usually receive PT less than other services that are important in the transition to adulthood including social support (housing and guardianship issues), employment, behavioral and occupational therapy, and pharmacotherapy (Aman, 2005; Shattuck, Roux , Hudson, Taylor, Maenner, & Trani, 2012)

GENERAL CONSIDERATIONS. PT interventions are designed to address patient/client and family/caregiver goals. Strategies must be appropriate for the individual's age, developmental level, and functional abilities. Motor learning principles are often incorporated into PT interventions for individuals with ASD to promote functional mobility and improve motor control and motor skills (Dowell, Mahone, & Mostofsky, 2009). These strategies include blocked or random practice schedules to promote motor skill acquisition and retention, different forms of feedback to provide the individual knowledge of performance or knowledge of response in gaining new motor skills, and whole and part practice to facilitate successful acquisition of discrete and complex motor tasks (Bhat, Landa, & Galloway, 2011).

In recent years, PT interventions have incorporated activity-based and fitness strategies to achieve PT goals and objectives and to promote health, fitness, and healthy weights in individuals with disabilities (Rowland, Fragala-Pinkham, Miles, & O'Neil, 2015; Srinivasan, Pescatello, & Bhat, 2014). Health promotion strategies are critical for youth with ASD because these children are 1.42 times more likely to be obese compared to children without obesity (Curtin, Anderson, & Bandini, 2010). Youth with ASD participate in less physical activity compared to peers with typical development and children with ASD participate in fewer activities and for shorter bouts compared to age-matched peers (Pan & Frey, 2006; Bandini et al., 2013).

General intervention strategies that physical therapists may use to improve health, function, and participation are provided in Table 13.3, Intervention Recommendations for Children with ASD. Goals of these interventions include: (1) improved participation in daily routines; (2) mastering new motor skills; (3) improved coordination, posture and balance; (4) enhanced reciprocal and bilateral tasks in play to promote motor and social skills (i.e., throwing and catching a ball with another person); (5) increased ability to imitate motor skills to learn new motor tasks and facilitate social interactions; and (6) increased health and fitness (Rowland, Fragala-Pinkham, Miles, & O'Neil, 2015; Glumac et al., 2014).

Because youth with ASD often have multiple sensorimotor challenges, it may be difficult to engage them in intervention sessions. It is important to tailor exercise programs to the individual's needs to promote and maintain adherence to exercise programs. Principles to consider in delivery of these programs include structure of the exercise environment and the physical therapist's approach to interact with the individual taking into consideration ways to provide feedback, instructions, and reinforcement (Srinivasan, Pescatello, & Bhat, 2014).

Considerations for infants and toddlers–birth to 3 years old. Physical therapists work with families and caregivers to increase a child's repertoire of motor skills and to promote participation in routines of daily life (Bhat, Bubela, & Landa, 2015). Therapists provide recommendations for parent-child play activities to improve infant and toddler motor skills, motor planning, and social interactions. Therapists provide support and guidance for structure, routines, and to adapt the environment to promote new skill acquisition and retention and positive behaviors in daily activities. Physical therapists may provide direct interventions to address body structure and function impairments such as strength, balance, and coordination. They often address activity limitations such as safe and efficient walking on flat surfaces (e.g., in classroom or cafeteria), uneven terrains (e.g., playground), and negotiating stairs and curbs. Strategies to promote imitation skills are important to improve motor development and social skills (e.g., singing songs while doing the actions to songs like "Head, Shoulders, Knees, and Toes," follow the leader, and animal walking games including crab, duck, and bear-walking) during indoor and outdoor play (Glumac et al., 2014).

Considerations for children ages 3–21 years. Physical therapists provide services to school-aged children in school or clinic settings. A students with ASD may receive special education services and may qualify for related services (e.g., physical therapy) based on the level of delay. Students in special education will have an individualized education program that defines service parameters (frequency, duration, goals, and objectives) (Effgen & Kaminker, 2014). If children with ASD have motor delays but no cognitive delays, they may qualify for related services in school under Section 504 of the Rehabilitation Act (Effgen & Kaminker, 2014; Kaminker, Chiarello, O'Neil, & Dichter, 2004).

School-aged children with ASD may have difficulty keeping up with their family members or other children at school, home, or on the playground. They may have difficulty walking up and down stairs due to decreased speed, endurance, or motor planning. In addition, children with ASD may have difficulty engaging in active play and sports during physical education classes or during recess or negotiating playground equipment (Srinivasan, Pescatello, & Bhat, 2014). These mobility issues may place limits on a child's ability to participate or socialize with other children. In the classroom setting, young children with ASD may have difficulty getting up and down from the floor during circle time, sitting at a desk for extended periods, or moving around in the classroom without bumping into other children or school furniture. Goals for children with ASD in the school setting may include being able to sit upright at a desk for extended periods, being able to access the school setting (i.e., classroom, school hallways, and school playground) safely and independently.

Activity-based interventions. Physical therapists often use activity-based or task oriented intervention strategies. Goals of activity-based interventions include increased strength and endurance fitness and promote activity and participation (Rowland, Fragala-Pinkham, Miles, & O'Neil, 2015). Task-oriented interventions often include direct teaching of specific motor skills. A motor task is broken down into smaller components and each component is taught individually and then steps are combined and practiced together to accomplish the entire task (Bhat, Bubela, & Landa, 2015). A cognitive approach also may be effective for improving motor skills in school-aged children with ASD. This approach entails combining the task-based intervention with a problem-solving framework to guide a child through the process of learning a new functional motor task. Cognitive interventions focus on teaching the strategies used for learning a new task so that patients/clients eventually transfer skills to new situations (Phelan, Steinke, & Mandich, 2009).

Physical therapists employed by school districts provide information and recommendations to parents and teachers to increase awareness about the impact of ASD on motor skills and functioning in school. Often, school-based physical therapists provide recommendations to promote inclusion activities to increase opportunities for socializing and modeling from same-aged peers among children with and without ASD. Physical therapists work with the interdisciplinary team in schools to reinforce social skills like self-regulation, listening, and taking turns during movement activities in physical education classes, on the playground before school or during recess, or during after-school programs (Glumac et al., 2014; Bhat, Bubela, & Landa, 2015). In clinic-based settings, therapists consult with family and community providers. Therapists in both settings make recommendations for home exercise programs and/or provide resources and ideas for active recreation to promote motor function and socialization (Glumac et al., 2014).

Intervention strategies depend on child's age and interests, functional mobility and school needs and parent, child, and teacher goals. For younger children who have difficulty with spatial awareness, using hula hoops, carpet squares, or specially placed seating (e.g., Nada Chair™ or camp chairs) can provide boundaries and identify personal space during circle time or when sitting on the floor during reading groups. Other examples of modifications include using ball chairs or "move and sit cushions" for children who have difficulty sitting still during classroom activities. Group classroom activities such as pairing a new vocabulary word with a specific yoga pose or movement activity such as "jumping jacks" can provide all children with a movement break during focused learning activities without singling out a child with autism. These whole-class movement breaks provide opportunities to reinforce movement skills needed to participate in social games and peer interactions (Bhat, Bubela, & Landa, 2015).

Community-based interventions. Community-based sports, mobility, and fitness programs provide opportunities for children and adults with ASD to participate in active recreation to promote fitness and functional mobility (Rowland, Fragala-Pinkham, Miles, & O'Neil, 2015; O'Neil, Fragala-Pinkham, Ideishi, & Ideishi, 2012). Fitness-related outcomes of exercise programs for children with ASD have been reported in land-based programs and aquatic-based exercise programs (Lang, Koegel, Ashbaugh, Regester, Ence, & Smith, 2010; Pan, 2011). Results suggest that both individual and group exercise programs improve strength, motor function, and aerobic fitness; however, individual sessions have better outcomes than group sessions (Sowa & Meulenbroek, 2012). Evidence indicates that children with ASD decrease stereotypic behaviors after participation in exercise interventions (Lang et al., 2010; Petrus, Adamson, Block, Einarson, Sharifnejad, & Harris, 2008). Components of exercise prescription include the frequency, intensity, duration, and type of intervention (American College of Sports Medicine, 2010).

Alternative therapies. Hippotherapy or therapeutic horseback riding is a physical and occupational therapy intervention strategy to improve function and participation in children with ASD (Gabriels et al., 2012). In hippotherapy, the horse's movements provide an unstable surface to promote trunk stability, postural balance, and control. Often, other activities are incorporated in hippotherapy sessions to promote motor skills, communication, and social interaction (e.g., mounting and dismounting sequences, riding skills, social-communication games when on the horse, grooming activities) (Gabriels et al., 2012). Evidence indicates that scores on the Vineland Adaptive Behavioral Scales-II improve in youth with ASD after hippotherapy in areas of motor control, postural stability, and adaptive behaviors (e.g., socialization, communication, receptive language, and coping skills) (Ajzenman, Standeven, & Shurtleff, 2013). Also, after hippotherapy, children with ASD have improved social function such as: sensory seeking, inattention/distractibility, sensory sensitivity, and sedentary behaviors (Bass, Duchowny, & Llabre, 2009).

CONSIDERATIONS FOR ADULTS 21 YEARS AND OLDER. Physical therapists work with adults with ASD to promote success in daily life. They recommend community resources to increase movement opportunities. They develop individualized exercise routines to promote motor coordination and walking skills. They work with each individual to help improve movement, function, and fitness to promote employment, function at home, and enjoy leisure activities (Glumac et al., 2014).

There is limited research that examines PT in adults with ASD and changes in function across the lifespan. This may be because adults with ASD exhibit increased prevalence of impairments in nonverbal communication and social reciprocity over time compared to impairments in functional motor skills, verbal communication, and repetitive or stereotypic behaviors (Shattuck et al., 2007). Moreover, adults with ASD receive transition services to promote independence in decision-making, personal responsibility, and financial independence so there may be a decreased focus and need for PT intervention (Shattuck et al., 2012).

Case Example

Jack is a nine-year-old boy with ASD (high functioning autism (HFA)) who is in the fourth grade in a public elementary school where he receives special education support services. He loves playing video games and watching the Boston Bruins on TV and attending his favorite local college hockey games. He lives with his parents and two older sisters.

History

Jack's mother reports that he was born at 42 weeks gestation without complications. She was concerned about gross motor milestones at 18 months of age and discussed concerns with the pediatrician. Jack rolled over at four months, sat independently at 10 months, started crawling on his belly at 12 months, but generally was content to sit and play with his toys. He would stand and take steps when held but did not cruise or initiate any walking on his own. She noted that he did not seem interested in other people or children and did not make attempts to communicate such as by pointing to objects or smiling in response to another person compared to her older daughters' development.

The pediatrician referred Jack to early intervention and he received a developmental assessment at 13 months of age. He demonstrated delayed gross motor, speech and communication skills, and started receiving weekly home visits by a physical therapist and a speech/language therapist weekly to assist the family with strategies to promote gross motor and communica-

Table 13.3
INTERVENTION RECOMMENDATIONS FOR CHILDREN WITH ASD

Intervention Strategies & Tactics	*Recommendations*
Environmental adaptations & instructions	1. Conduct interventions in the same physical space using familiar and predictable intervention activities (including equipment) and schedules. 2. Gradually introduce new activities. Build in time in the intervention so the child can adapt to new activities. 3. Have consistent personnel (therapists, assistants, coaches) conduct the interventions. 4. Be sure the intervention environment is at ambient temperatures (thermoneutral) because children have immature thermoregulatory systems. 5. Use visual cues (spot markers) so the child understands where to be when doing the exercises and activities 6. Adapt the environment to meet the child's needs. For children with hypersensitivity, avoid distractions, loud noises, and bright lights or be sure to provide modifications for the child such as sun glasses, ear phones, or head phones. 7. Use consistent verbal cues across therapy sessions with short and clear instructions. 8. Help the child to understand the progression of intervention activities and to anticipate transitions by using visual picture schedules or actual picture sequences of the interventions. 9. Combine verbal and visual instructions as much as possible. For example, use pictures with clear instructions such as "do this." 10. Use manual guidance as needed during the motor activities, especially when teaching a new task, but be sure to remove the guidance as soon as possible so the child does not rely on it. 11. To increase motivation, consider paired or group interventions for children with and without ASD to provide motor modeling for the child with ASD. 12. Use verbal reinforcement and gestures to provide motivating feedback (i.e., "good job" or high-fives). 13. To promote adherence to interventions, use the child's favorite sensory activities (i.e., stickers, small toys, healthy snacks) to provide a break and/or reward.
Intervention strategies & considerations	1. Use adaptive equipment to accommodate the child's motor needs such as a batting T in adaptive sports, adapted tricycles or bicycles, playground or sports balls with different textures or light weight. 2. Observe exercise intensity using heart rate monitors or pictorial scales of perceived exertion (i.e., OMNI, Robertson, 2000) for children who are hypersensitive and cannot tolerate wearing the monitor. Be sure to train the child in how to use a rating scale before using it to observe exercise intensity.

Table 13.3–*Continued*

3. Use scales to rate perceived exertion for children on antipsychotic medications because medications can affect resting and exercise heart rate and blood pressure (ACSM, 2010).
4. Consider individual sessions for children who are low functioning and group sessions for children who are high functioning.
5. Progress intervention activities and exercises gradually based on child's motor ability and response to exercise.
6. Give sufficient breaks and avoid overwhelming the child.
7. For exercise interventions, give sufficient time for warm-up and cool-down phases (Rowlands, Fragala-Pinkham, Miles & O'Neil, 2015).
8. Ask the child to communicate that an intervention activity or exercise needs to be stopped if the child demonstrates negative behaviors (i.e., tantrums, nonadherence, and self-injurious behaviors).
9. Be sure to collaborate with parents, caregivers, or teachers on behavioral plans for consistent approaches to address negative behaviors (Landa, 2007).
10. Encourage carry-over of intervention activities and exercises into the child's daily routine by providing parents or teachers with ideas and recommendations that may work in the home or school.
11. Use a variety of enjoyable activities that the child likes to help him or her be successful in participating in physical activity and exercise. Be sure to introduce the new activities slowly so that the child is not overwhelmed.

Adapted from: S. M. Srinivasan, L. S. Pescatello, & A. N. Bhat. (2014). Current perspectives on physical activity and exercise recommendations for children and adolescents with autism spectrum disorders. *Physical Therapy, 94,* 875–889.

tion skills. He attained independent walking on level surfaces at 20 months but still had decreased gross motor skills and balance. At three years of age, he was transitioned to a preschool program four mornings a week and received physical, occupational, and speech language therapy services two times per week for 30 minutes per session focusing on gross motor, fine motor, and communication skills in addition to education services. Jack's physical therapy preschool goals included walking up and down stairs in the school and on the playground structures with supervision; improving speed and ease of getting up off the floor after circle time, moving around on the playground and playground equipment (swing, slide, ladders, climbing net, and tricycle) with other children with supervision; improving gross motor skills such as running, jumping and ball skills for playing with other children.

The physical therapist worked on functional training by practicing motor skills such as getting up from the floor in the classroom, walking on the stairs and on the playground; strengthening activities including climbing, squatting down, and reaching overhead for toys, and using sports and games to also encourage core and leg strengthening; balance training on uneven or narrow surfaces on the playground and while kicking a soccer ball; and consultation with teachers and other school staff on ways to assist Jack with gross motor skills and participation in gross motor skills with other children in his preschool setting; and consultation with parents on ways to encourage gross motor skills.

At five years of age, he transitioned to kindergarten at his neighborhood school. He continued with speech therapy twice per week but was decreased to one time per week for occupational therapy and one time per month consultation services for physical therapy. At the end of kindergarten he was discharged from physical therapy services since he had achieved age appropriate gross motor skills and was keeping up with his peers in physical education class and on the playground during recess.

Current Issues

Jack is now in fourth grade and is functioning well academically in the areas of math and science but has some difficulty with reading and writing skills. He has a part-time, one-on-one classroom aide, special reading instruction 1 hour per week, and occupational therapy and speech/language services 1 time per week to focus on fine motor and communication skills. He also participates in a small group one time per week led by the speech therapist and focusing on social skills.

His fourth grade teacher was concerned that Jack is having difficulty keeping up with the other children on the playground and during weekly class field trips to the woods near the school for their science classes. Over the summer, Jack was having some issues with anxiety so he was started on a new medication which caused some issues with weight gain and may also be contributing to the problem. The physical education teacher also confirms that Jack requires frequent rests and modifications to participate in activities this year. The teacher discusses her concerns with Jack's family and they agree with the issues. A PT evaluation is requested.

PT Evaluation

PT examination findings were obtained by educational chart review and parent and teacher interview. The physical therapist observed Jack's mobility, activity, and participation in the classroom, on the playground, and in gym class. Jack has a one-to-one classroom aide to assist with organization of his school day.

TESTS AND MEASURES. Jack's functional skills were measured via teacher interview using the School Function Assessment. To examine Jack's fitness level, several tests were used: (1) the Fitnessgram PACER to determine aerobic capacity, (2) the Brockport isometric push-ups and modified curl-up for muscular endurance (Winnick & Short, 1999), (3) the BOT-2 for motor proficiency (Bruininks & Bruininks, 2005), and (4) BMI and waist circumference for body composition. The COPM was used to generate and rate Jack's individual goals to promote functional mobility and fitness (Law et al., 2005).

PT DIAGNOSIS. Jack's PT diagnosis was decreased motor skills, functional mobility and fitness were associated with decreased activity, participation and increased weight.

PROGNOSIS. Jack's motor skills, functional mobility, and fitness will improve in 12–14 weeks of PT 1x/week and the 14-week skating program 1x/week. It is anticipated that he will increase his activity level during PT sessions, at recess time, and in the community setting at home and by participating in the skating program after school and that he will improve his motor skills and balance and move towards a healthy weight.

PLAN OF CARE. Jack will receive direct PT intervention once a week to address motor control, fitness, and overall functional mobility. The physical therapist will work closely with the teacher, OT, and speech and language pathologist to ensure that Jack's motor skill interventions and opportunities are integrated with other classroom activities and services.

PT INTERVENTION. Jack will receive PT at school, once a week and he will be referred to the adaptive skating program to promote motor control, balance, and fitness. Also, he will have the opportunity for social participation and fun during the skating program.

This case illustrated the types of intervention strategies that a physical therapist may use in providing PT for a child with ASD at different ages and during different episodes of care and settings including early intervention, preschool, and school settings.

References

Aman, M.G. (2005). Treatment planning for patients with autism spectrum disorders. *Journal of Clinical Psychiatry, 66*(S10), 38–45.

American Academy of Child and Adolescent Psychiatry. (AACAP). (1999). Summary of the practice parameters for the assessment and treatment of children, adolescents, and adults with autism and other pervasive developmental disorders. *Journal of the Academy of Child & Adolescent Psychiatry, 38*(12), 1611–1615.

American College of Sports Medicine. (2010). ACSM's Guidelines for exercise testing and prescription (8th ed.). Philadelphia, PA: Lippincott Williams and Wilkins.

American Physical Therapy Association Board of Directors (APTA, BOD). (2014). Guidelines: Physical therapy documentation of patient/client management (BOD G03-05-16-41). Retrieved from http://www.apta.org/uploadedFiles /APTAorg/About_Us/Policies/Practice/DocumentationPatientClientManage ment.pdf

American Physical Therapy Association (APTA). (2014). *Guide to physical therapist practice 3.0.* Retrieved from http://guidetoptpractice.apta.org/

American Psychiatric Association. (2013). *Diagnostic and statistical manual of mental disorders* (5th ed.). Washington, DC: Author.

Ayres, A. J. (2014). *Sensory integration and praxis tests: SIPT manual.* Los Angeles: Western Psychological Services.

Ajzenman, H. F., Standeven, J. W., & Shurtleff, T. L. (2013). Effect of hippotherapy on motor control, adaptive behaviors, and participation in children with autism spectrum disorders: A pilot study. *American Journal of Occupational Therapy, 67,* 653–663.

Bandini, L. G., Gleason, J., Curtin, C., Lividini, K., Anderson, S. E., Cermack, S. A., Maslin, A., & Must, A. (2013). Comparison of physical activity between children with autism spectrum disorders and typically developing children. *Autism, 17*(1), 44–54.

Barry, M. J., & Edgman-Levitan, S. (2012). Shared decision making: The pinnacle of patient-centered care perspective. *New England Journal of Medicine, 366,* 780–781.

Bass, M. M., Duchowny, C. A., & Llabre, M. M. (2009). The effect of therapeutic horseback riding on social functioning in children with autism. *Journal of Autism & Developmental Disorders, 39,* 261–1267.

Bronfenbrenner, U. (1993). Ecological models of human development. In *International encyclopedia of education* (2nd ed., Vol. 3). Oxford: Elsevier. Reprinted in M. Gauvain & M. Cole (Eds.), *Readings on the development of children* (2nd ed., pp. 37–43). New York: Freeman.

Bhat, A. N., Landa, R. J., & Galloway, J. C. (2011). Current perspectives on motor functioning in infants, children, and adults with autism spectrum disorders. *Physical Therapy, 91,* 1116–1129.

Bhat, A. N., Bubel, D., & Landa, R. (2015). Autism spectrum disorders and physical therapy. In J. S. Tecklin (Ed.), *Pediatric physical therapy* (5th ed., pp. 403–423). Philadelphia: Lippincott Williams & Wilkins.

Bruininks, R. H., & Bruininks, B. D. (2005). *The Bruininks-Oseretsky test of motor proficiency (BOT-2)* (2nd ed.). Minneapolis, MN: Pearson Assessments.

Bryson, S. E., Zwaigenbaum, L., McDermott, C., Rombough, V., & Brian, J. (2008). The autism observation scale for infants: Scale development and reliablity data. *Journal of Autism & Developmental Disorders, 3,* 731–738.

Casanova, M., Buxhoeveden, D., Switala, A., & Roy, E. (2002). Minicolumnart pathology in autism. *Neurology, 58*(3), 428–432.

Cattaneo, L., & Rizzolatti, G. (2009). The mirror neuron system. *Archives of Neurology, 665*(5), 557–560.

Centers for Disease Control and Prevention (CDC). (2014). Prevalence of autism spectrum disorder among children aged 8 years: Autism and Developmental Disabilities Monitoring Network. *Morbidity and Mortality Weekly Report, 63*(SS 2), 1–21.

Cervantes, C. M., & Porretta, D. L. (2010). Physical activity measurement among individuals with disabilities: A literature review. *Adapted Physical Activity Quarterly, 27,* 173–190.

Chugani, D. C. (2005). Pharmacological intervention in autism: Targeting critical periods of brain development. *Clinical Neuropsychology, 2*(6), 346–353.

Cliff, D. P., Reilly, J. J., & Okely, A. D. (2009). Methodological considerations in using accelerometers to assess habitual physical activity in children aged 0–5 years. *Journal of Science and Medicine in Sports, 12*(5), 557–567.

Coster, W., Deeney, T., Haltiwanger, J., & Haley, S. (1998). *School function assessment.* San Antonio, TX: The Psychological Corporation.

Courchesne, E., Redcay, E., & Kennedy, D. (2004). The autistic brain: Birth through adulthood. *Current Opinions in Neurology, 17*(4), 489–496.

Croce, R., Horvak, M., & McCarthy, E. (2000). Reliability and concurrent validity of the Movement Assessment Battery for Children. *Perceptual Motor Skills, 93,* 275–280.

Curtin, C., Anderson, S. E., Must, A., & Bandini, L. (2010). The prevalence of obesity in children with autism: A secondary data analysis using nationally representative data from the National Survey of Children's Health. *BMC Pediatric, 10,* 1–5.

Dapretto, D., Davies, M. S., Pfeiffer, J. H., Scott, A. A., Sigman, M., Bookheimer, S. Y., & Iacoboni, M. (2006). Understanding emotions in others: Mirror neuron dysfunction in children with autism spectrum disorders. *Nature Neuroscience, 9*(1), 28–30.

Dole, R. L., & Chafetz, R. (2010). *Peds rehab notes: Evaluation and intervention pocket guide.* Philadelphia: F. A. Davis.

Dowell, L. R., Mahone, E. M., & Mostofsky S. H. (2009). Associations of postural knowledge and basic motor skill with dyspraxia in autism: Implication for abnormalities in distributed connectivity and motor learning. *Neuropsychology, 23*(5), 563–570.

Downey, R., & Rapport, M. J. K. (2012). Motor activity in children with autism: A review of current literature. *Pediatric Physical Therapy, 24,* 2–20.

Dumas, H. M., & Fragala-Pinkham, M. A. (2012). Concurrent validity and reliability of the pediatric evaluation of disability inventory-computer adaptive test mobility domain. *Pediatric Physical Therapy, 24,* 171–176.

Effgen, S. K., & Kaminker, M. K. (2014). Nationwide survey of school-based physical therapy practice. *Pediatric Physical Therapy, 26,* 394–403.

Folio, M. R., & Fewell R. R. (2000). *Peabody developmental motor scales examiner's manual* (2nd ed). Austin, TX: Pro-Ed.

Fournier, K. A., Hass, C. J., Naik, S. K., Lodha, N., & Cauragh, J. H. (2010). Motor coordination in autism spectrum disorder: A synthesis and meta-analysis. *Journal of Autism & Developmental Disorders, 40,* 1227–1240.

Gabriels, R. L., Agnew, J. A., Holt, K. D., Shoffner, A., Zhaoxing, P., Ruzzano, S., . . . Mesibov, G. (2012). *Research in Autism Spectrum Disorders, 6,* 578–588.

Glumac, L., Pallai, B., Tartick, K., Savard, L., Bake, M., Greeley, K., & Milkavich, L. (2014). *Physical therapist's guide to autism spectrum disorder,* APTA Move Forward Guide. Retrieved from http://www.moveforwardpt.com/SymptomsConditions Detail.aspx?cid= a6482e75-65c6-4c1f-be36-5f4a847b2042#.VQoS0CmY11I

Jansiewicz, E. M., Goldberg, M. C., Newschaffer, C. J., Denckla, M. B., Landa, R., & Mostofsky, S. H. (2006). Motor signs distinguish children with high functioning autism and Asperger's syndrome from controls. *Journal of Autism & Developmental Disorders, 36,* 613–621.

Kaminker, M., Chiarello, L., O'Neil, M. E., & Dichter, C. (2004). Decision making for service delivery in schools: A survey of pediatric physical therapists. *Physical Therapy, 84,* 919–933.

Kao, Y. C., Kramer, J. M., Liljenquist, K., & Coster, W. J. (2015). Association between impairment, function, and daily life task management in children and adolescents with autism. *Developmental Medicine and Child Neurology, 57*(1), 68–74.

King, G., Law, M., King, S., Hurley, P., Hanna, S., Kertoy, M., Rosenbaum, P., & Young, N. (2004). *Children's assessment of participation and enjoyment (CAPE) and preferences for activities of children (PAC).* San Antonio, TX: Harcourt Assessment, Inc.

Kramer, J. M., Coster, W. J., Kao, Y. C., Snow, A., & Orsmond, G. I. (2013). A new approach to the measurement of adaptive behavior: Development of the PEDI-CAT for children and youth with autism spectrum disorders. *Physical and Occupational Therapy in Pediatrics, 33*(3), 366–367.

Krebs, N. F., Himes, J. H., Jacobson, D., Nicklas, T. A., Guilday, P., & Styne, D. (2007). Assessment of child and adolescent overweight and obesity. *Pediatrics, 120,* 193–228.

Hayakawa, K., & Kobayashi, K. (2011). Physical and motor skill training for children with intellectual disabilities. *Perceptual Motor Skills, 112,* 573–580.

Landa, R. (2007). Early communication development and intervention for children with autism. *Mental Retardation & Developmental Disabilities, 13,* 16–25.

Landa, R., & Garrett-Mayer, E. (2006). Development in infants with autism spectrum disorders: A prospective study. *Journal of Child Psychology and Psychiatry, 47*(6), 629–638.

Lang, R., Koegel, L. K., Ashbaugh, K., Regester, A., Ence, W., & Smith, W. (2010). Physical exercise and individuals with autism spectrum disorders: A systematic review. *Research in Autism Spectrum Disorders, 4*(4), 565–576.

Law, M., Baptiste, S., Carswell, A., McColl, M., Polatajko, H., & Pollock, N. (2005). *Canadian occupational performance measure* (4th ed.). Ottawa, Ontario: CAOT Publications.

McKenzie, T. L. (2006). SOPLAY: System for observing play and leisure activity in youth. Retrieved from http://activelivingresearch.org/soplay-system-observing-play-and-leisure-activity-youth

MacDonald, M., Esposito, P., & Hauck, J. (2012). Bicycle training for youth with Down syndrome and autism spectrum disorders. *Focus: Autism and Other Developmental Disabilities, 27,* 12–21.

Ming, X., Brimacombe, M., & Wagner G. C. (2007). Prevalence of motor impairment in autism spectrum disorders. *Brain & Development, 29*(9), 565–570.

Minshew, N. J., Sung, K., Jones, B. L., & Furman, J. M. (2004). Underdevelopment of the postural control system in autism. *Neurology, 63,* 2056–2061.

Mostofsky, S. H., Powell, S. K., Simmonds, D. J., Goldberg, M. C., Caffo, B., & Pekar, J. J. (2009). Decreased connectivity and cerebellar activity in autism during motor task performance. *Brain, 132*(9), 2413–2425.

Mullen, E. M. (1995). *Mullen scales of early learning.* Circle Pines, MA: American Guidance Service.

O'Neil, M. E., Fragala-Pinkham, M., Ideishi, R. I., & Ideishi, S. K. (2012). Community-based programs for children and youth: Our experiences in design, implementation and evaluation. *Physical & Occupational Therapy in Pediatrics, 32*(2), 111–119.

O'Neil, M. E., & Palisano, R. (2000). Attitudes toward family-centered care and clinical decision making in early intervention among physical therapists. *Pediatric Physical Therapy, 12,* 173–182.

O'Neil, M. E., Fragala-Pinkham, M. A., Lennon, N., George, A., Forman, J., & Trost, S. G. (2015). Reliability and validity in measuring physical activity in youth with cerebral palsy who are ambulatory. *Physical Therapy, 95*(10), published ahead of print.

Pan, C. (2011). The efficacy of an aquatic program on physical fitness and aquatic skills in children with and without autism spectrum disorders. *Research in Autism Spectrum Disorder, 5,* 657–665.

Pan, C., & Frey, G. C. (2006). Physical activity patterns in youth with autism spectrum disorders. *Journal of Autism & Developmental Disorders, 36,* 597–606.

Petrus, C., Adamson, S., Block, L., Einarson, S., Sharifneja, M., & Harris, S. (2008). Effects of exercise interventions on stereotypic behaviors in children with autism spectrum disorder. *Physiotherapy Canada, 60,* 134–145.

Phelan, S., Steinke L., & Mandich A. (2009). Exploring a cognitive intervention for children with pervasive developmental disorder. *Canadian Journal of Occupational Therapy, 76*(1), 23–28.

Piper, M., & Darrah J. (1994). *Motor assessment of the developing infant.* Philadelphia: Saunders.

Potvin, M. C., Snider, L., Prelock, P. A., Kehayia, E., & Wood-Dauphinee, S. (2013). Psychometrics of the children's assessment of participation and enjoyment for those with high functioning autism. *American Journal of Occupational Therapy, 6*(2), 209–217.

Power, E., Code, C., Croot, K., & Sheard, C. (2010). Florida Apraxia Battery–Extended and Revised Sydney (FABERS): Design, description, and a healthy control sample. *Journal of Clinical and Experimental Neuropsychology, 32*(1), 1–18.

Presidential Youth Fitness Program. (2013). *Presidential youth fitness program physical educator resource guide.* Silver Spring, MD: National Foundation on Fitness, Sports and Nutrition. Retrieved from http://www.pyfp.org/.

Robertson, R .J., Goss, F. I., Boer, N. F., Peoples, J. A., Foreman, A. J., Dabayebeh, I. M., . . . Thompkins, T. (2000). Children's OMNI Scale of Perceived Exertion: Mixed gender and race validation. *Medicine & Science in Sports & Exercise, 32*(2), 452–458.

Rowland, J. L., Fragala-Pinkham, M., Miles, C., & O'Neil, M .E. (2015). The scope of pediatric physical therapy practice in health promotion and fitness for youth with disabilities. *Pediatric Physical Therapy, 27,* 2–15.

Reuben, D. B., & Tinetti, M. E. (2012). Goal-oriented patient care: An alternative health outcomes paradigm. *New England Journal of Medicine, 366,* 777–779.

Sallis, J. F., Buono, M. J., Roby, J. J., Micale, F. G., & Nelson, J. A. (1993). Seven-day recall and other physical activity self-reports in children and adolescents. *Medicine & Science in Sports & Exercise, 25*(1), 99–108.

Schmitz, C., Martineau, K., Barthelemy, C., & Assinante, C. (2003). Motor control and children with autism: Deficit of anticipator function? *Neuroscience Letters, 348,* 1–20.

Shattuck, P. T., Seltzer, M. M., Greenberg, J. S., Orsmond, G. I., Bolt, D., Kring, S., Lounds, J., & Lord, C. (2007). Changes in autism symptoms and maladaptive behaviors in adolescents and adults with autism spectrum disorder. *Journal of Autism & Developmental Disorders, 37,* 1735–1747.

Shattuck, P. T., Roux, A. M., Hudson, L. E., Taylor, J. L., Maenner, M. J., & Trani, J. F. (2012). Services for adults with an autism spectrum disorder. *Canadian Journal of Psychiatry, 57*(5), 284–291.

Sowa, M., & Meulenbroek, R. (2012). Effects of physical exercise on autism spectrum disorders: A meta-analysis. *Research in Autism Spectrum Disorders, 6,* 46–57.

Sparrow, S., Chiccetti, D. V., & Balla, D. (2005). *Vineland adaptive behavior scales* (2nd ed.). Minneapolis, MN: Pearson Assessments.

Srinivasan, S. M., Pescatello, L. S., & Bhat, A. N. (2014). Current perspectives on physical activity and exercise recommendations for children and adolescents with autism spectrum disorders. *Physical Therapy, 94,* 875–889.

Steiner, W. A., Ryser, L., Huber, E., Uebelhart, D., Aeschlimann, A., & Stucki, G. (2002). Use of the ICF Model as a clinical problem-solving tool in physical therapy and rehabilitation medicine. *Physical Therapy, 82*(11), 1098–1107.

Sullivan, K. J., Wallace, J., O'Neil, M. E., Musolina, G., Mandich, M., Studer, M. T., & Bottomly, J. M. (2011). A vision for 2050: Physical therapy as partners in the national health agenda. *Physical Therapy, 91*(11), 1–9.

Ulrich, D. (2000). *Test of gross motor development.* Framingham, MA, Therapro, Inc.

Trost, S. G. (2007). State of the art reviews: Measurement of physical activity in children and adolescents. *American Journal of Lifestyle Medicine, 1,* 299–314.

Trost, S. G., & O'Neil, M. E. (2014). Clinical use of objective measures of physical activity. *British Journal of Sports Medicine, 48*(3), 178–181.

Tudor-Locke, C., Pangrazi, R. P., Corbin, C. B., Rutherford, W. J., Vincent, S. D., Raustorp, A., Tomson, L. M., & Cuddihy, T. F. (2004). BMI-referenced standards for recommended pedometer-determined steps/day in children. *Preventive Medicine, 8*(6), 857–864.

Williams, D., Goldstein, G., & Minshew, N. (2006). Neuropsychologic functioning in children with autism: Further evidence for disordered complex information processing. *Child Neuropsychology, 12*(4–5), 279–298.

Wing, L., Gould, J., & Gillberg, C. (2011). Autism spectrum disorders in the DSM-5: Better or worse than the DSC-IV? *Research in Developmental Disabilities, 32,* 768–773.

Winnick, J. P., & Short, F. X. (1999). *The brockport physical fitness test manual: A health-related test for youth with physical and mental disabilities.* Champaign, IL: Human Kinetics.

World Health Organization (WHO). (2002). *Towards a common language for functioning, disability and health.* ICF. WHO, Geneva, Switzerland.

Chapter 14

USING BIG DATA TO DIRECT QUALITY IMPROVEMENT

Carl V. Tyler, Jr.

An Introduction to Big Data

What is Big Data? How is it currently being used? Importantly, how can it be applied to health information systems for use in quality improvement? This chapter is divided into three sections. The first section will acquaint the reader by defining Big Data, explaining its organization and characteristics, and include common uses for Big Data platforms. The second section will use the experience from the Learning Collaborative in Developmental Medicine from the Cleveland Clinic to illustrate its utility in quality improvement, and point out some methodological concerns in Big Data analytics. This section will also include examples of Big Data analytics that are related to health concerns for people with autism spectrum disorder (ASD). Lastly, this chapter includes a look to the future, and addresses the potential of Big Data to improve health care for people with ASD, through analytics and integration into quality improvement projects.

Definition of Big Data

As it relates to health systems, Big Data refers to continuously produced, high volumes of clinical and health service data requiring specialized computerized platforms to accrue, manage, and utilize that data for clinical, administrative, and research purposes. Because of the wide variety, types and sources of contributing information, Big Data platforms require complex capacities to integrate that data into forms that can be interpreted and utilized in intended ways. To the three words typically applied to describe Big

Data–"high volume, velocity, and variety," one of the leading health information management companies in the United States, the creators of Explorys®, have suggested the additional core features of "veracity" and "value" (Explorys, n.d.).

Characteristics and Organization of Big Data

Primary sources of Big Data typically include clinical data documented in electronic health records (EHRs), claims data for healthcare cost reimbursement, and pharmaceutical data. Electronic health record data provides information about medical diagnoses, procedures, pharmacotherapies, diagnostic laboratory, and imaging test orders and results, referrals, and biophysical data such as vital signs (Tyler, Schramm, Karafa, Tang, & Jain, 2010). Of particular relevance to ASD is the potential for big data systems to merge genetic information with other health and service information (Denny, 2012; Hoffman, 2007; Weber, Mandl, & Kohane, 2014).

Big Data contains both structured, coded data (e.g., linked to diagnoses or procedures) and unstructured narrative text such as ambulatory encounter clinical notes, inpatient admission and progress notes, and discharge summaries. The complex task of extracting structured information from narrative text is possible through an array of methods termed natural language processing tools (Jensen, Jensen, & Brunak, 2012).

Analytic Platforms for Big Data and Their Key Functions

Big Data platforms have to perform complex functions in order for clinicians, administrators, researchers, and others to make sense of the data. There are several functions including: Critical integrating functions, standardizing functions, ontologies, and analytic functions. These are described below.

Big Data platforms have critical integrating functions. These include a means to identify when data from different sites and sources is linked to the same individual.

Standardizing data includes correctly uniting the same pieces of information, which appear, and are labeled in different ways. For example, Explorys identified no less than 17 different ways that the single blood test HgbA1c, a measure of blood glucose control in people with diabetes, appeared in their data.

Big Data platforms must have an organizing set of hierarchical structures with defined relationships between these structures, called ontologies, to logically organize the data and to allow query or retrieval from the Big Data repository. Many Big Data systems rely on the underlying clinical terms, concepts, and hierarchies defined by the Systematized Nomenclature of Medicine-Clinical Terms (SNOMED-CT®) (SNOMED, 2015).

Analytic functions include correctly linking data by patient, provider, site of care, test, diagnosis, and/or treatment, within specified timeframes. Analytic capacity needs to allow for deidentification of protected health information for population level analytic purposes, as well as the ability, with proper authorization, to reidentify patients for research, clinical care, and quality improvement purposes. Finally, information derived from Big Data platforms must be sufficiently specific and valid to intelligently direct actions that lead to improved health care.

Big Data Management Companies

Explorys typifies the scale of leading Big Data management companies in the United States. Founded as an innovation spinoff from the Cleveland Clinic in 2009, Explorys' healthcare partners include some of the most prominent healthcare systems in the United States, together accounting for over $63 billion in care. With over 275 billion clinical, financial, and operational data elements, spanning 48 million unique patients, 340 hospitals and over 300,000 providers, Explorys' secure cloud-computing platform is being used by 23 major integrated healthcare systems to identify patterns in diseases, treatments, and outcomes. This network includes Cleveland Clinic, Trinity Health, St. Joseph Health System, Catholic Health Partners, Adventist Health System, and many others with patients in all 50 states (Explorys, n.d.).

Common Uses of Big Data

Utilization of big data has often focused on patients and services related to common and high cost conditions, such as diabetes and heart disease, and services included in commonly employed measures of healthcare quality, such as Healthcare Effectiveness and Data Information Set (HEDIS) criteria (Barrington, 2014; Safran et al., 2007).

However, the large and diverse populations whose information is captured by Big Data also allows for investigation of health and services provided to people with rarer conditions, or ones whose care is not well assessed through commonly employed quality measures. People with developmental disabilities typify one such subpopulation, whose care quality is insufficiently characterized through standard quality measures alone. The following real-life example demonstrates how Big Data was utilized to inform the work of a multistakeholder quality improvement and educational group called the Learning Collaborative in Developmental Medicine.

Quality Improvement Initiative: The Learning Collaborative in Developmental Medicine

The Learning Collaborative in Developmental Medicine was a multistakeholder, educational and quality improvement collaborative, which aimed to improve the care of adults with intellectual and other developmental disabilities (IDD) at the health system level (Tyler & Werner, 2014). This was a year-long quality improvement initiative internally funded by the Medicine Institute of the Cleveland Clinic. The group met on a bimonthly basis for four hours with one-hour telephone conference call planning meetings on alternating months.

Each face-to-face session focused on a single subgroup of people with IDD. Each meeting included a presentation by content experts, self-advocates, family members or service providers, advocacy organizations, and healthservice providers. In addition, for each subgroup discussed, deidentified population level analyses of Big Data (limited to Cleveland Clinic patients) were presented. The Learning Collaborative group members incorporated those data analyses into their discussions about ways to improve health through patient care tools for use by self-advocates, families, service, and healthcare providers.

The deidentified health and service data reviewed by the Learning Collaborative participants pertained to adults with IDD who received care through the Cleveland Clinic between 2007 and 2013. Data included demographics, diagnoses, laboratory studies, biophysical data, procedures, and pharmacotherapies. Searches were conducted via a web-based server developed by Explorys. Analyses were reported as health system population count and proportion estimates. Explorys collaborators served as consultants to the Learning Collaborative to optimize use of Explorys functionalities for these specific purposes.

Big Data Analyses Pertaining to Health Care of Adults with Down Syndrome

The following analyses refer to a cohort of adults with Down syndrome who received health care through the Cleveland Clinic between 2007 and 2013. Table 14.1 depicts the demographic characteristics of this cohort. Table 14.2 illustrates common comorbid physical and mental health characteristics specifically relevant to people with Down syndrome, and compares their rates, termed "population proportion estimates (designated in the tables as "PPN")" to population prevalence (designated in the tables as "PREV"), derived from the medical literature. Discrepancies in rates of comorbidities between the health system data (population proportion estimates) and the medical literature

Table 14.1
DEMOGRAPHIC CHARACTERISTICS OF
COHORT OF ADULTS WITH DOWN SYNDROME

Age (in years)	Count	Proportion (PPN)*
15–19	60	4
20–24	150	12
25–29	110	9
30–34	120	9
35–39	120	9
40–44	140	9
45–49	150	11
50–54	150	12
55–59	120	9
60–64	80	6
65–69	30	2
Race/Ethnicity		
African-American	120	9
Caucasian	870	71
Hispanic/Latino	20	1

*PPN as population proportion estimates are not numerically equal to count percentages.

(population prevalence) were interpreted as possible failures of screening, diagnosis, and/or documentation in the electronic health record.

These Big Data analyses suggested that among adults with Down syndrome, clinicians adequately recognized and documented comorbid thyroid disease and myelopathy. Rates of comorbid mental health conditions of depression, obsessive-compulsive disorder and dementia were also congruent with those reported in the medical literature. In contrast, there appeared to be deficits in screening, diagnosis and/or documentation of visual and hearing impairments, celiac disease, osteoporosis, obesity, and ASD. While these analyses represented crude, unadjusted estimates of comorbid conditions, they provided general target areas for the multistakeholder team to focus their quality improvement efforts.

Methodological Issues in Big Data Analytics

End-users of Big Data need to appreciate the state of the emerging science around managing and interpreting Big Data. The ways that core analytic platform functions outlined above are addressed (or not addressed) represent potential areas of bias and error in the interpretation of Big Data

Table 14.2
COMORBID CONDITIONS IN COHORT OF ADULTS WITH DOWN SYNDROME
COMPARED TO PREVALENCE DOCUMENTED IN MEDICAL LITERATURE

Condition	Count	PPN*	Prev (%)	Interpretation
Sensory				
Hearing loss	130	11	50	Underscreening/dx/documentation
Vision disorder	110	9	4	Underscreening/dx/documentation
Medical				
Hypothyroidism	510	42	30–40	Adequate screening
Hyperthyroidism	30	2	1	Adequate screening
Celiac disease	30	2	10	Underscreening
Gout	80	7	Unknown	Unknown
Osteoporosis	70	6	20–50	Underscreening/dx/documentation
Obesity	200	18	50	Underscreening/dx/documentation
Myelopathy	20	2	1–2	Adequate diagnosis
Mental Health				
Depression	150	12	2–10	Adequate diagnosis
OCD	40	3	2–5	Adequate diagnosis
Anxiety	50	4	Unknown	Unknown
Dementia	130	11	4–13	Adequate diagnosis
Autism	20	2	2–10	Possible underdiagnosis

*PPN = Population Proportion Estimates, Prev = Prevalence as documented in medical literature, Dx = Diagnosis.

analyses. For example, in a recent study of comorbid conditions in people with ASD utilizing data from several health systems within the same geographic region, investigators did not identify when data from different sites and sources were linked to the same individual (Kohane et al., 2012).

The sensitivity of electronic health record (EHR) data varies widely according to the type of information. Sensitivity is highest for prescribing and diagnostic test data, while it is lowest for lifestyle, social, educational, and economic information (Thiru, Hassey, & Sullivan, 2003). Unfortunately, these later domains that are poorly captured in EHRs are critical environmental and psychosocial determinants of health and quality of life in people with ASD. Data exchanges that link EHR data to public health and other databases have the potential to address some of these inherent limitations to EHRs (Guilbert et al., 2012).

In a review of data quality assessment of EHR data reused for research, Weiskopf and Weng (2013) characterized five dimensions of EHR data quality as completeness, correctness, concordance, plausibility, and currency. They also delineated EHR data-quality assessment methods into the following seven categories: Comparison with gold standard, data element agreement, data source agreement, distribution comparison, validity checks, log review, and element presence.

Researchers, health policy and health system leaders desiring to utilize information from Big Data sources are well-advised to talk with clinical informatics specialists who are knowledgeable about the specific Big Data platform they intend to access and who can address the data quality and data quality assessment issues outlined above. Similarly, conversations with frontline clinicians and others who enter clinical information into the EHRs of participating health system networks can provide critical insight into the quality and limitations of the data from a "frontline" perspective (Bowman, 2013; Phillips & Fleming, 2009).

Methodological questions inherent to any cohort analysis include how the ASD cohort will be defined, issues of sensitivity and specificity, and an appraisal of the advantages, disadvantages, and limitations to the methods employed to define the cohort. Similar questions apply when defining any comparison cohorts.

Applying Big Data Analytics to ASD

The following series of analyses exemplify the analytic capacity of one of the core applications developed by Explorys, termed Enterprise Performance Management: Explore, which allows deidentified population level analyses of Big Data from participating health system networks to be conducted within seconds.

A cohort of 39,540 individuals who carried a diagnosis of autistic disorder was identified. Stratification by age yielded a subset of 14,400 adults. Subsequent analyses reported below were conducted on this adult subset. While 92% of this adult cohort had a healthcare encounter within the past five years, only 63% had been seen within the past year, suggesting that a significant proportion of the cohort may not receive regular health care on an annual basis.

In general, approximately 20% of ASD is associated with a molecular genetic anomaly, some of which are recognizable clinical syndromes (Rosti, Sadek, Vaux, & Gleeson, 2013). In this cohort, about 1% bore a comorbid diagnosis of fragile X syndrome, a frequency consistent with published case series (Reddy, 2005). Further analyses stratified by this and other ASD-associated clinical syndromes are feasible.

A series of queries related to common physical conditions relevant to people with ASD was conducted. For example, gastrointestinal issues are common in people with ASD (Buie et al., 2010; Carbone, 2013; Hsiao, 2014). Thirty-four percent of the cohort had at least one healthcare encounter in which a gastrointestinal disorder was listed as a diagnosis. Under each category of gastrointestinal disorder, further specification through a SNOMED-based ontology is possible.

In a similar fashion, a query about comorbid epilepsy was conducted. Twenty-one percent of the cohort had at least one healthcare encounter in which epilepsy was a listed diagnosis. This value is comparative to pooled estimates of comorbid epilepsy of 23.7% and 8.9% in studies of people with ASD, with and without intellectual disability (Tuchman, Hirtz, & Mamounas, 2013). Five percent of the total cohort had at least one encounter in which an antiepileptic drug allergy was diagnosed.

Comorbid allergic conditions are an area of intense clinical interest, scrutiny, and concern in people with ASD (Angelidou et al., 2013; Kotey, Ertel, & Whitcomb, 2014). Thirty-nine percent of this cohort was diagnosed at least once with an allergic condition; 13% of the total cohort had specifically an IgE-mediated allergic condition.

Sleep disturbances are a significant neurobehavioral issue in people with ASD (Nicolaidis, Kripke, & Raymaker, 2014; Tani, Lindberg, Nieminen-von Wendt, von Wendt, & Alanko et al., 2003). Twelve percent of this cohort carried a comorbid sleep disorder diagnosis; 5% were specifically diagnosed with sleep apnea.

In addition to comorbid diagnoses, the Explore platform allows examination of pharmacotherapeutic patterns. Particularly relevant to people with ASD are the use of psychopharmaceutical agents and the recognition of attendant adverse drug effects (Frighi et al., 2011; Murray, Hsia, Glaser, Simonoff, & Murphy et al., 2014). Thirty-two percent of the cohort received at least one prescription for antipsychotic medicine; 18% received at least one prescription for an atypical antipsychotic medication. In a separate query for potential adverse side effects from these agents, 5% of the total cohort bore a diagnosis of movement disorder, and 1% was specifically diagnosed with a drug-induced movement disorder. The above analyses are a small sampling of the range of health and health services relevant to people with ASD that can be examined through currently available deidentified population-level Big-Data applications.

Selecting Outcomes

A great deal of future work is necessary to fully tap the potentialities of Big Data to improve the healthcare of people with ASD. Validation studies are needed to assure that the ASD population is accurately captured by Big Data information systems. Once ASD cohorts can be accurately defined, commonly employed existing healthcare quality measures (e.g., HEDIS) can then be applied to these cohorts. In addition, quality outcome measures appropriate and relevant to people with ASD and their care providers need to be adapted from existing measures or developed and tailored to the functionalities of EHRs and Big Data information management systems (Payakachat, Tilford, Kovacs, & Kuhithau, 2012). In an on-going manner, emerging knowledge about ASD needs to be integrated into existing analytics. There is also a need to systematically utilize Big Data in an exploratory fashion to identify comorbid physical and mental health conditions not yet linked to ASD in general, or linked to specific clinical syndromes, or molecular genetic subsets of ASD. As recently demonstrated in an electronic health record time-series analysis by Doshi-Velez, Ge, and Kohane (2014), some comorbidities may cluster in specific ways in this population.

Integration into Quality Improvement (QI)

Carefully constructed clinician education and other EHR-integrated supports are needed to serve dual functions of more detailed ASD-relevant documentation and improved health care. In an iterative fashion, the improved quality of ASD-relevant documentation through these clinical supports can further enhance the value of Big Data-derived enhancements to health care. Clinical decision supports can guide improved recognition and management of comorbid conditions and enhance the quality of psychopharmacotherapeutic interventions. At local and health system-wide levels, caregiver education and referrals for community-based supports also need to be integrated into the EHR.

Other Applications of Big Data Information Systems

The use of deidentified population level Big Data derived from data merged from multiple healthcare systems, as presented above, represents just one of many methods to utilize Big Data to improve the health care of people with ASD. Adapting models of continuously learning health systems, individual clinics and health systems can develop short-cycle QI projects to test the impact of specific clinical support strategies, utilizing additional capacities of Big Data applications to examine health care at clinic, provider, and patient-specific levels (Schneeweiss, 2014). Multistakeholder, practice-based research networks and learning collaboratives such as the Learning Collaborative in Developmental Medicine described above, with representatives from the self-advocacy, advocacy, service and health service communities, are key to more fully understanding the human lives represented by

Table 14.3
LEVELS OF ANALYSIS FOR RESEARCH RELATED TO PEOPLE
WITH DISABILITIES AND RELATED QUESTIONS OR OUTCOMES

Level	*Common Questions or Outcomes of Interest*
Impact of public policy, geographic variation	• Who gets services? • How does prevalence vary?
Effect of organized programs	• Who uses services? • Where are people treated? • Is there a change in amount of services used? • Is there a change in use of other services? Cost of care?
Specific interventions directed at the ability	• Changes in body function and structure, dis-activities and participation • Quality of life
Specific interventions directed at a given medical problem, not necessarily related to the disability, for people with a disability	• Typical condition-specific outcomes for the problem • Generic outcomes (e.g., function, quality of life) • Costs • Utilization of second-order services (e.g., hospitals, emergency rooms)
Comprehensive program designed to integrate medical and social services	• Prevention of conditions secondary to the disability • Prevention of conditions secondary to the disability • Typical condition-specific outcomes for the problem • Generic outcomes (e.g., function, quality of life) • Costs • Utilization of second-order services (e.g., hospitals, ERs)

*Reprinted with permission from the Agency for Healthcare Quality and Research (AHRQ). Source: Butler, M., Kane, R. L., Larson, S., Jeffrey, M. M., & Grove, M. (2012). Closing the quality gap: Revisiting the state of the science. In *Quality improvement measurement outcomes for people with disabilities.* Rockville, MD: Agency for Healthcare Research and Quality (US). (Evidence Reports/Technology Assessments, No. 208.7) In Introduction. Available from: http://www.ncbi.nlm.nih.gov/books/NBK114205/ or in printable format at http://www .effective-healthcare.ahrq.gov/ehc/products/336/1280/EvidenceReport208_CQGDisabilities_Final Report_20121015.pdf

Big Data and to generating real-world, sustainable solutions to the complex health and service needs of people with ASD (Tyler & Werner, 2014).

The Agency for Healthcare Research and Quality Evidence Report "Quality Improvement Measurement of Outcomes for People with Disabilities" (2012) cogently summarized the state of research related to quality improvement in the healthcare of people with disabilities (see Table 14.3) (Butler, Kane, Larson, Jeffery, & Grove, 2012).

Strategic utilization of Big Data can assist with the development, tracking, and refinement of QI measures. From the level of the population to that of the individual, there is a critical need to identify and develop process and outcome measures meaningful to people with ASD, their families and support providers, and their healthcare providers.

Conclusions

Evolving analytic platforms are enabling the use of continuously collected health system data—Big Data—to examine and improve the health and healthcare of people with ASD. Partnerships between the disabilities community, clinicians, informatics specialists, and researchers are necessary to assure that these data are used effectively with a clear vision of both its potentialities and its limitations.

References

Angelidou, A., Alysandratos, L. D., Asadi, S., Zhang, B., & Francis, L., Vasiadi, M., . . . Theoharides, T. C. (2011). Brief report: "Allergic symptoms" in children with autism spectrum disorders. More than meets the eye? *Journal of Autism & Developmental Disorders, 41,* 1579–1585.

Barrington, R. (2014). Navigating an ocean of information: How community care of North Carolina uses data to improve care and control costs. *North Carolina Medical Journal, 75*(3), 183–187.

Bowman, S. (2013). Impact of electronic health record systems on information integrity: Quality and safety implications. *Perspectives in Health Information Management, 10*(Fall), 1–19, Available at http://www.ncbi.nlm.nih.gov/pmc /articles/PMC3797550/

Buie, T., Campbell, D. B., Fuchs, G. J. 3rd, Furuta G. T., Levy, J., VandeWater, J., . . . Winter, H. (2010). Evaluation, diagnosis, and treatment of gastrointestinal disorders in individuals with ASD: A consensus report. *Pediatrics, 125,* S1–S18.

Butler, M., Kane, R. L., Larson, S., Jeffrey, M. M., & Grove, M. (2012).Closing the quality gap: Revisiting the state of the science. In *Quality improvement measurement outcomes for people with disabilities.* Rockville, MD: Agency for Healthcare Research and Quality (US). (Evidence Reports/Technology Assessments, No. 208.7) In Introduction. Available from http://www.ncbi.nlm.nih.gov/books

/NBK114205/ or in printable format at http://www.effectivehealthcare.ahrq.gov /ehc/products/336/1280/EvidenceReport208_CQGDisabilities_FinalReport _20121015.pdf

Carbone, P. S. (2013). Moving from research to practice in the primary care of children with autism spectrum disorders. *Academic Pediatrics, 13,* 390–399.

Denny, J. (2012). Chapter 13: Mining electronic health records in the genomics era. *PLOS Computational Biology, 8*(12), 1–15.

Doshi-Velez, F., Ge, Y., & Kohane, I. (2014). Comorbidity clusters in autism spectrum disorders: An electronic health record time-series analysis. *Pediatrics, 133,* e54–63.

Explorys®. (n.d.). Explorys. Retrieved from www.explorys.com Last accessed January 12, 2015.

Frighi, V., Stephenson, M. T., Morovat, A., Jolley, I. E., & Trivella, M., Dudley, C. A., . . . Goodwin, G. M. (2001). Safety of antipsychotics in people with intellectual disability. *The British Journal of Psychiatry, 199*(4), 289–95.

Guilbert, T. W., Arndt, B., Temte, J., Adams, A., Buckingham, W., Tandias, A., . . . Hanrahan, L. P. (2012). The theory and application of UW eHealth-PHINEX, a clinical electronic health record–Public Health Information Exchange. *Wisconsin Medical Journal, 11,* 124–133.

Hoffman, M. A. (2007). The genome-enabled electronic medical record. *Journal of Biomedical Informatics, 40,* 44–46.

Hsiao, E. Y. (2014). Gastrointestinal issues in autism spectrum disorder. *Harvard Review of Psychiatry, 22,* 104–111.

Jensen, P. B., Jensen, L. J., & Brunak, S. (2012). Mining electronic health records: towards better research applications and clinical care. Nature Reviews. *Genetics 13*(6), 395–405.

Kohane, I. S., McMurry, A., Weber, G., MacFadden, D., & Rappaport, L., Kunkel, L., . . . Churchill, S. (2012). The co-morbidity burden of children and young adults with autism spectrum disorders. *PLoS One, 7,* e33224.

Kotey, S., Ertel, K., & Whitcomb, B., (2014). Co-occurrence of autism and asthma in a nationally-representative sample of children in the United States. *Journal of Autism & Developmental Disorders, 44,* 3083–3088.

Nicolaidis, C., Kripke, C. C., & Raymaker, D. (2014). Primary care for adults on the autism spectrum. *The Medical Clinics of North America, 98,* 1169–1191.

Payakachat, N., Tilford, J. M., Kovacs, E., & Kuhlthau, K. (2012). Autism spectrum disorders: A review of measures for clinical, health services and cost-effectiveness applications. *Expert Review of Pharmacoeconomics & Outcomes Research, 12*(4), 485–503.

Phillips, W., & Fleming, D. (2009). Ethical concerns in the use of electronic medical records. *Modern Medicine, 106,* 328–333.

Reddy, K. (2005). Cytogenetic abnormalities and fragile-X syndrome in autism spectrum disorder. *BMC Medical Genetics, 6*(3), 1–16.

Rosti, R. O., Sadek, A. A., Vaux, K. K., & Gleeson, J. G. (2013). The genetic landscape of autism spectrum disorders. *Developmental Medicine & Child Neurology, 56,* 12–18.

Safran, C., Bloomrosen, M., Hammond, W. E., Labkoff, S., Markel-Fox, S., Tand, P.C., & Detmer, D. E. S(2007). Toward a national framework for the secondary use of health data: An American Medical Informatics Association White Paper. *Journal of the American Medical Informatics Association, 14*(1), 1–9.

Schneeweiss, S. (2014). Learning from big health care data. *The New England Journal of Medicine, 370*(23), 2161–2163.

SNOMED Clinical Terms® (SNOMED CT®) (2015) *US National Library of Medicine.* Retrieved from http://www.nlm.nih.gov/research/umls/Snomed/snomed_main .html

Tani, P., Lindberg, N., Nieminen-von Wendt, T., von Wendt, L., Alanko, L., Appelberg, B., & Porkka-Heiskanen, T. (2003). Insomnia is a frequent finding in adults with Asperger syndrome. *BMC Psychiatry, 3*(12), 1–10. Available at http://www.ncbi.nlm.nih.gov/pmc/articles/PMC270035/

Thiru, K., Hassey, A., & Sullivan, F. (2003). Systematic review of scope and quality of electronic patient record data in primary care. *British Medical Journal, 326*(7398), 1070.

Tuchman, R., Hirtz, D., & Mamounas, L. A. (2013). NINDS epilepsy and autism spectrum disorders workshop report. *Neurology, 81*(18), 1630–1636.

Tyler, C. V., Schramm, S., Karafa, M., Tang, A. S., & Jain, A. (2010). Electronic health record analysis of the primary care of adults with intellectual and other developmental disabilities. *Journal of Policy and Practice in Intellectual Disabilities, 7*(3), 204–210.

Tyler, C. V., & Werner, J. J. (2014). Community-engagement strategies of the Developmental Disabilities Practice-based Research Network (DD-PBRN). *Journal of the American Board of Family Medicine, 27*(6), 831–838.

Weber, G. M., Mandl, K. D., & Kohane, I. S. (2014). Finding the missing link for big biomedical data. *Journal of the American Medical Association, 311*(24), 2479–2480.

Weiskopf, N. G., & Weng, C. (2013). Methods and dimensions of electronic health record data quality assessment: enabling reuse for clinical research. *Journal of the American Medical Informatics Association, 20,* 144–151.

Section 4

MONITORING PATIENT OUTCOMES: RESEARCH AND POLICY DEVELOPMENT

Chapter 15

MEASURING AND EVALUATING OUTCOMES OF THE HEALTHCARE ENCOUNTER

JUDITH S. MILLER, MEGHAN N. DAVIGNON,
TERISA P. GABRIELSEN AND ERON Y. FRIEDLAENDER

Introduction

How do we know if we are improving healthcare encounters for our patients with autism spectrum disorder (ASD)? For some individuals, an excellent healthcare experience might mean that staff took extra time to deliver care at the patient's pace, helping him or her get through a medical procedure without additional sedation, and addressing some of his or her long-standing anxiety associated with going to the doctor. For other patients, an excellent healthcare experience might be one during which staff accurately determine if a patient will be able to tolerate the procedure without sedation, providing it quickly and efficiently so the patient and the family may have as positive an experience as possible.

These two scenarios might both yield successful encounters for very different reasons. From a measurement perspective, however, it can be difficult to identify metrics that can be viewed consistently as indicators of success across such unique, complex encounters. Furthermore, while both scenarios are designed to positively impact future healthcare encounters, the different strategies used may need to be matched to the particular patient and type of encounter, rather than applied universally.

This chapter highlights the complexities of measuring the healthcare experience for individuals with ASD, and provides a framework to help researchers and clinicians identify meaningful metrics. The chapter combines a social ecological theory and a tiered intervention strategy to demonstrate two important concepts, which integrate well with the rich information provided in other chapters. First, an individual's healthcare experience is never isolated; it is influenced by a series of social systems including the family, healthcare team, hospital, and larger community. And second, tiered interventions target the right level of patient need. General strategies aim to improve the experience for all patients, while moderate levels of support help patients at risk for difficulty during a healthcare encounter, and high levels of individualized support are needed for those few patients who have the most challenges.

While the focus of this chapter is on healthcare encounters, rather than overall health outcomes, the two topics are related and influence each other in a bidirectional manner. Particularly when we discuss measurement variables, we will include examples relevant to both the healthcare experience and health outcomes, and we encourage the reader to carefully consider the distinction between a healthcare encounter and a health outcome in their research and quality improvement projects.

What Is a Good Healthcare Experience for an Individual with ASD?

Most people would agree that a good healthcare experience means high quality care at reasonable cost and accessibility. Of course, individual perceptions of "high quality" and "reasonable" vary widely. Families of children with ASD have often experienced long waits for specialty evaluations, and a lack of support for care coordination despite very complex clinical needs. Parents have also likely experienced multiple healthcare encounters with a variety of professionals, in a variety of settings, some of which have gone much smoother than expected, and others that were surprisingly difficult. Thus, over time, parent expectations of what is high quality and reasonable care may evolve into something that would be unrecognizable to non-ASD parents. For some families, wait periods of "only" six months for a specialty appointment may be viewed as fast service, hospital procedures that involve use of holding or restraints may be commonplace, and high levels of child distress during part or all of the healthcare encounter may be the rule rather than the exception. It is perhaps not surprising, then, that many individuals with ASD have unmet healthcare needs (Kogan, Strickland, Blumberg, Singh, Perrin, & vanDyck, 2008).

From the provider's perspective, high quality care with reasonable cost and accessibility is the goal for all patients, and is continuously a moving target. Continuous quality improvement strategies and the tracking of relevant metrics are critical, but often focus on large groups of patients. This may not capture the successes and failures occurring during healthcare encounters of patients with ASD. Few healthcare providers receive specific training with special needs populations, but some of the most progressive work on helping individuals with ASD is being done in the dental community (Davit, Hundley, Bacic, & Hanson, 2011; Megargel & Broder-Fingert, 2012), where specific training certification in special needs patients can be obtained from the Special Care Dentistry Association (SCDA).

Furthermore, from a community perspective, individuals with disabilities and special needs have long had to advocate for equality, educating society about how to include and provide support for individuals with special needs. Cultural, political, religious, and societal values create a lens through which individuals with special needs are viewed, valued, and treated by the community, healthcare institutions, and healthcare workers. This impacts how well or how poorly an individual with ASD experiences a healthcare encounter.

Integrating an Ecological Systems Perspective with Tiered Interventions to Improve Outcomes

The social ecological perspective reminds us that individuals with ASD are not encapsulated; their families, healthcare providers, service systems, and community will influence their development, behavior, health, and health care encounters. A tiered interventions perspective reminds us that not all individuals with ASD share the same health risks or respond to the same interventions; some patients with ASD will do well with universal considerations, some are at risk and need monitoring or some extra support, and some have extremely difficult encounters and require more intensive intervention. Together they provide a more comprehensive framework for studying the healthcare experience.

The Social Ecological Perspective

Social ecological models, first introduced by Bronfenbrenner (1979), outlined the various systems within which an individual child develops. According to Bronfenbrenner the five systems in his model influence each other in multidirectional ways. This social ecological model has been adapted to a wide variety of topics beyond child development, including health (Grzywaca & Fuqua, 2000). We adapted Bronfenbrenner's (1979) and the CDC's four-tiered model (Dahlberg & Krug, 2002) to examine how these complex interactions (individual, family and health care team, hospital and clinic and community) shape an individual's overall health care experiences and outcomes (see Figure 15.1). There are multiple variables and methods to consider when

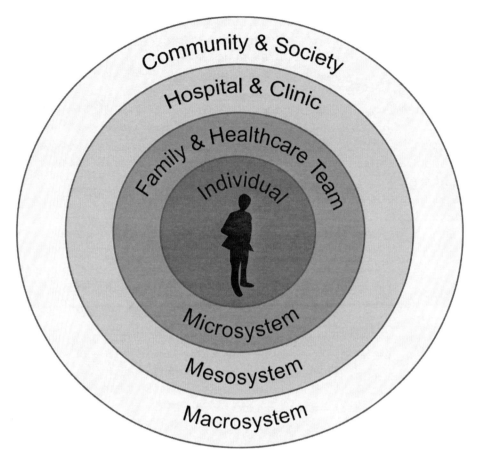

Figure 15.1. A social ecological model illustrating the complex interactions among individuals, society, institutions, and community shape the healthcare experiences and health outcomes of individuals with autism spectrum disorder. The figure was adapted using concepts presented in Bronfenbrenner, U. (1979) and the Center for Disease Control and Prevention's four-tiered model by Dahlberg & Krug (as cited in Krug, Dahlberg, E.G., Mercy, J. A., Zwi, A. B., & Lozano, R. (Eds.). (2002).

measuring improvement in any of the domains of individual, families and healthcare team, hospitals and clinics, and communities and society.

Domain: Individuals

In this domain we consider how individual differences impact the healthcare encounter. Individuals with ASD are heterogeneous. Beyond basic demographic variables (e.g., age, sex, physical size, and strength), individuals with ASD vary widely in intelligence, communication skill, and personality. Furthermore, expressive language and receptive language may not be even, and while most children with language delays comprehend more than they can express, some individuals with ASD show more expressive language (especially naming vocabulary) than receptive skills (Hudry et al., 2014; Maljaars, Noens, Scholte, & van Berckelaer-Onnes, 2012). Some individuals with ASD have particular difficulty with abstract language and interpret what is said concretely and literally. They also may struggle to interpret nonverbal cues correctly, which can impact what they understand from hospital staff.

VARIED RESPONSES TO CHANGE. Individuals with ASD vary on how well they tolerate new situations and changes in routine. In general, most individuals with ASD have some difficulty with novel situations, transitions, or changes to routine, but some are able to tolerate change with preparation, while others become extremely distressed and even aggressive in reaction to relatively minor changes in routine. Sensory overstimulation also varies in ASD, with some individuals showing hypo and/or hyper-sensitivities to lights, sounds, textures, pain, background noise, etc. Many parents report that their child with ASD has an excellent memory for locations, and can locate an office or area of the hospital visited years ago, or can remember positively- or negatively-specific healthcare experiences.

Domain: Families and Health Care Team

In this domain, we consider how differences among families and within health care teams may impact a healthcare encounter. Families with ASD experience high levels of stress, financial strain, and an increase in their own mental and physical health problems than their non-ASD counterparts (Cidav, Marcus, & Mandell, 2012; Karst & Hecke, 2012). Size and makeup vary, and extended family members can be a source of support or stress (or both). Families also differ in financial resources, health literacy, tolerance for discomfort in their child, and their ability to manage their child's distress and possible difficult behaviors. Furthermore, some parents, but not all, are comfortable taking an active part in healthcare encounters to help their child cope and/or help the care team improve the chances of success around procedures like physical exams, vital signs, venipuncture, and other treatments.

Healthcare teams vary in size and provider makeup. But more importantly, they vary in training, expertise, level of comfort working with individuals with ASD, and volume of patients with ASD regularly served. Teams that provide ongoing follow-up care may approach patient care differently than those who are providing a time-limited service. Team members also differ in how their encounters with patients might promote behavioral difficulty or distress, as well as whether team membership is consistent or varies from day to day. For example, a patient will react differently depending on the type of participation or cooperation needed for the treatment.

Domain: Hospitals and Clinics

Clinics and hospitals vary in size, type of care provided, expectation for ongoing care, support for staff around caring for patients with developmental disabilities, and resources and expertise managing difficult behaviors. The mix of patient demographics and payers may drive certain models of care. Furthermore, hospitals may differ in missions as either training institutions, or as a secondary or tertiary care centers. The hospital's position as a local provider, regional center of specialty care, or as an academic institution can influence the types of patients seen and the models of care promoted. The strength of individual disciplines and services within the hospital, such as nursing, Child life, behavioral health, and other allied health professionals determine the expertise available when patients with ASD and related disorders present to the hospital. The presence and engagement of such teams have the potential to ease distress and avoid difficult encounters.

Domain: Communities and Societies

In this domain, we consider how the community and social context contribute to the healthcare encounter. Communities and societies vary in attitudes and views on individuals with special needs. Private versus socialized healthcare influences the types of services available to all citizens. Laws and policies around individuals with special needs, children, and the underserved influence the social safety nets available, which can add or decrease general stress levels for individuals and families. Educational services for individuals with ASD influence overall growth and development, and can range from being a positive influence to creating significant stress and upheaval when education teams and families disagree on educational strategies. Additionally, cultural and societal views and attitudes about children with ASD and special needs can be a source of support or stress for families. Many families have experienced negative encounters in public when their children display ASD-related behaviors that are disruptive. They may live in chronic stress about how to keep their child with special needs safe and productive in a society that either idealizes individualism, shames disability, or that frequently fails to protect vulnerable and diverse populations.

A Tiered Intervention Perspective

Tiered interventions perspectives have been applied widely to education (Fletcher & Vaughn, 2009) and public health (Frieden, 2010). Our adapted model uses a 3-tiered pyramid structure (see Figure 15.2. Tiers of Intervention for Hospital Settings).

Applied here, tier one hospital-wide interventions utilize universal strategies, like health education materials, to improve the experience for all patients. At tier two, patients identified as higher risk for a difficult healthcare encounter can be provided with some targeted support to reduce potential difficulties in a healthcare experience. Finally, at tier three, interventions are indicated for a small number of patients requiring high levels of individualized support during a healthcare encounter to ensure safe and high quality care. Developing interventions at each tier informs quality of care for all patients, including those with special needs. Use of a tiered model assumes screening or assessment, which will be addressed later in the chapter.

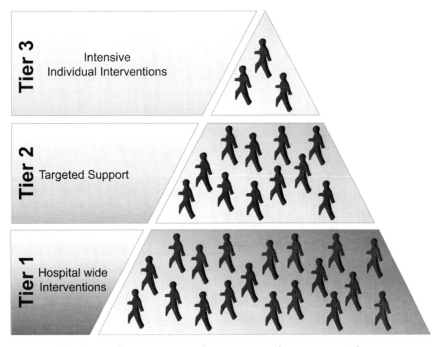

Figure 15.2. The figure illustrates tiers of intervention for patients with autism spectrum disorder cared for in hospital settings. The figure is adapted from the 5-tiered public health impact pyramid depicted widely in education (Fletcher & Vaughn, 2009) and public health (Frieden, 2010).

TIER ONE–HOSPITAL WIDE INTERVENTIONS. Most people rely on preparation, coping skills, and staff training when engaging healthcare systems for services, independent of whether they have a disability. For example, many hospitals provide preparation information for all families about what to expect, and what to bring to the hospital. Organizational strategies to provide preparation materials and methods that are accessible, feasible, understandable, and relatable for all patients and the hospital personnel are likely to provide sufficient support for the majority of individuals with ASD.

Healthcare staff, in general, should be versed in using common coping strategies for all patients, such as distraction methods, evidence-based fact-sharing, reassurance, and/or flexibility in order to provide effective care. Informed providers know when to dictate instructions using simple language, warn about transitions, offer positive reinforcement, allow for frequent breaks, recognize when directives are overwhelming, and attempt to limit unstructured time. These strategies are effective for all patients, not just patients with ASD. Many patients with ASD require no additional accommodations or adaptations during medical encounters when well-implemented tier one interventions are in place.

Likewise, general staff training about child development, individual differences among children and families, and a family-centered approach that encourages caregiver participation helps improve care for all patients, not just those with special needs. Staff who are able to integrate this into their own practice will see benefits for all their patients.

TIER TWO–TARGETED SUPPORT. Simple accommodations such as priority scheduling, additional preparation opportunities (e.g., practice visits), environmental adaptations, and communication tools can reduce the risk of a more difficult encounter. Preparation materials that have been put into formats helpful for children with ASD (e.g., Social Stories™; Gray, 2010) may help relay expectations and structure interactions. Social Stories explain the sequence of an action or activity using simple illustrations with or without accompanying text. In addition, some children use specific picture systems at home or at school, which can be easily adapted to hospital-based care. Among these are if/then cards, or visual schedules (Waldrop, n.d.). If/then cards display two images linking an action to a reward if the given action is completed. Visual schedules organize a series of words or pictures to represent the steps of a given process.

Flexibility and simple accommodations in the care environment often reduce anxiety enough to gain compliance and support safe interactions. For example, some children with ASD seek out (or avoid) certain sensations or movements. When possible, respecting and working around soothing self-stimulatory behaviors as well as minimizing triggers for agitation can facilitate a more rewarding and cooperative experience.

TIER THREE–INTENSIVE INDIVIDUAL INTERVENTIONS. A minority of children with ASD demonstrate escalating problem behaviors. Behavioral support around compliance with procedures and tolerance for medical devices may need to be specifically provided, and highly individualized behavioral strategies may need to be taught to caregivers in order to manage chronic medical conditions after discharge. Agitation plans (guidelines for the use of anxiolytics and support for agitation) are also critical. In some cases, the families or caregivers can provide information about the individual's current medications, factors that can lead to distress, activities that are particularly calming or provide good distraction, dietary preferences, etc., which can be extremely helpful in creating an effective set of strategies for working with the individual in the healthcare setting.

An Example of Identifying Gaps in Care

At The Children's Hospital of Philadelphia (CHOP), we recently completed a systematic investigation of facilitators and barriers to hospital-based procedural care from both parent and staff perspectives (Davignon, Friedlaender, Cronholm, Paciotti, & Levy, 2014). The key concept of individualized care when needed pervaded all themes. One parent said, "It's about knowing that child. . . . All about individual care. And again that's a reflection of how much information the parents can really give the doctors." Parents requested personalized care and recognized the need to provide information to the healthcare team that would help them really get to know their child as an individual.

Stakeholders described two main approaches to improve outcomes: Previsit preparation strategies, and flexibility regarding patient flow and the physical environment. Specifically, quality outcomes were linked to an individualized approach by a well-prepared care team (knowledgeable about ASD) who worked with informed, prepared families. Well-prepared providers understand: (1) How to approach and communicate with children with ASD, (2) the importance of recognizing an individual child's needs and challenges, and (3) the value of a proactive plan to address identified needs across the care team. Study participants requested that the healthcare team "be alerted" before their child is seen so the healthcare team were prepared to meet their special needs, and they would "know what you are dealing with" (Davignon et al., 2014). One nurse pointed out that the entire healthcare team and family needed to address the unique needs of the child being seen and each (e.g., physician, nurse practitioner, nurse, child life therapist, family member) would contribute to a holistic plan of care (Davignon et al., 2014).

Informed, prepared parents have detailed knowledge of upcoming encounters, use this knowledge to prepare themselves and their child, and problem-solve with staff around their child's challenges. One parent said,

> If I knew the things that they needed to accomplish, and then I could say, "okay, first we should do this or first we should do that" . . . I think that would have helped, because . . . I know the pace that she's going to go at, or I know what difficult thing to maybe tackle first (Parent) (Davignon et al., 2014 p. 212).

Unfortunately, most providers expressed difficulty communicating with this population, particularly those with limited verbal skills. Providers described little experience with alternative forms of communication to improve interactions, and limited skills with children who are agitated and exhibit challenging behaviors. Some examples included: "I [was] just thrown into the fire. I don't think that I had any sort of training for it. I've learned here from experience" (Nurse) (Davignon et al., 2014, p. 211). Providers recognized the lack of knowledge among staff members in communicating with ASD children, and reflected that it was not due to a lack of motivation, but a lack of knowledge; they just did not know.

Deficits in educational preparation and managing challenging behaviors have the potential to influence confidence when providing quality care for ASD patients. As one doctor reported, because of limited educational preparation in the care of ASD patients, he didn't feel "confident" in his skills as a physician or regarding being a "good" doctor to patients with ASD.

Preparing providers for an individual child's needs was central to improved outcomes and was consistent with other literature (Johnson & Rodriguez, 2013; Souders, Freeman, DePaul, & Levy, 2002; Nordahl et al., 2008). The following two comments are illustrative:

> You might not take the time beforehand to . . . review everything until you bring them back because you're focused on "let's get this patient back in the room and get their vital signs started," and then you're . . . looking up their history as you're meeting them. So I wouldn't mind having some sort of red flag to–Hey Stop–and look everything up, read the chart before you even go get them [Nurse] (Davignon et al., 2014, p. 210).

Another would find it helpful to have specific information in the chart that would indicate whether this patient may be at risk for a difficult encounter. The parent said:

> I wonder if there almost could be . . . a branch point specific to kids with autism. . . . Things like specific questions about... will they cooperate to get a weight or

an IV . . . making sure staff know early on if the child has any history violent outbursts, so that when they're going to take a vital sign they're not surprised. [Other professional] (Davignon et al., 2014, p. 211).

However, we identified some disagreement about who should initiate this communication, such as families or staff. Moreover, once needs had been identified, few standardized systems existed to support the development of proactive care plans and communication within care teams.

On the other hand, sometimes clinical staff do not routinely solicit parent input. One parent recalled:

> I think for me, when they did the MRI, they didn't really give me a lot of information on how they were [going to] sedate him. . . . I was very upset, because . . . they just come around from the side, he's . . . laughing, and then he's [got a mask shoved over his face]. . . . So I felt like the most terrible parent in the world, like someone was trying to smother my child (Davignon et al., 2014, p 211).

Lack of a uniform system of communication to circulate detailed information about a visit and provide preparatory guidance to the parents limits shared decision-making, which is an Institute of Medicine priority for improving patient-centered care (Institute of Medicine, 2001). Additionally, better outcomes have been associated with targeted parent-child preparation (Davit et al., 2011; Seid, Sherman, & Seid, 1997).

Measuring Outcomes from an Integrated Perspective

Measuring healthcare outcomes is not a simple matter. Single variables often do not capture the complexity of real-life challenges and successes during a healthcare encounter, and general variables, like overall satisfaction, cannot easily be translated into action steps for future improvement activities. Thus, once a meaningful topic has been identified (e.g., care of patients with ASD within a particular hospital unit, or use of primary care by adults with ASD), it is then important to consider both the variables that will best represent the outcome to be studied, as well as the variables that would help rule out alternative explanations for those outcomes.

Another challenge to the study of individuals with ASD is that often we must rely heavily on the observations of family and staff members if patients are unable to communicate directly. The Agency for Healthcare Research and Quality outlines some helpful guidance questions to consider when selecting a measure of outcome (National Quality Measures Clearinghouse, 2014), to which we have added some additional questions for this unique population.

Are the Outcome Measures to Be Used for Quality Improvement?

For groups looking to improve their own practice, quality improvement involves identifying an area for improvement, selecting measures of those areas, obtaining a baseline assessment, and remeasuring to assess the effect of improvement efforts. For accountability studies, measures are chosen to reflect what is valuable to the accountability organization, and often have to be collected in a manner that can be consistent across several institutions. Outcomes of accountability studies might be tools for helping consumers compare outcomes of different healthcare systems, performance-based payments, or certifications for professionals or the organization. Finally, research is aimed at developing new knowledge that is generalizable to a wide range of patients or settings. This often includes large data sets that merge multiple sources of data, and could include program evaluation, or assessing the effect of policy changes on health outcomes.

At What Point in an Episode of Care Is the Outcome Measured?

A healthcare encounter can start well and end poorly, or *vice versa.* In order to study specific aspects of the encounter, it is often necessary to think carefully about when the outcome is measured. In our own work, when trying to improve the process of intravenous line (IV) placement, we found it necessary to gather feedback immediately after the IV placement and before other parts of the encounter in order to reduce the chance that later aspects of the encounter would influence perceptions of how well the IV placement went. Conversely, if one were to measure the effects of a negative healthcare experience on future utilization, it would be important to take a longitudinal perspective and perhaps measure utilization months or even years into the future.

What Other Organizational and Nonhealth Factors May Influence the Outcomes?

As discussed throughout this chapter, a healthcare encounter occurs within the context of an individual, family, healthcare team, clinic, and larger community. Careful consideration of these systems can ensure that study results provide information that can be used to improve care, rather than simply identifying problems that may have multiple contributors.

Can One Clearly Define the Influences?

Like the question above, this is aimed at understanding alternative explanations for study results. Our integrated, social ecological perspective and tiers of intervention framework can help identify possible systems, organizations, staff, and other factors that may also influence the outcome of a healthcare visit.

What Is the Appropriate Comparison?

The healthcare experience of individuals with ASD might be compared to that of patients in the general population, or patients with chronic medical conditions, or patients with developmental disorders. In some cases, it may be appropriate to compare the experience of individuals with ASD to that of underserved populations who also experience barriers to health care. The experience within a particular unit or clinic could be compared before and after improvement efforts. The outcome of an individual might be compared to their prehospital health state. Availability of services in a geographic area might be compared to other disorders with similar population prevalence, or to disorders with a similar level of healthcare involvement.

What May Be Inferred about ASD Health Care?

It is always helpful to consider the "so what" question throughout design of a project, and then again during the implementation and interpretation phases. The variables of highest interest often are not feasible to collect in a complete and systematic manner, and next-best variables are used which may alter the conclusions we can draw from the study. Sometimes, the most accessible variables are measures of the healthcare process rather than an individual's healthcare experience or health state. Process variables, such as readmission rates, length of stay, and discharge placement are often used as "proxies" for an individual's health state or actual health outcome. Their use can provide important information so long as the study team remains aware of the limits of inferring an actual outcome from a process variable. See Table 15.1 Variables and Methods for Studying Outcomes for considerations of methods and variables to consider in studying outcomes of the healthcare encounter and experience.

Research Methods to Consider

There is a plethora of research methods that could be appropriate to study the healthcare experience and health outcomes. The use of large, merged data sets to study many important aspects of health and healthcare utilization is discussed elsewhere in this book. Traditional methods like randomized control trials are helpful, but can be difficult to conduct if there is a relatively low volume of patients with ASD or if the participants with ASD differ

Table 15.1
VARIABLES AND METHODS FOR STUDYING OUTCOMES

System Level	Elements to Consider	Possible Measureable Outcomes	Possible Methods
Individual	-Age -Sex -Baseline health state -Developmental level -Ability to communicate (comprehensive and/or expression) -Ability to cooperate with procedures -Tolerance for novel environments and stimuli -Ability to swallow pills -Co-occurring medical conditions -Co-occurring behavioral disorders -Effect of previous health-care experiences	-Access to care (all types) -Use of preventive care -Timeliness of treatment -Management of pain -Satisfaction with care -Traumatic care experiences -Cost of care -Quality of care -Health outcomes	-Group comparisons to determine if patients with ASD are experiencing different health care than individuals with other development disabilities, chronic conditions, or healthy contols. -Narrative medicine to elucidate individual healthcare perspectives. -Focus groups, individual interviews or surveys to identify mediators or moderators of health outcomes.
Family	-Size and makeup -Social resources -Financial resources -Health literacy -Ability to manage child's baseline health state -Ability to manage child's baseline behavioral state -Ability to access medical and behavioral support if needed -Extent to which they have been prepared for the clinic/hospital visit	-Satisfaction with care -Feasibility of access -Ability to manage care after discharge -Discharged to home or care facility -Extra costs (financial, time, emotional) associated with health care in ASD -Extent of care management required by the family	-Narrative medicine to understand the family experience -Focus groups of the family's experiences and worries for the future -Group comparisons to families with other developmental disorders, chronic conditions, or healthy controls.
Care team	-Size and makeup -Disciplines represented -Responsibility for ongoing care management -Familiarity and expertise with ASD	-Staff satisfaction -Work-related staff injuries -Training and professional development -Staff burnout or engage-ment with patients with ASD	-Narrative medicine -Studies of pre- and post-improvement efforts -Focus groups -Surveys pre- and post-training

Table 15.1–*Continued*

	-Confidence that they can manage child's medical and behavioral needs -Ability to access additional support if needed -Expertise/feasibility of helping children learn skills to tolerate procedures -Volume of patients with ASD/DD		
Unit or Clinic	-Size and makeup -Type of care and procedures provided -Physical environment -Volume of patients with ASD/DD -Workflow -Team communication strategies -Use of EHR tools -Approach to family-centered care -Use of preparatory information provided to families -Use of specific care plans for special needs patients	-Extra resources (staff, time, etc.) needed for care -Disruption to workflow, (related to patient and staff concerns)	-Pre- and post-intervention comparisons -Use of preparatory materials by families and staff
Hospital	-Size and location -Volume of specific procedures -Volume of patients with ASD receiving specific procedures -Disability friendly environment -Policies and procedures around safety events, restraint use, special needs patients -Available resources for psychiatric and/or behavioral consultation and support	-Extended stays -More invasive or costly procedures -Safety risks or events -Use of restraints -Use of extra hospital resources (e.g., behavioral consultations, Child Life) -Costs associated with any of the above	-Pre- and post-intervention comparisons

continued

Table 15.1–*Continued*

Larger Community	-Population demographics -Geographic setting (urban v. rural) -Proximity to centers of ASD expertise -Quality of health care generally -Social safety nets -Attitudes and culture around health care -Attitudes and culture around ASD	-Effects of health care on quality of life, productivity, poverty, economy, etc. -Costs associated with health care (or lack of) for citizens with ASD	-Large, merged datasets across communities

widely on variables that may contribute to the success or challenge in a healthcare encounter (e.g., level of intellect, language, behavioral challenge, anxiety).

Community-Based Participatory Research

Community-based participatory research (CPBR) is a collaborative approach to research that involves full partnership between the community and researchers, ideally from study inception through implementation and dissemination. The problem is defined by the community, the issue is studied in a collaborative and action-oriented manner, and the goal is an outcome that can be used by the community. Similar efforts to directly include the input and perspectives of individuals with disabilities have also been endorsed by businesses seeking to increase their ability to meet the needs of employees with disabilities (Jorgensen, 1989; Levy, 2013).

Medical Anthropology

Medical anthropology methods would focus on developing an understanding of the healthcare experience from the eyes of individuals with ASD and other stakeholders. As providers, we have become sensitive to how those with ASD are different. We do not yet understand why individuals with ASD experience thoughts, sounds, feelings, and words differently. Deeper appreciation for the experience of ASD rather than our interpretation would enable healthcare systems to structure meaningful interactions and provide sound, efficient, comprehensive care (Bagatell, 2010).

Narrative Medicine

Narrative medicine aims to "recognize, absorb, interpret, and act on the stories and plights of others" (Charon, 2001, p. 1897). While population-based studies offer a sound evidence base to inform the care delivered to individual patients, narrative medicine in turn suggests that an appreciation for a series of singular experiences reflects a more global perspective. In other words, it "illuminate(s) the universally true by revealing the particular" (Charon, 2001, p. 1898). Narrative medicine demands grounded, authentic engagement, promotes patient-centered care, and complements the much larger body of quantitative and qualitative experience to date on quality service delivery to people with ASD.

Researchers use semistructured interviews to obtain in-depth information about a given subject of interest (e.g., perceptions of facilitators and barriers to procedures used to sedate children with ASD). An interview guide is used to direct interviews with participants and obtain information on a list of topics of interest to the researchers. The interviews are transcribed verbatim, coded, and analyzed for major themes. Analysis is an iterative process, which begins following the first interview and continues until the point of thematic saturation, which is the point at which no significant new information is being obtained. Typically, somewhere between eight and 15 interviews per group of interest (e.g., parents of children who are under six years and non-verbal) need to be conducted to reach this point. Themes are then compared and contrasted across interviewed groups (Creswell, 2013; Hesse-Biber & Leavy, 2006).

Focus Groups

Focus groups gather participants to discuss a topic of interest (e.g., what is the group's opinion of tools created to help facilitate interactions with children with ASD). Frequently this technique is used to gauge stakeholder opinions regarding surveys, proposed programs, or to help interpret results of prior research. The meeting is usually recorded, transcribed verbatim, and coded for themes. Again, the aim is to reach thematic saturation for each group whose opinion is of interest (e.g., providers, parents, and administrators). Typically, at least three focus groups should be conducted to reach this point (Morgan, 1998).

Participant Observation

Participant observation is useful for obtaining in-depth information about a setting or scenario of interest from a more objective perspective (Jorgensen, 1989). For example, a child, his or her family, and the medical staff are observed from admission to discharge. Notes are taken about the setting, time, actions, and words of those present in the environment. The researcher takes field notes, which are later transcribed and coded for analysis of themes. In certain scenarios, this may include audio and video recordings as well. Observations are continued to the point of thematic saturation (Jorgensen, 1989; Creswell, 2013).

Strategies to Improve Healthcare Experiences for All

Groups looking to improve the healthcare experience for patients, families, and staff should first do some initial evaluation to determine where to focus efforts. If there are very few tier one strategies in place to improve the experience for all patients, then that will be an important area to focus. For tier two strategies, we describe below some of the specific efforts we have made at CHOP that may be relatively easy for other groups to also implement.

Patient and Family Preparation Materials

The CHOP has educational and preparation materials on our website (www.chop.edu), aimed at all children, including those with special needs. They often follow formats similar to those with which families with ASD and related disorders may already be familiar (e.g., Social Stories, visual schedules, and desensitization activities). Several units and clinics have also expanded their own websites to provide additional preparatory information for all families, including access to in-person, previsit care planning, or tours to become familiar with the environment before the visit.

General Staff Training in ASD

At CHOP we developed a specific on-line training module about ASD to help increase awareness and competency. We also provide specific trainings to individual units during their regularly scheduled in-service training times. In addition, we enhanced our hospital's "KIDS CARE" strategy (**K**nock, **I**ntroduce yourself, **D**iscuss the plan, **S**crub your hands, **C**heck ID bands, **A**ssess pain, **R**eturn in a timely manner, **E**xplain what you are going to do prior to doing it) for children with ASD and special needs (Figeuroa-Altman, Bedrossian, Steinmiller, & Wilmot, 2005).

Identifying Patients at Risk for a Difficult Encounter

We recommend implementation of a screening questionnaire at the time of scheduling patients for any appointment or interface (outpatient, inpatient, emergency department, and preoperative). The following three-question screener has been piloted in a busy procedural care unit as well as an outpatient subspecialty clinic. It was easy to administer in less than one minute by nonclinical staff, acceptable to parents, and helpful to staff, as measured by phone call length and a brief survey. It included a yes or no response to the following question: (a) Is there a behavioral diagnosis or developmental delay that staff should be aware of? (b) Does your child have special communication needs? And, (c) Does your child struggle to sit still for a haircut, dentist appointment, or doctor's exam?

Children whose parents endorse any of the above three items are identified in the medical record in an easily recognizable location on the patient banner, indicating they may need a unit-specific follow-up assessment to help inform a plan of care accommodation as necessary. Ideally, this plan of care would remain in place for future hospital encounters, and be accessible to families, so families can help their child experience consistent levels of care across healthcare settings. Making this information visible to medical assistants, technicians, phlebotomists, nurses, and physicians improves the frontline encounters with these patients as soon as they arrive at the hospital, and represents a potentially "meaningful use" of the electronic health record.

An Example of Tiered Interventions and Staff Education

We introduced a novel clinical pathway to help providers organize and structure a patient encounter. The pathway offers a focused review of defining characteristics within this population, practical considerations, and the matching of targeted interventions with patients across a range of behaviors. It also catalogues resources for staff including templates to create if/then cards, visual schedules, and tip sheets; recommendations for environmental modifications to patient care areas, tools to improve accuracy of pain assessment, discrete modifications to bedside care, and methods to more successfully share information among providers and with families.

An Example of Research: Pain Assessment in Patients with ASD

Accurate pain assessment is essential to providing quality health care. Current methods for pain assessment may not be helpful for children with ASD who struggle to communicate about their own experience. We completed an investigation designed to illuminate barriers to pain assessment in children with ASD and describe novel methods to communicate with children about their experience of pain. Specifically, we sought to identify a pain vocabulary familiar to this population, and to better develop our understanding of frames of reference for pain among individuals with ASD.

We performed a qualitative, descriptive study using semistructured interviews, including interactive, electronic technology, among children with ASD experiencing acute pain following a surgical procedure. We asked participants what words they used to talk about pain, ways they communicated pain, and what helped make their pain better. In addition, children were asked to draw their pain onto the outline of a body on an electronic table and interpret pain or hurt on a series of expressive digital images of children with a variety of emotions. Investigators also explored understanding of graded response and reliability of different pain assessment tools (poker chips as representative manipulatives, Wong/Baker Faces Scale and a Numeric Rating Scale) among participants. We found that most patients were able to talk about their pain, and found it helpful to use a concrete visual guide like the outline of a body when describing the pain. Many children struggled to grade their pain on a scale, and in many cases the patient's body language and facial expressions did not match the pain score or description of intensity.

Preliminary findings from our pain assessment study suggested to us that: (1) It is essential to use words familiar to the child; (2) children depend on their parents to help communicate their feelings and needs with staff; (3) describing pain is often preferred to using a number scale; (4) most participants were able to talk about their pain and how it feels; (5) locating pain, either on themselves or using an electronic image of a human outline, is a favored technique to help describe pain; (6) facial expressions and body language often do not match pain scores or descriptors of pain intensity; and (7) most children understand the concept of a graded response.

Translation of Principles across the Lifespan

The principles of an integrated social/ecological systems approach and tiers of intervention apply at any age. The same social systems (i.e., family, healthcare team, unit, hospital, community) are present throughout the lifespan. Families of individuals with ASD are often highly involved in all aspects of health care, particularly for adults with lower cognitive skills but very often for individuals with ASD who are higher functioning. Adults with ASD may struggle with navigating complex social service systems, or with solving the myriad of novel problems that arise when trying to make and keep a healthcare appointment, or with being able to follow through with healthcare instructions. Many times, adults with ASD appreciate and benefit from the same preparation materials and strategies used to help children with ASD tolerate healthcare procedures, with minor modifications to make the content or delivery more age–or developmentally appropriate. This includes using adult examples and pictures in preparation materials, including additional age-appropriate options for distraction activities, preparing educational materials in both a lower-literacy and higher-literacy format to accommodate different developmental levels.

As is true for all adults and children, the effects of previous negative experiences can be hard to remediate. Unfortunately, individuals with ASD often remember with clarity the unpleasant aspects of any healthcare encounter, which can then lead to problems and an increased likelihood of future encounters being difficult. At any age, the long-term effects of previous traumatic healthcare experiences should not be discounted. Providing opportunities for children and adults with ASD to overcome anxiety around doctor visits, and to tolerate healthcare procedures is an investment in their future health. Tools to help healthcare staff facilitate care, including general training and patient-specific information ahead of the encounter and/or documented in the medical record, can help teams individualize care.

Conclusion

Improving the healthcare experience for individuals with ASD can improve both their health and their ability to access health care throughout their life. A framework that integrates a social ecological systems perspective with a tiered intervention perspective highlights how healthcare experiences are influenced by the individual, family, healthcare team, clinic, hospital, and society at large. Interventions to improve the healthcare experience can be tiered to provide general improvement for all patients, assistance for those at risk of a difficult encounter, and individualized intervention for those patients with the highest need. Healthcare experiences may often need to be studied qualitatively, and we provided several guiding questions to help narrow the possible variables that could be studied.

References

Bagatell, R. (2010). From cure to community: Transforming notions of autism. *Ethos*, *38*, 33–55.

Bronfenbrenner, U. (1979). *The ecology of human development: Experiments by nature and design*. Cambridge, MA: Harvard University Press.

Charon, R. (2001). The patient-physician relationship. Narrative medicine: A model for empathy, reflection, profession, and trust. *Journal of the American Medical Association, 286*(15), 1897–1902.

Cidav, Z, Marcus, S. C., & Mandell, D. S. (2012). Implications of childhood autism for parental employment and earnings. *Pediatrics, 129,* 617–623.

Creswell, J. W. (2013). *Qualitative inquiry and research design: Choosing among five approaches* (3rd ed.). Thousand Oaks, CA: Sage.

Dahlberg, L. L., & Krug, E. G. (2002). Violence-a global public health problem. In E. Krug L. L. Dahlberg, J. A. Mercy, A. B. Zwi, & R. Lozano (Eds), *World report on violence and health* (pp. 1–56). Geneva, Switzerland: World Health Organization.

Davignon, M. N., Friedlaender, E., Cronholm, P. F., Paciotti, B., & Levy, S. E. (2014). Parent and provider perspectives on procedural care for children with autism spectrum disorders. *Journal of Developmental & Behavioral Pediatrics, 35,* 207–215.

Davit, C. J., Hundley, R. J., Bacic, J. D., & Hanson, E. M. (2011). A pilot study to improve venipuncture compliance in children and adolescents with autism spectrum disorders. *Journal of Developmental & Behavioral Pediatrics, 32,* 521–525.

Figeuroa-Altman, A. R., Bedrossian, L., Steinmiller, E., & Wilmot, S. M., (2005). KIDS CARE: Improving partnerships with children and families: A model from The Children's Hospital of Philadelphia. *American Journal of Nursing, 105*(6), 72A–72C.

Fletcher, J., & Vaughn, S. (2009). Response to Intervention: Preventing and remediating academic difficulties. *Child Development Perspectives, 3,* 30–37.

Frieden, T. R. (2010). A framework for public health action: The health impact pyramid. *American Journal of Public Health, 100,* 590–595.

Gray, C. (2010). *The new social story book, revised and expanded 10th anniversary edition.* Arlington, TX: Future Horizons, Inc.

Hesse-Biber, S. N., & Leavy, P. (2006). *The practice of qualitative research.* Thousand Oaks, CA: Sage.

Hudry, K., Chandler, S., Bedford, R., Pasco, G., Gliga, T., Elsabbagh, M., Hohnson, M. H., & Charman, T. (2014). Early language profiles in infants at high-risk for autism spectrum disorders. *Journal of Autism & Developmental Disorders, 44,* 154–167.

Institute of Medicine. (2001). *Committee on quality of health care in crossing the quality chasm: A new health system for the 21st Century.* Washington, DC: National Academy Press. Retrieved from https://www.iom.edu/Reports/2001/Crossing-the-Quality-Chasm-A-New-Health-System-for-the-21st-Century.aspx

Johnson, N. L., & Rodriguez, D. (2013). Children with autism spectrum disorder at a Pediatric hospital: A systematic review of the literature. *Pediatric Nursing, 39,* 131–141.

Karst, J. S., & Van Hecke, A. V. (2012). Parent and family impact of autism spectrum disorders: A review and proposed model for intervention evaluation. *Clinical Child & Family Psychology Review, 15,* 247–277.

Kogan, M. D., Strickland, B. B., Blumberg, J. J., Singh, G. K., Perrin, J. M., & vanDyck, P. C. (2008). A national profile of the health care experiences and family impact of autism spectrum disorder among children in the United States, 2005–2006. *Pediatrics, 122*(6), 1149–1158.

Jorgensen, D. L. (1989). *Participant observation: A methodology for human studies.* Thousand Oaks, CA: Sage.

Maljaars, J., Noens, I., Scholte, E., & van Berckelaer-Onnes, I. (2012). Language in low-functioning children with autistic disorder: Differences between receptive and expressive skills and concurrent predictors of language. *Journal of Autism & Developmental Disorders, 42,* 2181–2191.

Megargel, E., & Broder-Fingert, S. (2012). Autism and hospitals: A difficult match. *Academic Pediatrics, 12,* 469–470.

Morgan, D. L. (1998). *Planning focus groups.* Thousand Oaks, CA: Sage.

National Quality Measures Clearinghouse. (2014). Selecting health outcome measures for clinical quality measurement. Retrieved from http://www.quality measures.ahrq.gov/tutorial/HealthOutcomeMeasure.aspx

Nordahl, C. W., Simon, T. J., Zierhut, C., Solomon, M., Rogers, S. J., & Amaral, D. G. (2008). Brief report: Methods for acquiring structural MRI data in very young children with autism without the use of sedation. *Journal of Autism & Developmental Disorders, 38,* 1581–1590.

Seid, M., Sherman, M., & Seid, A. B. (1997). Perioperative psychosocial interventions for autistic children undergoing ENT surgery. *International Journal of Pediatric Otorhinolaryngology, 40,* 107–113.

Souders, M. C., Freeman, K. G., DePaul, D., & Levy, S. E. (2002). Caring for children and adolescents with autism who require challenging procedures. *Pediatric Nursing, 28*(6), 555–562.

Special Care Dentistry Association (SCDA). *SCDA Mission and vision.* Retrieved from www.scdaonline.org

Waldrop, K. (n.d.). *Using visual structure for medical appointments.* Retrieved from http://teacch.com/resources/teacch-articles-on-educationalapproaches/Doctor_Dental_appointmentvisualstructure.pdf

Chapter 16

RESEARCH AND POLICY DEVELOPMENT

LINDSAY SHEA, DAVID S. MANDELL AND CRAIG NEWSCHAFFER

Integrating Services: A Matter of Policy

The idea of integrated care for individuals with psychiatric and developmental disabilities is decades old (Mandell, Guevara, & Pati, 2006). In the mid-1980s, the high rates of institutionalization of children and adolescents with these disabilities led to a dramatic increase in funding for community-based mental health services that "wrapped around" the child and family. These services had an emphasis on care coordination and integrating care for the purpose of addressing disparate needs. It was believed that such an approach was better suited for the complexity of care often required for these individuals. At the same time, pediatricians began to promote the idea of a medical home, wherein care would be coordinated from the pediatrician's office and integrated across different systems in which children with special needs received care (Kuhlthau et al., 2011). Recently, the idea of a medical home for children with autism spectrum disorder (ASD) has gained currency (Hyman & Johnson, 2012), as has the idea of a medical home for adolescents with special health care needs who are transitioning to adulthood (Lemly, Weitzman, & O'Hare, 2013).

In this chapter, we examine selected models of integrated health and service care delivery and include a description of the efforts underway in Pennsylvania, a national leader in policy and program development for constituents with ASD. To address the dearth of published data and research in adults with ASD, we include a number of designs that use comparative effectiveness research (CER) and argue for establishing and testing policies that support integrated delivery models and research efforts. Finally, we provide useful and straightforward guidelines for policy advocacy and recommend robust studies to accompany new efforts to integrate care for individuals on the autism spectrum.

Integrated Care Needs of Adults with ASD

Although an exact population count of people with ASD currently does not exist, it is estimated that about 1.5 million people and approximately 1% of adults in in the U.S. have an ASD (Nicolaidis, Kupke, & Raymaker 2014). People spend the majority of their lives as adults, and consequently, considering the integrated healthcare needs of adults with ASD is therefore a priority. Given the lack of an evidence base to establish their needs and varying and changing presentations, determining best practice for health care for adults with ASD is exceptionally challenging. Adults with ASD experience increased rates of chronic illnesses including: epilepsy, gastrointestinal issues, nutritional problems, metabolic syndrome, sleep disturbances, anxiety, and depression (Levy et al., 2010; Nicolaidis et al., 2014). Unmet healthcare needs in the areas of preventative services, including health screenings and dental care, have been identified (Bruder, Kerins, Mazarella, Sims, & Stein, 2012; Rich, Lipson, Libersky, & Parchman, 2012; Nicolaidis et al., 2014). Researchers have also reported that adults with ASD experience lower satisfaction in healthcare encounters, lower self-efficacy, increased utilization of emergency departments, and numerous barriers in accessing healthcare and supportive social services (Bruder et al., 2012; Nicolaidis et al., 2014; Rich et al., 2012).

The lack of an evidence base has also contributed to gaps in the training of professionals who care for, and the training of informal caregivers of, adults living in community settings (Brugha et al., 2011; Bruder et al., 2012). In Bruder and colleagues' study (2012), about two-thirds (67%) of primary care physicians (PCPs) in the U.S. state of Connecticut reported a need for training on providing care to adults with ASD. Researchers and care providers have asserted that person-centered medical homes will be better positioned to meet the needs of the adults with ASD (Bruder et al., 2012; Nicolaidis et al., 2014; Rich et al., 2012), although an evidence base will still be critical to do so. They also reported an interest in acquiring this knowledge.

Medical Homes and Pediatric Populations

Medical homes and systems of care were developed to integrate and coordinate care from one office. The American Academy of Pediatrics (AAP) in 1967 introduced the concept of a medical home as centered on the child's medical records. The AAP further developed the model to better meet care and service needs from a primary care perspective that included family-centered, accessible, culturally effective, coordinated, comprehensive, and compassionate care. Practitioners, families, advocates, and policy makers recognized that children with complex needs required a level of case management not available through traditional services. These integration efforts were consistent with the values of many of the people involved and seemed intuitively to address a pressing need. Perhaps as a result, there were few rigorous tests of these models (Kuhlthau et al., 2011).

In 2014, Hadland and Long (2014) conducted a systematic review of the literature on the medical home presence relation to three outcome measures: primary care services, health care utilization, and child well-being. Children with a medical home were more likely to receive preventive medical care, anticipatory guidance, and developmental screening; a higher health-related quality of life; and were less likely to seek care in the emergency department. There are no equivalent programs for adults.

We now find ourselves in the position of needing to develop new models of integrated care, especially for the growing number of adults diagnosed with autism. A challenge to progress on this task is the lack of evidence around if or how pediatric interventions will work in adult populations (Piven & Rabins, 2011).

Evidence of Value in Pediatric Medical Homes

Early randomized trials of the pediatric models for example, identified greater satisfaction among families and showed higher utilization of services, but clinical and functional outcomes were no better in the experimental group than in the control group (Bickman, 1996; Bickman, Summerfelt, & Noser, 1997). More recently, Powell and colleagues (2014) conducted a systematic review of strategies for implementing mental health interventions. Positive outcomes included improved health status, family-centered care, and improved family functioning. Yet, Hadland and Long (2014), reported that the medical home apparently did not offer a protective effect with regard to preventable hospitalizations. Both teams of researchers agreed that we must learn from earlier efforts to integrate care for children and build on decades of research that new programs must be accompanied by policies and resources that promote their adoption and successful implementation (Powell, Proctor, & Glass, 2014).

Policy Issues

Research reports on adults with ASD lag behind those on children with ASD. The difference in the number of research reports includes those on strategies to facilitate seamless and successful transition from pediatric to

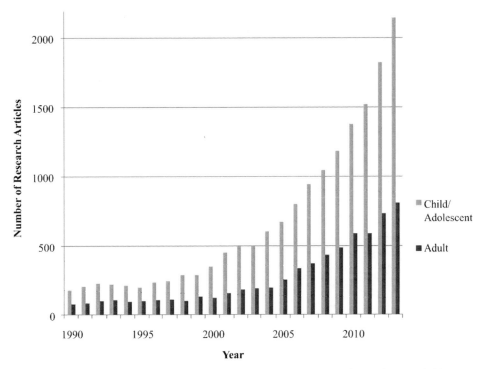

Figure 16.1. Illustration of the number of autism-specific research articles on children or adolescents versus adults, by year.

adult care, and integrated health care. Figure 16.1 illustrates the disparity.

A 2014 Huffington Post article suggested that the field of autism should "mind the policy gap" (Vahabzadeh, 2014). While there are important and specific policy gaps as children with ASD approach the transition into adulthood, an established base of evidence to guide their care once they reach adulthood is significantly lacking. With few exceptions, this indicates that "minding the policy gap" should be reconsidered as a warning for a more permanent policy cliff. This evidence base is critical to establish reimbursement rules (Bryson & Ostmeyer, 2014), set practice guidelines to ensure quality of care, and set qualifications standards for care providers.

ASD Medicaid Policy

An important system of care for individuals with ASD of all ages in the US is Medicaid (or Medical Assistance). Medicaid is a program jointly funded and operated by the federal government through the Centers for Medicare and Medicaid Services and by states. Children, individuals, and families can be eligible for health insurance through the Medicaid system if they meet disability or income criteria or for other reasons, including being eligible due to foster care. Medicaid is the payer of last resort if and when services are not covered through private insurance or another insurance mechanism. Medicaid has historically been an important system of care for individuals with ASD since private health insurance has limited coverage for individuals with ASD or excluded it altogether.

The Medicaid system in the US has relative flexibility in meeting the varying needs of states and of specific groups in need of services, like ASD. For example, Medicaid allows states to run waivers, which are exceptions to the traditional Medicaid eligibility rules for special groups. However, as of 2013, only 10 Medicaid waivers for children with ASD existed in the US (Warfield, Chiri, Leutz, & Timberlake, 2014). A recent report on the state of the states for individuals with ASD lists more than 30 waivers across the life-span for people with ASD. This list also included waivers for general developmental disabilities that may not focus on the provision of care to individuals with ASD specifically (L & M Policy Research LLC, 2014) .

PARTICIPANT-DIRECTED FRAMEWORK. Of the 10 Medicaid waivers specifically for children with ASD, four utilize a participant-directed framework (Warfield et al., 2014). Participant-directed is also referred to as consumer-directed or self-directed in some states. The Centers for Medicare and Medicaid Services (2014) defined participant-directed as services a participant in a Medicaid program, or their representative, have authority over and take direct responsibility for managing with a system of supports. Self-direction is designed to promote individual choice and control over delivery of services through waivers and may include control over the budget for their services as well (Centers for Medicare and Medicaid Services, 2014).

This provision is important given the wide range of presentations and symptoms observed in individuals on the autism spectrum. Parents and family caregivers are often the child's or dependent's representative and they drive the configuration(s) of care for these patients. This allows for family caregivers to structure services around their individual's strengths and needs, and to incorporate the needs of their family with the treatment plan. In a participant-directed framework, families may even be empowered to hire and fire provider(s) of services for their child. One study of a participant-directed, ASD-specific waiver for young children in Massachusetts found that families experienced less stress and reported a positive impact on family functioning (Warfield et al., 2014) in this configuration. A second study of the same waiver found similar results with parents reporting increased satisfaction and confidence in determining their child's care in a self-directed waiver (Timberlake, Leutz, Warfield, & Chiri, 2014).

In considering policy mechanisms that may include elements such as self-directed care for optimally delivering integrated health care, family-professional relationships are likely a key factor in influencing outcomes and program success (Blue-Banning, 2004; Keen, 2007). A participant-directed framework serves whole families. Complementary research has found that families most often reported needing more information on services, family support, and respite care (Hodgetts, Zwaigenbaum, & Nicholas, 2015).

Unfortunately, almost no research exists to determine if or how these results might translate into programs or waivers for adolescents transitioning into adulthood. One study to evaluate the implementation of a social skills curriculum for adolescents with ASD in a mental health setting outlined several of the components for effective clinical implementation, but touched only briefly on the policy components or mechanisms necessary for replication (Bryson & Ostmeyer, 2014). The clinical and policy demands of putting these programs and mechanisms in place are particularly challenging given the amplified needs of adolescents facing the transition into adulthood, regardless of disability or ASD-specific status, and a lack of ASD-specific training among community mental health center clinicians (Brookman-Frazee, Drahota, & Stadnick, 2012).

Integrated health care has also been woven into health policy in the US through the Affordable Care Act (ACA). Although elements of the ACA invest concretely in integrated health care, the interpretation and implementation of the ACA have yet to be determined and executed (Croft & Parish, 2013).

ASD Insurance Mandates

About half of the states in the US have passed ASD-specific insurance mandate laws to improve access to services for children through the private insurance system. Research on these mandates is mixed regarding impact and effectiveness. One study compared the characteristics of the states that passed an ASD-specific insurance mandate to those that had not. Oddly, the researchers found that states that were in most need of such a mandate due to restricted access to services were the least likely to pass an ASD-specific mandate. The researchers also noted that less needy states were more likely to pass a mandate and thus highlighted the potential policy duplication of this mechanism (Johnson, Danis, & Hafner-Eaton, 2014). For example, other federal policy mechanisms through both the judicial and the legislative branch including the Olmstead decision in 1999 and the Mental Health Parity and Addiction Equity Act of 2008 have been aimed at providing access and funding for services in similar ways (Salzer, Kaplan, & Atay, 2006).

Researchers have reported that ASD-specific insurance mandates may create a cumulative advantage in states rather than help to compensate for weak policy access infrastructure in states that need it to provide access and funding for services to children with ASD (Rzhetsky et al., 2014). Also, Rzhetsky and colleagues (2014) observed a varying effect of mandates on ASD prevalence which suggested that implementation of the mandates may not increase access as uniformly within or across states as was intended.

ASD-specific insurance mandates have, to date, not included required access to services for adults with ASD and, in fact, they rarely require access through the transition into adulthood. Finally, implementation of these mandates has not been studied and could be problematically linked to the enforcement entities and their political affiliations, which can vary over time, and across states.

Pennsylvania State: Model of Success

In the absence of guiding policy and research, state governments have been forced to determine how to define and implement integrated health care for individuals with ASD and their families. Many states have undertaken ASD task force initiatives to engage their communities. Several states have formed units at the state level to help form and implement ASD-specific policy and programs, although the structure of these units varies considerably across states.

Pennsylvania has emerged as a national leader by constructing policy and programs to help meet the needs of individuals with ASD, their families, and the providers of services to these groups. Pennsylvania was among the first US states to institute a state-level entity focused on ASD, which evolved into the Pennsylvania Bureau of Autism Services. When established, the Bureau of Autism Services provided technical assistance on ASD to state-level entities, held statewide training conferences, and administered one of the first waivers specifically for adults with ASD in the US (Pennsylvania Department of Human Services, 2015a). In addition, the website has content that is adult-specific (Pennsylvania Department of Human Services, 2015b). Two specific programs were exceptionally novel: the Autism Services, Education, Resources, and Training (ASERT) Collaborative and the Adult Community Autism Program (ACAP).

ASERT Collaborative

The ASERT Collaborative (www.paautism.org) is a competitive grant mechanism awarded to three regional sites with the mission of working to improve the lives of Pennsylvanians with ASD. The ASERT Collaborative was formed to support the Bureau of Autism Services in reaching into the corners of Pennsylvania (Lubetsky, Handen, Lubetsky, & McGonigle, 2014). The ASERT Collaborative uses data from multiple sources to identify and meet the needs of the residents of Pennsylvania's vast geographical area and diverse county characteristics (47 of Pennsylvania's 67 counties are rural, although the nation's fifth largest city, Philadelphia, is also in Pennsylvania). The ASERT Collaborative is divided into three regions to cover the western (led by the University of Pittsburgh), central (led by Penn State University), and eastern (led by Drexel University) areas of Pennsylvania. Three initiatives of the ASERT Collaborative and the Bureau of Autism Services have gathered data to help identify the needs and priorities of Pennsylvanians living with ASD and their families. They are Pennsylvania Autism Needs Assessment, Pennsylvania Autism Census, and the Adult Community Autism Program.

PENNSYLVANIA AUTISM NEEDS ASSESSMENT. A statewide Autism Needs Assessment survey available online and in paper versions, as well as in English and Spanish, was conducted in 2009. This initiative resulted in over 3,500 survey responses, 149 of which were self-reported by individuals with ASD. All versions of the complete survey, aggregate results, and topically focused reports are available at www.paautism.org/needsassessment. The ASERT Collaborative uses the Pennsylvania Autism Needs Assessment to strategize high yield projects and programs to maximize impact for Pennsylvanians living with ASD and their families.

A primary need identified in the needs assessment was social skills groups for adolescents and adults. To help meet this need, the central region ASERT Collaborative, led by Dr. Michael Murray from Penn State University, generated a curriculum for social skills groups and those social skills groups are currently rolling out across the Commonwealth of Pennsylvania at all three ASERT Collaborative sites. Implementation of this initiative is also targeted at community partners who will be able to use the curriculum to implement and bill for social skills groups as a service in the future.

A need identified by the Pennsylvania Autism Needs Assessment was for training of first responders and emergency room personnel to help providers support individuals with ASD who may be in crisis or in need of acute medical help. The western region ASERT Collaborative, led by Dr. John McGonigle, compiled a First Responder and Emergency Department Personnel training program (McGonigle et al., 2014) which has been implemented by the Pennsylvania Department of Health in their training curriculum for first responders statewide.

PENNSYLVANIA AUTISM CENSUS. The Pennsylvania Autism Census Report (available at www.paautism.org/census) was first issued in 2009 and, as a complement to the Pennsylvania Autism Needs Assessment, provides an administrative count of individuals with ASD of all ages being served in Pennsylvania. The Pennsylvania Autism Census Report was led by Dr. Lindsay Shea, ASERT Collaborative Eastern Region Director, and is the first of its kind in the US to provide detailed information on the systems providing services to individuals with ASD. In particular, the Pennsylvania Autism Census Project provided a glimpse into the characteristics of adults with ASD including their county of residence and other demographic information. This type of detailed information is critical in assisting policymakers to determine policy and program needs and is an important tool for individuals with ASD and their families to use to advocate for and demonstrate their needs, and the needs of their communities. A new version of the Pennsylvania Autism Census Report with data from additional years and systems is available at www.paautism.org/census.

ADULT COMMUNITY AUTISM PROGRAM. The Adult Community Autism Program (ACAP) is a unique managed care program designed to provide integrated health care to Pennsylvanians living with ASD. ACAP provides physical, behavioral, and community services to adults age 21 or older who are eligible for Medicaid and have an ASD diagnosis. Additional eligibility criteria can be found through the Pennsylvania Department of Public Welfare Bureau of Autism Services at www.autisminpa.org. In 2013 and 2014, the ASERT Collaborative Eastern Region partnered with the Bureau of Autism Services to conduct qualitative focus groups with ACAP participants, their family members, the ACAP service provider direct care staff, and program administration. Initial findings from those focus groups reflected the challenges of implementing a managed care program for adults with ASD and highlighted the need for streamlined communication. A full report on this project will be available through the ASERT Collaborative at the www .paautism.org website.

Future Research: Comparative Effectiveness

As innovative ideas around integrated healthcare services for individuals with ASD, such as the ACAP program highlighted above, move into practice, there will be increased opportunities to engage in comparative effectiveness research (CER) around these approaches. An Institute of Medicine (IOM) committee defined CER as the generation and synthesis of evidence that compares these benefits of alternative methods to prevent, diagnose, treat, and monitor a clinical condition or to improve the delivery of care (Institute of Medicine, 2006). The purpose of CER is to assist consumers, clinicians, purchasers, and policy makers to make informed decisions that will improve health at both the individual and population levels. The IOM further reported on national priorities for CER; the three highest among 28 priorities are health delivery, disparities, and disabilities (IOM, 2009).

Funding for Comparative Effectiveness Research (CER)

CER is more than a novel catch phrase. In 2010, the Affordable Care Act (ACA) created a new nonprofit, nongovernment organization, the Patient Centered Outcomes Research Institute (PCORI), fully supported by federal funding, whose mission is to increase CER. In FY 2015, PCORI intended to fund $475 million in CER with proposed annual commitments in the hundreds of millions for the next several years (http://www.pcori.org/blog/target -continuing-focus-pcoris-research-portfolio). The National Institute of Health (NIH) has a CER Coordinating Committee monitoring NIH's considerable ongoing investment in CER, and the Agency for Healthcare Research and Quality (AHRQ) also has an extensive CER portfolio. Federal research funders are clearly investing heavily in this work and there is evidence that key stakeholders in the US healthcare system believe that moving forward the findings from CER will increasingly inform priority-setting and decision-making.

The National Pharmaceutical Council conducts an annual survey of healthcare stakeholder about their attitudes toward CER. In 2014, 59% of the respondents felt that CER was very important to the industry and, though only 16% reported that CER had an impact on their decision-making in the past year, and 92% thought CER would have an impact on their decision-making within the next five years (Hofelch, West, Walker, Schur, & Adams, 2014).

Research Designs Using CER

The major classes of approaches in CER are large-scale observational studies and large-scale pragmatic trials. Note that scale is central to CER approachs because there is an inherent desire for findings to generalize broadly and, while large studies can have problems with generalizability, they are less-likely to involve highly-selected study populations than smaller sized ventures. In the context of integrated care for individuals with ASD, the "treatment condition" under study would be an approach, strategy, or system intended to foster integration of care. The two major designs are observational CER and pragmatic trials.

OBSERVATIONAL CER. In the observational design, pertinent outcomes for individuals with ASD who have experienced an integrated care approach would be contrasted to those who have not. The process dictating who received and who did not receive integrated care is not under the control of the researcher and reflects whatever forces in the population move individuals into one versus another treatment condition. The inherent challenge here is that the individuals being compared are not "exchangeable"—that as a group they differ systematically from each other in ways that influence their probability of good or bad outcomes. Observational CER tends not to involve primary data collection but often capitalizes on large existing administrative data systems maintained by healthcare providers or payers. These data sources can support large-scale studies and try to find ways to leverage large sample size and commonly the availability of data from multiple health care encounters per individual to overcome the challenge of potential nonexchangeability of study subjects. For example, the development of the statistical analytic technique of propensity score adjustment mirrors the rise of CER (Borah, Moriarty, Crown, & Doshi, 2014).

CER and behavioral health. With respect to behavioral health in general, the preponderance of large-scale observational CER completed to date have focused on the effectiveness of pharmacologic treatments because these treatments are commonplace and expensive and because administrative data can reliably identify individuals who have or have not received such treatment.

Before observational CER can be extended to examine integrated care in ASD, there will need to be some dissemination of such programs into practice and a way to detect the delivery of integrated care in available administrative data sets. For example, if Medicaid programs move toward funding integrated care for individuals with ASD through waiver mechanisms, there would need to be ways (within the Medicaid data systems) to distinguish waiver participants from nonparticipants. Those specifically receiving an integrated care model should be identifiable. If this becomes possible, the administrative data will have to capture data on the outcomes of interest. These systems are amenable to assessing certain aggregate cost and utilization outcomes that would be relevant for policy development. However, these systems are unlikely to capture the variables of satisfaction with care, quality of life, or core ASD symptom changes over time. There is, however, the potential for these data sources to capture certain important adverse events including both directly measurable outcomes like inpatient psychiatric hospitalization stays and more complex outcomes such as polypharmacy for which there have been algorithms developed to detect such occurrences using administrative healthcare claims data (Spencer et al., 2013).

Demonstration programs. Although it may be some time before large, readily accessible administrative data sets can support full-scale observational CER on integrated care options for individuals with ASD, there are some approaches that can occur now. For example, smaller scale studies can be designed simultaneously with the launch of demonstration programs–and these can set the stage for larger future observational CER. These require developing a strategy to extract the most relevant administrative data from individuals participating in demonstration programs and contrasting these to comparison groups. A model for this approach is provided by a recent analysis (Grimes et al., 2011) of the Mental Health Services Program for Youth (MHSPY). The MHSPY is a demonstration project in Massachusetts, funded through blended streams of public agency dollars, to create and support a clinical care management entity to deliver integrated mental health and social services to Medicaid-eligible children with serious emotional disturbance. Here, Medicaid data from the first 100 participants in the demonstration were contrasted to a group of 20,000 like aged children–all subjects in the demonstration and comparison group had a previous history of psychiatric hospitalization or residential treatment.

The analysts used CER techniques, like propensity score matching, and, though the small sample size of the demonstration group limited the statistical power of analyses, interesting preliminary results were generated. Findings suggested that participation appeared to protect against psychiatric hospital readmission in the younger participants but not in the older participants and, perhaps more importantly, a model for doing more robust analyses on larger samples in the future was established.

PRAGMATIC TRIALS. The second major CER approach is pragmatic trials. A trial is distinguished from an observational study because research participants are randomly assigned to a treatment condition by the investigators and thus, on average, the treatment groups will be similar and exchangeable. Random assignment is the most powerful tool available to promote causal inference in research studies and, consequently, trials are considered critically important in CER. However, randomized studies are often implemented on smaller samples selected either for convenience (i.e., participants are patients at an academic medical center) or to further promote exchangeability (i.e., restriction to one or another age or gender group) and where a treatment condition can be optimally delivered under very controlled circumstances. The problem is that with this selection and ideal, often resource-intensive, delivery of treatment comes limitations in generalizing study findings to other, larger, more-representative populations where the treatment will be delivered under real-world circumstances.

Explanatory and pragmatic trials. In 1967, a distinction was made between so-called "explanatory" and "pragmatic trials" with the former referring to smaller trials done with more selected populations under ideal treatment delivery circumstances and the latter referring to randomized studies to larger populations under real-world conditions (Schwartz & Lellouch,

1967). Frameworks and tools (see, for example, (Thorpe et al., 2009; Tosh, Soares-Weiser, & Adams, 2011) have been developed to help evaluate post hoc whether completed trials tend more toward explanatory or pragmatic, but are also useful when planning such studies. The CER approach, while not discounting explanatory trials, favors pragmatic trials generating evidence relevant for bringing approaches to scale in diverse communities. PCORI has recently released calls for studies that used pragmatic trials approaches testing approaches "improving health system level approaches to managing care" (PCORI, 2015).

Integrated versus standard care. The inherent difficulty in mounting pragmatic trials and evaluating approaches like integrated care strategies for individuals with ASD is finding ways to randomize subjects to the appropriate conditions, in this case, "integrated" versus "standard" care. Such studies will likely be reliant on group, as opposed to individual, level randomization where different providers are randomly moved to integrated approaches while others continue with current practice. Outcomes are still evaluated at the subject level and the clustering of subjects in different practices is accounted for statistically. A challenge in fielding these studies often comes from the desire to give all participating providers an opportunity to have access to the new approach.

Stepped-wedge randomization. Study designs like stepped-wedge randomization have been developed to address this (Keriel-Gascou, Buchet-Poyau, Rabilloud, Duclos, & Colin, 2014). In a stepped-wedge design, all participating providers start operating under standard practice and then are moved into the intervention condition at different, randomly determined, times. Subject outcomes are monitored throughout the entire study period. Stepped-wedge and other group-randomized pragmatic trial approaches typically emphasize shorter-term outcomes since effects need to be observable over what are typically short follow-up periods. Pragmatic trials of integrated care approaches in ASD have yet to be implemented, but such studies have been done for other conditions (see, for example, the Kruis et al. (2014) study assessing integrated care approaches in COPD).

As providers, payers, and regulators move further along in the development and implementation of integrated care approaches for ASD, attention should be paid from the outset to creating opportunities for research. Well before it is feasible to field large-scale observational or pragmatic trials, the planning of smaller studies can be a means of bringing together practitioners and academics in order to build relationships, more fully understand barriers to, and opportunities for, study implementation and data collection, and generate preliminary data that may still have tangible impact in the public and private sectors.

Influencing Policy-Making

A research base is critical to identifying the necessary components of integrated health care for individuals with ASD. However, it is not the only component. Advocacy and influence in policy making are vital to informing the creation and implementation of integrated health care for individuals with ASD as well. Providers play an important role in influencing policy-making since they are uniquely positioned at the front line of emerging issues and interface with individuals with ASD, their families, the systems of care, and other providers daily. Even after successful legislation is passed, continued advocacy to ensure effective and efficient implementation is needed. Ongoing monitoring is required to ensure integrated health care is enacted in ways that maximize the support of individuals with ASD and their families.

Training on advocacy and the idea of advocacy may carry individualistic responsibility that can feel overwhelming to healthcare providers. Training messages placing responsibility for advocacy for patients on providers' lack a focus on the full network of providers caring for an individual who may also be engaged to help advocate both for that specific patient and more broadly in advocating for wider system change. Considering the broader network of providers available for partnerships to most effectively advocate can help providers feel supported and weave in multiple perspectives to help maximize advocacy efforts (Hubinette, Dobson, Voyer, & Regehr, 2014; Shaw, 2014).

An option for healthcare providers is to engage the academic research community in supporting their efforts in advocacy to document and communicate their experiences and needs. Partnerships with academic entities can lead to reciprocal infusion of expertise in analytic methods and cutting-edge strategies for providers, and for the providers' real-world experiences to help make academic research relevant and meaningful. However, research has previously found that academically-based researchers thought they were more engaged with the ASD community than the community itself reported (Pellicano, Dinsmore, & Charman, 2014).

Healthcare providers can also engage the individuals with ASD and their families directly in advocacy efforts. Conversations with individuals with ASD and their families around their experiences and their needs may provide natural bridge for suggestions such as contacting and meeting with local legislators and seeking advocacy training. Accompanying individuals with ASD and their families on these visits could be especially valuable for healthcare providers since the combined presentation of the barriers being faced is particularly illustrative to policymakers.

Strategies for Engaging Policymakers

There are several strategies that healthcare providers can employ when engaging policymakers individually, or along with other providers, individuals with ASD, or their families. These are described below.

PAIR QUALITATIVE AND QUANTITATIVE. Individual stories are incredibly powerful in describing how a system is succeeding or failing. When these stories are paired with quantitative data describing how many other people are or might be experiencing the same thing, their value increases exponentially. Consider contacting an academic expert, provider organization, or other group who might have data to support your story. Always consider how data play a role since it helps to communicate the experiences of many people.

UNCOVERING KNOWLEDGE GAPS. Policymakers come from a wide variety of backgrounds but, for the most part, very few are or have been providers of direct services. Even ASD may be a new topic entirely for them. Start with the basics and do not become weighed down in the details. After you put together your talking point or your one page handout for a policymaker, review it later and ask others to do the same to help make sure you are not including too much detail or making assumptions about how much they might know about the issue.

BREVITY AND EFFICIENCY. It can be difficult to figure out how to compile most effectively materials that tell your story, or even how to tell your story in a concise way that most directly communicates your points. Consider advocacy training to help you whittle your message and try to stick to one-page documents and 30-second or less talking points. When you have everyday experiences and passionate beliefs about your needs, it can be challenging to remember the person you are talking to does not need or necessarily want to hear all of the details. Your most effective message delivery will be short and to the point.

PURSUASIVENESS. Policymakers work in jobs where they have to be elected and re-elected. Imagine if your job was based on how popular you were in your community, in your region, in your state, or even in the entire nation. Policymakers view their responsibilities and approach very differently because their jobs are very different from almost any other job. Headline news, for the good or the bad, infiltrates communities and heavily influences how people view policymakers and, most importantly, how they vote (Blake, Bonk, Heimpel, & Wright, 2013). Remember this perspective when you prepare to meet with a policymaker and especially in how you put together materials for the policymaker and his/her staff. It is important not to fabricate your experiences or story but pulling compelling details can help trigger the reaction policymakers need to pay attention. Also, news stories help, so if you are experiencing success as a provider, reach out to news outlets.

INCLUSIVENESS. Policymakers need to visit their communities and most policymakers enjoy being around their constituents. Being with the people they represent and hearing their stories is a top reason most policymakers become policymakers in the first place. Invite them to your provider place of business to see your story firsthand, to an ASD support group meeting, or even engage individuals with ASD and their families and visit the policy-maker's office for a visit. Anything you can do to help make your story real and relevant will help it stick with the policymaker when they need to think about priorities, cast a vote, or tap into your experience and expertise in forming new policy.

Policymakers have teams of people who support them and often these teams play critical roles in policy decision-making. A policymaker may not be able to meet with you directly but may send a representative or a chief of staff. It is important to remember that these team members play important roles in the policy process and their time is valuable, too. Team members from various policymakers often interact so if a policymaker is not focusing on your issue, he or she might be able to refer you to another policymaker who is in an even more important position of power on the issue. Ask for and take him or her up on these connections.

EXPANSIVENESS. Policymakers exist at all levels. Although broad policy flows down from the federal level, states often have flexibility in how they interpret and implement policy directives. States also have their own repre-sentatives and senators who cast important votes in how state policy is formed. The same flow can reach to counties and even to more local munic-ipalities. As you consider engaging policymakers, remember that there are many options for where you might begin. None of these pathways are wrong and it might take a few tries to find the path that most directly leads to the impact you seek.

PERSISTENCE. Policymakers are people first, and sometimes you will not form an apparent bond with a specific policymaker or his/her staff. If you do not find a connection on your first visit to a policymaker, keep trying. Give it some time and then schedule another visit. Consider trying alternate strate-gies to convey your information. If you talked through your first visit, con-sider constructing a one-page document that outlines briefly your experi-ences and most important points. One research study out of Australia found that sometimes connections with policymakers can be based on factors out of your control (Haynes et al., 2012). Consider alternate strategies like social or mass media to tell your story, too.

Conclusion

Policy formation and implementation require a well-formed base of evidence to optimally inform content and to successfully roll out to communities. While the evidence on how best to advocate for the needs of people with ASD is growing rapidly, significant gaps remain. ASD as a relative newcomer to the healthcare environment in which counterparts in developmental disabilities, such as intellectual disability, and mental health, such as depression, and schizophrenia, have received more and longer public attention and consequently benefitted from policies to improve care. It has only been about two decades since ASD advocacy and awareness began to increase, but much has already been accomplished and advocates have promising ideas for comparative effectiveness studies and how these might favorably change the way care is provided to people on the autism spectrum. The path has been identified and the journey begins with well-planned research and well-intentioned advocacy.

References

Bickman, L. (1996). Implications of a children's mental health managed care demonstration evaluation. *Journal of Mental Health Administration, 23*(1), 107–117.

Bickman, L., Summerfelt, W. T., & Noser, K. (1997). Comparative outcomes of emotionally disturbed children and adolescents in a system of services and usual care. *Psychiatric Services, 48*(12), 1543–1548.

Blake, A., Bonk, K., Heimpel, D., & Wright, C. S. (2013). Effective communications strategies: Engaging the media, policymakers, and the public. *Child Welfare, 92*(2), 217–233.

Blue-Banning, M., Summers, J. A., Frankland H. C., Nelson L. L., & Beegle, G. (2004). Dimensions of family and professional partnerships: Constructive guidelines for collaboration. *Exceptional Children, 70,* 167–184.

Borah, B. J., Moriarty, J. P., Crown, W. H., & Doshi, J. A. (2014). Applications of propensity score methods in observational comparative effectiveness and safety research: Where have we come and where should we go? *Journal of Comparative Effectiveness Research, 3*(1), 63–78.

Brookman-Frazee, L. I., Drahota, A., & Stadnick, N. (2012). Training community mental health therapists to deliver a package of evidence-based practice strategies for school-age children with autism spectrum disorders: A pilot study. *Journal of Autism & Developmental Disorders, 42*(8), 1651–1661.

Bruder, M. D., Kerins, G., Mazarella, C., Sims, J., & Stein, N. (2012). Brief report, the medical care of adults with autism spectrum disorders: Identifying the needs. *Journal of Autism & Developmental Disorders, 42*(11), 2498–2504.

Brugha, T. S, McManus, S., Bankart, J., Scott, F., Purdon, S., Smith, J., . . . Meltzer, H. (2011). Epidemiology of autism spectrum disorders in adults in the community in England. *Archives of General Psychiatry, 68*(5), 459–465.

Bryson, S. A., & Ostmeyer, K. F. (2014). Increasing the effectiveness of community mental health center social skills groups for children with autism spectrum disorder: A training and consultation example. *Administration and Policy in Mental Health and Mental Health Services Research, 41*(6), 808–821.

Centers for Medicare and Medicaid Services. (2014). Self-directed services. Retrieved 10/25, 2014, from http://www.medicaid.gov/Medicaid-CHIP -Program-Information/By-Topics/Delivery-Systems/Self-Directed-Services.html http://www.medicaid.gov/Medicaid-CHIP-Program-Information/By-Topics /Delivery-Systems/Self-Directed-Services.html

Croft, B., & Parish, S. L. (2013). Care integration in the patient protection and Affordable Care Act: Implications for behavioral health. *Administration and Policy in Mental Health and Mental Health Services Research, 40*(4), 258–263.

Grimes, K. E., Schulz, M. F., Cohen, S. A., Mullin, B. O., Lehar, S. E., & Tien, S. (2011). Pursuing cost-effectiveness in mental health service delivery for youth with complex needs. *Journal of Mental Health Policy and Economics, 14*(2), 73–83.

Hadland, S. E., & Long, W. L. (2014). A systematic review of the medical home for children without special health care needs. *Maternal Child Health Journal, 18,* 891–898.

Haynes, A. S., Derrick, G. E., Redman, S., Hall, W. D., Gillespie, J. A., Chapman, S., & Sturk, H. (2012). Identifying trustworthy experts: How do policymakers find and assess public health researchers worth consulting or collaborating with? *PLoS One, 7*(3), e32665.

Hodgetts, S., Zwaigenbaum, L., & Nicholas, D. (2015). Profile and predictors of service needs for families of children with autism spectrum disorders. *Autism, 19*(6), 673–683.

Hofelch, A., West, K., Walker, K., Schur, C., & Adams, A. (2014). Comparative effectiveness research and the environment for healthcare decision-making. Retrieved from http://www.npcnow.org/system/files/research/download/2013-npc-cer -survey-booklet-final.pdf

Hubinette, M., Dobson, S.,Voyer, S., & Regehr, G. (2014). 'We' not 'I': Health advocacy is a team sport. *Medical Education, 48*(9), 895–901.

Hyman, S. L., & Johnson, J. K. (2012). Autism and pediatric practice: Toward a medical home. *Journal of Autism & Developmental Disorders, 42*(6), 1156–1164.

Institute of Medicine (US) Committee on Crossing the Quality Chasm: Adaptation to Mental Health and Addictive Disorders. (2006). *Improving the quality of health care for mental and substance-use conditions.* Washington DC: National Academies Press.

Johnson, R. A., Danis, M., & Hafner-Eaton, C. (2014). US State variation in autism insurance mandates: Balancing access and fairness. *Autism, 18*(7), 803–814.

Keen, D. (2007). Parents, families and partnerships: Issues and considerations. *International Journal of Disability, Development & Education, 54,* 339–349.

Keriel-Gascou, M., Buchet-Poyau, K., Rabilloud, M., Duclos, A., & Colin, C. (2014). A stepped wedge cluster randomized trial is preferable for assessing complex health interventions. *Journal of Clinical Epidemiology, 67*(7), 831–833.

Kruis, A. L., Boland, M. R., Assendelft, W. J., Gussekloo, J., Tsiachristas, A., Stijnen, T. . . . Chavannes, N. H. (2014). Effectiveness of integrated disease management for primary care chronic obstructive pulmonary disease patients: Results of cluster randomised trial. *British Medical Journal, 349,* g5392.

Kuhlthau, K. A., Bloom, S., Van Cleave, J., Knapp, A. A., Romm, D., Klatka, K., . . . Perrin, J. M. (2011). Evidence for family-centered care for children with special health care needs: A systematic review. *Academic Pediatrics, 11*(2), 136–143.

L & M Policy Research, LLC. (2014). *Autism spectrum disorders (ASD): State of the states of services and supports for people with ASD.* Washington, DC. Retrieved from http://www.medicaid.gov/medicaid-chip-program-information/by-topics/long-term-services-and-supports/downloads/asd-state-of-the-states-report.pdf

Lemly, D. C., Weitzman, E. R., & O'Hare, K. (2013). Advancing healthcare transitions in the medical home: Tools for providers, families and adolescents with special healthcare needs. *Current Opinion in Pediatrics, 25*(4), 439–446.

Levy, S. L., Giarelli, E., Lee, L. Schieve, L. A., Kirby, R. S., Cunniff, C., . . . Rice, C. (2010). Autism spectrum disorder and co-occurring developmental, psychiatric, medical conditions among children in multiple populations of the United States. *Journal of Developmental and Behavioral Pediatrics, 31,* 267–275.

Lubetsky, M. J., Handen, B. L., Lubetsky, M., & McGonigle, J. J. (2014). Systems of care for individuals with autism spectrum disorder and serious behavioral disturbance through the lifespan. *Child & Adolescent Psychiatric Clinics of North America, 23*(1), 97–110.

Mandell, D. S., Guevara, J. P., & Pati, S. (2006). The search for coordinated, continuous community-based care: How the parallel efforts of the Medical Home and Systems of Care can inform each other. In W. H. Fisher (Ed.), *Research in community and mental health, Vol. 14–Research on community-based mental health services for children and adolescents.* Oxford, UK: Elsevier.

McGonigle, J. J., Migyanka, J. M., Glor-Scheib, S. J., Cramer, R., Fratangeli, J. J., Hegde, G. G., . . . Venkat, A. (2014). Development and evaluation of educational materials for pre-hospital and emergency department personnel on the care of patients with autism spectrum disorder. *Journal of Autism & Developmental Disorders, 44*(5), 1252–1259.

Nicolaidis, C., Kripke, C. C., & Raymaker, D. (2014). Primary care for adults on the autism spectrum. *Medical Clinics of North America, 98*(5), 1169–1191.

Patient-Centered Outcomes Research Institute. (2015). Large pragmatic studies to evaluate patient-centered outcomes–Winter 2015 Cycle. Available at http://www.pcori.org/announcement/large-pragmatic-studies-evaluate-patient-centered-outcomes-winter-2015-cycle

Pellicano, E., Dinsmore, A., & Charman, T. (2014). Views on researcher-community engagement in autism research in the United Kingdom: A mixed-methods study. *PLoS One, 9*(10), e109946.

Pennsylvania Department of Human Services. (2015a). Bureau of Autism Services. Available at http://www.dhs.state.pa.us/dhsorganization/officeofdevelopmental programs/bureauofautismservices/index.htm

Pennsylvania Department of Human Services. (2015b). Autism services, Available at http://www.dhs.state.pa.us/foradults/autismservices/index.htm

Piven, J., & Rabins, P. (2011) ASD in older adults: Toward defining a research agenda. *Journal of the American Geriatrics Society, 59*(11) 2151–2155.

Powell, B. J., Proctor, E. K., & Glass, J. E. (2014). A systematic review of strategies for implementing empirically supported mental health interventions. *Research on Social Work Practice, 24*(2), 192–212.

Rich, E., Lipson, D., Libersky, J., & Parchman, M. (2012). *Coordinating care for adults with complex care needs in the patient-centered medical home: Challenges and solutions. White Paper* (Prepared by Mathematica Policy Research under Contract No. HHSA290200900019I/HHSA29032005T). AHRQ Publication No. 12-0010-EF. Rockville, MD: Agency for Healthcare Research and Quality.

Rzhetsky, A., Bagley, S. C., Wang, K., Lyttle, C. S., Cook, E. H., Jr., Altman, R. B., & Gibbons, R. D. (2014). Environmental and state-level regulatory factors affect the incidence of autism and intellectual disability. *PLoS Computational Biology, 10*(3), e1003518.

Salzer, M. S., Kaplan, K., & Atay, J. (2006). State psychiatric hospital census after the 1999 Olmstead Decision: Evidence of decelerating deinstitutionalization. *Psychiatric Services, 57*(10), 1501–1504.

Schwartz, D., & Lellouch, J. (1967). Explanatory and pragmatic attitudes in therapeutical trials. *Journal of Chronic Diseases, 20*(8), 637–648.

Shaw, D. (2014). Advocacy: The role of health professional associations. *International Journal of Gynaecology and Obstetrics, 127*(Suppl 1), S43–S48.

Spencer, D., Marshall, J., Post, B., Kulakodlu, M., Newschaffer, C., Dennen, T., . . . Jain, A. (2013). Psychotropic medication use and polypharmacy in children with autism spectrum disorders. *Pediatrics, 132*(5), 833–840.

Thorpe, K. E., Zwarenstein, M., Oxman, A. D., Treweek, S., Furberg, C. D., Altman, D. G., . . . Chalkidou, K. (2009). A pragmatic-explanatory continuum indicator summary (PRECIS): A tool to help trial designers. *Journal of Clinical Epidemiology, 62*(5), 464–475.

Timberlake, M. T., Leutz, W. N., Warfield, M. E., & Chiri, G. (2014). "In the driver's seat": Parent perceptions of choice in a participant-directed Medicaid waiver program for young children with autism. *Journal of Autism & Developmental Disorders, 44*(4), 903–914.

Tosh, G., Soares-Weiser, K., & Adams, C. E. (2011). Pragmatic vs explanatory trials: The pragmascope tool to help measure differences in protocols of mental health randomized controlled trials. *Dialogues in Clinical Neuroscience, 13*(2), 209–215.

Vahabzadeh, A. (2014). How autism highlights health care challenges. Retrieved 10/24, 2014, from http://www.huffingtonpost.com/arshya-vahabzadeh/autism-health-care_b_4290175.html

Warfield, M. E., Chiri, G., Leutz, W. N., & Timberlake, M. (2014). Family well-being in a participant-directed autism waiver program: The role of relational coordination. *Journal of Intellectual Disability Research, 58*(12), 1091–1104.

Chapter 17

ASK THE EXPERTS

ELLEN GIARELLI AND JENNIFER PLUMB

On November 8, 2014, an all-day conference on "Creating Integrated Healthcare for People with Autism Spectrum Disorder" was held on the campus of Drexel University. There were four sessions comprising presentations and panel discussions. The sessions focused on the epidemiology, etiology, diagnosis, associated features, and special needs of people with ASD and how these interface with medical problems as they arise over the lifespan. Each session ended with question and answer sessions with the panelists. This chapter includes selected questions posed to the panelists in each session and their responses. The conference was supported by a grant from the National Institutes for Health Agency for Health Research and Quality, and Drexel University.

The moderators were: Jean Ruttenberg, Diana Robins, PhD, Margaret O'Neil, PhD, and Paul Shattuck, PhD.

Session I: What Is the Scope/Breadth of the Problem: Integrating Care for People with ASD?

During session 1, the speakers provided an overview of the public health problem of autism spectrum disorder (ASD) including a description of the natural history, etiology, rising prevalence, risk factors, and core features. This was followed by an analysis of the state of healthcare services provided across service settings. Session I panel members were James Connell, PhD; Jennifer Harrison Elder, PhD, FAAN; Jennifer Pinto-Martin, PhD, M.PH; and Catherine Rice, PhD who was the Keynote Speaker.

Moderator

Dr. Pinto-Martin, will the case inclusion criteria for the Study of the Epidemiology of Early Development (SEED), funded by the National Center on Birth Defects and Developmental Disabilities, Centers for Disease Control and Prevention need to be adjusted now that there are new criteria for the diagnosis of autism spectrum disorder, in the DSM-5.

Dr. Pinto-Martin. No, the SEED is using DSM-IV and will continue to use DSM IV, because that's how we've been enrolling children all along. I guess a subsequent issue will be how data analysis will change. At this time, we are not sure. We might look at what the differences will be had we used DSM-5. But we have so much to do with the data that we are already collecting. A decision on that issue will be several years in the future.

Moderator

Nonverbal learning disabilities (NVLD) are not included under ASD. Asperger's syndrome and nonverbal learning disability share characteristics. What is the panel's comment on why NVLDs are not included?

Dr. Rice. When we're talking about the diagnostic criteria for ASD we are referring to the Diagnosis and Statistical Manual (DSM) of the American Psychiatric Association. We're looking at psychiatrically-focused, medically-defined conditions. The DSM has not included nonverbal learning disability as a separate or specific disorder. In my own work as a developmental physiologist, I've struggled to find out more on the origin, the definition and the diagnostic classification under which nonverbal learning disorder actually exists. I think it's been used in practice–particularly in school settings–rather than in a diagnostic situation. Clinically, children with nonverbal learning disorder look a lot like those with Asperger's syndrome. It may be a different label for some similar characteristics and constitute a "pulling out" of specific features rather than looking at the whole clinical picture.

Moderator

There was a study that associated autism rates with the proximity of pregnant women to farms that used certain pesticides (organophosphates)? Can you address this?

Dr. Pinto-Martin. The only way we can understand whether any environmental factor has a real attributable risk for autism spectrum disorders is by conducting large controlled studies. Such studies should include careful assessment, not only of the exposer itself but careful characterization of the cases in the study. There are many published studies that are poorly done, quickly conceptualized, and included a broad range of poorly characterized exposers related to a perhaps poorly characterized sample of individuals with autism. The cases may not even have a gold standard diagnosis. We need to be cautious when new findings are reported and remind people that any new finding requires validation in a well done study before we do anything about it. Unfortunately, even when we have good data, it is difficult to translate these data into a public health message that is understandable, acceptable, and resonates with the consumer. We have a service to perform, which is to warn people about arriving at a quick conclusion when they see something in the media. In general, we need to tell them to be patient and to wait for a thorough scientific evaluation.

Moderator

In epidemiological studies, genetic factors are often identified. Do you think that environmental factors are being neglected?

Dr. Pinto-Martin. Oh, no, not neglected at all. It's just that we don't have good data yet to really be able to pin down either the environmental or the genetic cause or causes. That's why the SEED is so important.

Moderator

Given the critical importance of biological rhythms in development, is it possible that disturbed maternal circadian rhythms during pregnancy is a contributory or causal factor in ASD?

Dr. Pinto-Martin. I know of no studies that have addressed this issue and have no data to which I can refer. There are so many interesting hypotheses and that is one of them. There are some studies about sleep patterns in children with autism but also in their parents. That may be an interesting starting place to just look at what's known at least about postbirth sleep patterns. I would say to you: design a study.

Dr. Rice. Can I just add one thing? I think this issue speaks to the need for a collaborative relationship between the healthcare provider (HCP) and the patient or family member. It should be characterized by open, bidirectional communication so that parents may feel comfortable saying to their HCP, "You know I just heard about a new theory. I'm concerned about that. What do you think?" If parents or family members voice that concern, it can be addressed.

Moderator

There is a lack of knowledge about ASD among healthcare providers, in particular, nurse practitioners and physicians. What are the incentives that one might offer to healthcare providers to encourage them to seek additional training to prepare to care for this population?

Dr. Connell. From my experience, funders are limited in their ability to prescribe specific kinds and amounts of services to the provider agencies. Provider agencies are complex systems with complicated operating budgets, varying levels of expertise and knowledge of evidence-based programs, and knowledge of the community resources that provide the most effective care. Furthermore, there is, regrettably, disagreement about the clinical models. For example, applied behavioral analysis (ABA) or Floortime, at the provider level, and funding may come from a number of sources (including Medicaid, school districts, etc.) that pay for different types of service. Looking at system change within organizations is complex. From a behavioral economic perspective, incentivized rate structures will support the use of evidence-based services such as ABA. For example, a funder could incentivize a rate structure in which additional funds are offered when specific types of services are implemented and benchmarks are met. I think that generates, within the organization, motivation to not only train their staff but to meet those benchmarks. Furthermore, there are existing and exploratory CPT codes that staff members in a medical office can use for behavioral services and care coordination. I work with many "care navigators" in my clinical practice. Social workers and nurse practitioners (NP) are uniquely equipped with the proper training in behavioral supports. NPs, in particular, are focused on the family in a holistic way, and if their training programs offered courses that focused on autism intervention and community supports, such as the ones in the Drexel and Penn nursing programs, NPs can be enormously beneficial to the individual and the family as they navigate community providers and resources.

Moderator

On one set of slides we saw a booklet about introducing children with ASD to the medical care to prepare them for a healthcare visit or procedure. I did not see a similar instructional tool to use with adults on the spectrum. Are you aware of a teaching aid that is specifically designed for adults?

Dr. Rice. There are a variety of resources out there for adults as well. For example, there are social stories geared toward an adult with autism that take them through the steps of certain procedures and include visual aids. I think some of the emergency room and hospital-based interventions that have been developed are much more adult focused. Teaching tools are often prepared with a cognitive or developmental level in mind, and therefore one prepared for a child may be in some ways suitable for an adult with ASD who has an intellectual disability or receptive language difficulties.

Dr. Connell. In Pennsylvania, for example, there are several excellent resources available on the website www.PAautism.org in addition to a call-in help line. There's a resource component to the website that provides information about how to think about the problems adults on the spectrum might have upon entering a physician's office and ways to sort of plan for the visit.

Moderator

Talk further about the unique stressors impacting families of adults, and the supports that would benefit them.

Dr. Harrison Elder. I have observed that there is a conspicuous lack of structured supports and places to go for the adults with autism, who may have skills but really still continue to need supports. Even someone who may be appropriate for a college setting still needs supports in that setting. Others need much more such as 24/7 care. So the family is stressed. What should be done with this person? Keeping them active, alert, and involved is a huge challenge. But one of the biggest stresses that I've heard more clinically is just the constant worry about what's going to happen when the parent can no longer take care of him or her. What is the future going to hold? Who is going to care for this person like I do? And the financial and emotional stress of worrying about that takes such a huge toll.

Moderator

Several panel members mentioned the gap between diagnosis and access to services or supports. Has anybody thought about any kind of concept that would parallel the visiting nurses association to address that gap so that families are supported during times of extreme stress?

Dr. Connell. There are discussions of care navigation models that are useful across the lifespan. A care navigator would be present from diagnosis through transition and adult planning to help coordinate services and help the parents plan each step in life-long care. We could be years away from having testable models that can be scaled to serve all those who need comprehensive services.

Moderator

What I have observed in multidisciplinary agencies are providers who are not required to use evidence-based methods, and not sufficiently documenting care and outcomes. A great deal of emphasis is placed on making the records look good for agency inspectors. But the actual provision of services is sorely lacking. Will the panel address this phenomenon?

Dr. Connell. I think it's actually a little bit worse than that. As soon as you start talking about reinforcement-based plans, that is, according to some state agencies, considered a "restrictive intervention." I like to point out that we all work under that system. It operates on all of our lives. So, while one could perhaps say it's a restrictive intervention, it is, in fact, a restrictive intervention we are all exposed to. I think a bigger question is can we agree on what the evidence-based strategies are? A more pressing issue is: Can we think about how to implement them? A person-centered approach will not infringe on the rights of an individual, and will ensure that people with ASD can have access to the larger community by building skills necessary for success as a member of the community. The limitation of the use of evidence-based intervention prevents that from happening.

Moderator

One of the things that we know about autism is this challenge of generalization and it gets a little bit more challenging as they reach their adult years. And yet a lot of our models are center-based, office-based, when the issues are happening in the community and elsewhere. Any response?

Dr. Rice. That's an excellent point that I think has to be part of the intervention continuum. Practice needs to be as inclusive as possible and include going out to the actual settings where you want the person to utilize those skills.

Dr. Harrison Elder. That would be a good use of coaches. The University of Florida is a large campus, and we have a number of students who are on the spectrum and high functioning. They struggle with the everyday activities. We plan to train these individuals using coaches and measure some of the outcomes; the things that are of most importance to the student's success. Interestingly, we have had some of students participate in focus groups where they asked, "Why do we want to cure it, that's part of our identity."

Moderator

This question concerns the hospital visit; there is a paucity of information so that if a parent or a mother/father wanted to learn more about, you know, autism. Hospitals do not seem to be equipped to manage the needs of patients with autism spectrum disorder.

Dr. Pinto-Martin. This speaks to the need for training people who work in hospitals about the specific challenges of this group of patients. Dr. Giarelli has started a post-baccalaureate certificate program at Drexel University, and we have one at the University of Pennsylvania for nurse practitioners. I think these efforts will start to change the tide if the people who are working in the hospitals recognize the importance, then they'll have the information available.

Moderator

What are your thoughts on the use of nontraditional mental health treatment approaches that are particularly sensitive to nonverbal communication and sensory sensitivity such as music, movement, art, dance therapy?

Dr. Connell. Tailored therapies are great. We are just starting to learn about how these modalities can be effective. Do they directly decrease the core systems of ASD, such as reduce the occurrence of problem behavior, increase social or communication skills, increase academic performance, generate new friends? I'm not sure. I think we have to see where the research goes with that.

Moderator

Complementary and alternative therapies are controversial. What do you recommend we tell patients who ask us (nurses) about these treatments? And, if a patient's (family) admits to the use of CAM, what should we do about medication dosage adjustment?

Dr. Harrison Elder. This is an excellent question since the use of complementary and alternative medicine (CAM) is wide-spread, and seems to be growing in popularity. Thus, all parents should be questioned about CAM use, or intended future use, as part of the patient history and progress reports at subsequent visits. This is particularly important because some CAM may interact with prescribed medications. Also, many CAM lack empirical validation and some are very expensive. That said, I remember an illustrative comment from a mother about CAM, "I am a professional and well-educated but more importantly, I am a mother of a child with autism. If I wait for science to tell me if a treatment is effective or not, like the GFCF diet for instance, my child with be grown. I must make decisions now!" Knowing that there continues to be a lag time, sometimes longer than 10 years, between the introduction of a CAM treatment and published data regarding its use, it is best to urge families to consider the following: (1) Is there credible evidence that the CAM is safe, and perhaps more important, not potentially harmful? (2) Can they financially afford it without affecting the family's overall quality of life and/or ability to engage in other recommended evidence-based treatments? (3) Do they have the time and resources to systematically document the use and relevant outcomes so these can be communicated with their primary healthcare provider? Well-educated nurses are in excellent positions to point families to credible resources and guide them in making these important decisions.

Session 2: What Are the Barriers to Effective, Safe, Coordinated, Patient-Centered, and Timely Care?

In this session, the speakers presented an approach to examining barriers and facilitators of effective, safe, coordinated, patient-centered, and timely care across acute care settings. Panelists addressed questions related to strategies to integrate knowledge of the special needs, strengths, and limitations of people with ASD into the delivery of health care services. The panelists were Renee Turchi, MD, MPH, FAAP; Marcia R. Gardner PhD, RN, CPNP, CPN; Margaret C. Souders, PhD, CRNP; and Elizabeth Pfeiffer, PhD.

Moderator

Health care providers are interested in sensory processing and how that may contribute to the development of these behavioral problems, and anxiety. Are there any objective measures of sensory processing differences that could be useful?

Dr. Pfeiffer. Measurement is a big concern especially with the ASD population and we rely heavily on parent reported and patient reported outcomes. Interestingly, some of the work that we are doing right now in our research is looking at physiological measurement and trying to get concurrent validity with some of the parent reported outcomes. We just started that process. Much more research is needed.

Moderator

Are there any initiatives on a national level for the integration of a medical home, with education and other systems to improve communication or to develop a model to follow?

Dr. Turchi. Yes, there are initiatives both nationally and locally. One of the things that I didn't get a whole lot of time to talk about was that we have a state-wide medical home program here in Pennsylvania, working at the practice level, pediatric primary care, and as well as now working with family physicians and internal medicine to address the transition of care. Our program is the Pennsylvania Medical Home Initiative (www.pamedicalhome .org), housed at the Pennsylvania Chapter of the American Academy of Pediatrics. Our work is funded by the Pennsylvania Department of Health (Title V) and we work with pediatric and adult primary care practices across the entire Commonwealth of Pennsylvania to foster practice transformation and medical home. To date, we have worked with over 150 practices. The national parent organization is the American Academy of Pediatrics for pediatricians and they have a center for medical home implementation funded by HRSA at the national level. As part of the national work, I'm part of a work group looking at resident education around the medical home. There are some subgroups that are looking at integration of mental health into primary care, specifically in the pediatric arena.

Moderator

Do the findings of the sleep studies on children with ASD translate to adults? What specific recommendations do you have for caretakers of adults with ASD who do have sleep dysfunction, and if we know more specifics about the types of sleep dysfunction we see in adults with ASD?

Dr. Souders. I have not specifically done research with adults, but my colleagues across the United States, spearheaded by Beth Mallow, have included adults in their studies, and individuals with ASD have just as high levels of sleep problems. The predominant problem is insomnia, which is difficulty falling asleep and staying asleep. And as we know, insomnia is also associated with other psychiatric disorders, and as adults mature, a lot of them often in addition to the ASD have a depression, they have anxiety, and they may have a mood disorder. These are associated with insomnia, and so we have a lot of work to do. In addition to melatonin as a medication that may improve sleep, I would recommend cognitive behavioral therapy for insomnia.

Moderator

Dr. Souders, you proposed some clear approaches to kind of creating a positive sleep environment. But what happens when the individual with ASD is hospitalized? What can we do to encourage sleep there?

Dr. Souders. I think that it's hard for individuals in the hospital to sleep in general. Vital signs every four hours, getting your blood drawn at 6 AM . . . those are things that are very important to change just in general for all people who are admitted to the hospital. I think there are data coming out saying that people who sleep in the hospital are the people who actually get out of the hospital earlier. Sleep at night is wonderful for your heart, for your blood pressure, for your immune system. And there are data coming out of the West Coast that says that if you actually did not sleep more than six hours and you get a flu vaccine, you may not build an immune response, looking at college students. So in general, if you sleep well, you're more likely to heal. That's just in the general population. So we know that it's so hard to have kids with ASD in the hospital, but I think that the goal is for us to empower families, and when you show up, just like you've been mamma bear for your kids across all your developmental therapies, you need to say, "I want my child to have a quiet time. The quiet time is going to start at eight. What can we do to change the vital signs? What can we do to change when the person's going to come and draw the blood? And how can we come up with a system so that when they do fall asleep, we're not going to wake them up for a procedure."

Moderator

Dr. Gardner, how do you recommend people start to integrate ASD knowledge into the nursing curriculum?

Dr. Gardner. That's a challenge in any kind of health care education system, because there are competing priorities about what is needed in a healthcare curriculum, and there is a limited amount of time to cover the essential concepts for safe and effective care. However, autism prevalence statistics demonstrate that care for this population already is, and will continue to be, a challenge for clinicians. We need to be sure that nurses, the largest group of healthcare providers in the healthcare system, are well-prepared as new graduates to care for people with ASD in multiple settings. This applies to graduates of both prelicensure programs and advanced practice–nurse practitioner-programs. All clinicians will encounter people on the spectrum. So, the starting point is to make the information as available as possible to faculty, so that they can prepare their students with best practices for the care of people on the autism spectrum. ASD is typically taught in pediatrics, but we need to include ASDs in courses on the care of adults, because the children with ASD, in few years, will be found in adult healthcare settings. Their nurses have to understand their behaviors and know how to care for them. Planned clinical experiences with both children *and* adults are needed. In addition, we do not have enough continuing education about nursing care for people with autism. Clinicians are not necessarily incentivized to learn about autism, and we don't have mandatory continuing education about the disorder the way that we do about child abuse or infection control. So, we have to bring educational opportunities to the conferences that clinicians and nursing faculty are likely to attend, to heighten their awareness. It doesn't matter where they practice or what their roles are.

Moderator

Physical symptoms or medical problems may be difficult to recognize, particularly in nonverbal or minimally verbal individuals. Challenging behavior might impede the comprehensive medical examination. What happens when the specialist you're working with is not willing to address symptoms? And, how to advocate for your patient if you disagree with what a specialist is suggesting.

Dr. Turchi. I have a patient, an older male who has autism, and for him getting a blood pressure is really traumatic, but he has some underlying cardiac issues, and so we talk with cardiology regularly to determine if the measure is really necessary or if it is just routine and part of a protocol. Care must be individualized and each healthcare professional must use his or her best judgment in the context of the patient's actual needs. Sometimes we need to revert back to the basics and actually talk to our colleagues over the phone/ in person and not just email or message them briefly in our electronic health record. We also try to do a face-to-face or teleconference even for 15 minutes with several specialists and include the community providers as well. We decide what is the most critical thing that must be done in the visit that moment. I am thinking about one of the first times I saw a patient who was new to my practice. Things had been going great. When a second medical assistant came in, the little guy flew up onto the table and just stood there. The visit completely stopped. His mom shared that at his previous practice they had four people come in and hold him down to give him the vaccinations. He remembered and reacted. We absolutely underestimated the sort of memory he had. And how traumatic just pulling up to the office was for him, let alone being in an examination room. First, I triage what I really need to do in the physical exam and work with the patient and family to see what we can do together and what we can coordinate with other procedures, visits, or tests. That is what patient- and family-centered care is really about.

Session 3: Data Needs: How Can We Assess and Monitor Patient Outcomes?

In session 3, the speakers described patient outcome measures and other indicators of successful implementation of integrated patient care services. Participants discussed how to improve the quality and consistency of data sources available for cross-service setting and cross-provider evaluation. The

panel explored ways to incorporate assessments into electronic medical record keeping. The participants examined way to standardize indicators and
data collection methodologies within and across clinical service settings. The
panelists were Judith Miller, PhD; Carl V. Tyler, Jr., MD, CMD, MS; and
Romy Nocera, PhD.

Moderator

Dr. Tyler, could you speak more about the multiple stake-holder initiative regarding the use of Big Data that took place and how that process hap-
pened?

Dr. Tyler. It was a learning collaborative. We selected a topic. The expert consultant gave a presentation, and then we looked at that data on that
topic. People with whatever developmental disability we were focusing on
that day were present for the entire morning. They presented their own perspectives, including family members.

Moderator

Dr. Miller, many outcomes you mentioned are important and relevant.
What efforts have been made to address culturally important variables?

Dr. Miller. Different cultures do things differently. I have a colleague
who spent time in New Zealand and he came back transformed because of
the way they integrated the care given to individuals with severe mental illness, usually psychosis, but often intellectual disability. They did not stress
themselves out about getting a ton of intervention. They did not stress about
making sure the individual spent a lot of time at school or a lot of time at
work. They focused on integrating that person in the family and giving him
or her a role within the family and making sure he or she was happy. That
reduced the overall stress level for the family, and may have raised everyone's quality of life. It was a very different approach. There is little research
on this topic. I think cultural awareness not only about the healthcare experience but also about how we approach individuals with autism, in society, is
lacking. For example, if there's a stigma associated with a disability, or if
there's a difference in the kind of social support based on cultural factors,
outcomes will vary. If there are different expectations for that individual
because of his or her gender, or age, or station in life, the interpretation of
the patient's needs will also differ. Outcomes will be valued differently to
individuals based on the cultural setting in which they find themselves.

Moderator

Dr. Nocera, how do you encourage emergency room staff to view patients with ASD differently?

Dr. Nocera. I put together a questionnaire and sent it out to the faculty and residents. I didn't get a huge response rate, but among the people who did respond, depending on where they were in their career if they were, for example, a first-year resident might have seen one patient. The experienced staff might have seen several patients with ASD. No one had specialized training, and currently there's nothing that I'm aware of that is immediately implemented as soon as a patient with ASD comes through the door. I often find that professionals don't want to be viewed as not knowing how to deal with that patient, especially if they are a resident and they're being graded on their functioning. But I have not heard of or seen that in our emergency department, thankfully. But, I was distressed by the report of one study in which emergency department physicians simply refused to treat ASD patients.

Moderator

Dr. Tyler, what efforts are being made to include outcome measures that allow for understanding of lifestyles, social, educational, etc.?

Dr. Tyler. They should be an intrinsic part of electronic health record data collection and analysis. Some data are better captured by clinicians, and some data are very unreliably captured. We have a system that integrated languages. At one clinic, the language preference it's defaulted to Croatian which is actually very funny because my wife is Serbo-Croatian and we speak Serbo-Croatian. So it's defaulted to Croatian to indicate how well and how poorly clinicians are flipping the language tab to the appropriate primary language, and most patients are speaking patients are speaking Croatian served by the Cleveland Clinic.

Moderator

Dr. Miller, in your opinion, should an expert in ASD be called in as part of the standard of care?

Dr. Miller. In an ideal world, we would know that not all patients with autism are going to have a hard time in the hospital, and there would be enough training of the general staff to use some of the tier-two interventions without a lot of help because they've done it before and they've been trained. At this point, however, most healthcare facilities don't have that and often what you see is a hospital culture where there is someone—some go-to person that people know can work well with patients who might have a difficult time. So everyone knows "Nurse Beth" is good with this population, so they call Nurse Beth whenever someone with ASD is scheduled. Well that might work most of the time, but it doesn't build capacity in the other staff members, and unfortunately there's not always a "Nurse Beth" around when you need her.

Session 4: How Should We Influence Policy-Making, Prioritize Lines of Inquiry, and Form Teams?

In Session 4, the speakers described innovative study designs, creative uses of existing data, and novel analytical approaches to better elucidate the complex causal pathways that might explain disparities in health care and health outcomes. The participants discussed approaches to developing policies and to advocating for system change. Participants shared ideas for collaborative research devoted to understanding the factors responsible for and potential solutions to mitigate health disadvantages. The panelists were David S. Mandell, ScD; Craig Newschaffer, PhD; and Lindsay Shea, DrPH.

Moderator

What are some of the policy barriers to achieving more integrated care for people with multiple issues?

Dr. Mandell. I think the primary one is funding, and there are two types of funding. One is like "Where's Waldo." There are different entities out of whose pockets funding for different things is coming. This creates fragmentation and reduced the potential to integrate care that might exist if the funding sources were connected. So that's the concurrent funding issue. There's also a sequential funding issue which is that if one does a better job of providing care to individuals with autism, one can realize an economic benefit. If the system providing efficient care is not the system reaping any of the reward, then the incentive to engage in integrated care is removed. So, for example, if I'm doing a better job of managing behavior in school in a way that reduces contact with the criminal justice system and reduces inpatient hospitalization, how is that recognized and therefore incentivizing me to continue? The same principle can be applied to integrated health care.

Dr. Shea. I think that the policy issues are several-fold. They hinge, certainly, on funding and structure. I think that the evidence base is also a problem because we have some standards around how we might structure policy. In Pennsylvania the ACAP model is a unique program that provides integrated health care to adults living with autism.

Dr. Newschaffer. "Integrated health care" is not a well-understood specific process. I see the term as a piece of jargon we use to refer to a range of activities. If you approach a policy maker and say, "We want integrated health care," they have no idea what you're talking about. I think part of our challenge as practitioners and researchers is to be very, very specific about what we are asking for and very, very specific about what we think the end goal will be. And unless we can do that effectively, we are going to have a difficult time advocating for any kind of meaningful change.

Moderator

Dr. Newschaffer, do you have any recommendations or thoughts about how to better coordinate university efforts across multiple healthcare settings that could be used to design larger cluster randomized control designs using multiple health care settings? Collaborations?

Dr. Newschaffer. First of all, I think that there are power [sample size] issues with implementing group-randomized designs. However, often these limitations are not as bad as you might intuitively think, and there are ways to plan adequately-powered designs using a manageable number of clusters. Of course, statistical power also depends on how much variability you think there will be, both within and across clusters. There are ways to do powerful and effective studies without having to put together a national network to get the study size that you need. So scale is a consideration, but I don't think it's an impediment to these kinds of designs. But, of course, there is a range of larger established healthcare delivery networks that do have advantages in terms of putting together these kinds of studies. Maybe finding ways to partner researchers with these systems will be part of the solution to moving this forward. I'm thinking about Dr. Tyler's presentation and some of the other initiatives that I know about. There is indeed opportunity to leverage electronic records. Electronic records probably don't have all of the data elements that we would want for this type of research, but they can be much richer than an insurance claims database. Electronic records tend to include text fields that are ripe for extraction using modern text mining methods. And because of the technology that is being used to capture data in EMRs—these records are getting richer and richer. I have even seen large randomized trials where most of the primary outcomes have been pulled from fairly sophisticated EMR systems.

Moderator

Under what circumstances does research evidence become more or less salient to policy makers?

Dr. Mandell. There was a study out of Australia that interviewed policy makers and academic researchers. In general, both groups agreed that research can shape policy before, during, and after it's formed. I also recall that a third of both groups thought that research was more often used to justify a point that a policy maker had already decided they were going to pursue.

Moderator

We are finding now in the public arena that the resources that are available to us to fund support services are becoming increasingly dear while the demands for supports and services is increasing. It's becoming necessary for us to demonstrate advocacy in terms of where we are directing resources and dollars. Research on the factors that improve health outcomes for people with autism must continue and will generate data that can be presented to local legislators as evidence for the need for policy change. Funding is needed to support this work.

Appendix

RESEARCHABLE IDEAS AND
TOPICS FOR DISCUSSION

Big Data

1. What are efficient methods to identify and validate ASD cohorts in big data information systems?
2. What are the pitfalls and potentialities of using big data related to persons with ASD?
3. How can practice-based researchers utilize big data to target health system innovations to improve the health care of persons with ASD?
4. How can big data be tapped to create quality of healthcare standards specific to persons with ASD?
5. How can the information gained from big data be integrated with clinician, caregiver, and self-advocate experience to yield a richer understanding of the health and health care of persons with ASD?
6. What are some of the unique limitations and precautions with using big data to examine health and healthcare quality related to persons with ASD?
7. What clinical and bioinformatics infrastructure developments would foster the use of big data for improving the health care of persons with ASD?

Emergency/Acute Care

1. What are the characteristics of urgent care provided to adults with ASD?
2. Individuals with ASD use emergency department (ED) services with greater frequency than those without ASD. In addition to the potential for atypical presentations, communication difficulties, and high incidence of psychiatric comorbidity, what are the educational needs of the ED team?

3. What are the most effective response strategies for healthcare team in the ED?
4. Describe both immediate and long-term environmental modifications that may be made to improve the patient's experience with emergency medical care?
5. Conducting research and inclusion of the person with ASD is critically important to understanding effectiveness of interventions. Obtaining informed consent is paramount in ensuring fair treatment of participants. What are the best ways to assess the individual with ASD regarding informed consent to participate in a research study?

Epidemiology

1. What is the prevalence and severity of common medical conditions (i.e., Heart disease, cancers, diabetes) among adults with ASD?
2. What is the prevalence and severity of sleep and eating disorders among adults on the autism spectrum?

Family Caregiving

1. Describe the roles of different healthcare providers in helping families of children with autism spectrum disorder (ASD) obtain the earliest possible diagnoses and ascertain the most appropriate forms of early intervention.
2. How can empirically valid treatments for ASD be integrated with the delivery of medical care across service settings?
3. Discuss the roles of all family members optimizing the delivery of primary, secondary, tertiary preventions for patients with ASD.

Forming Collaborations

1. What is the ideal structure and process for interdisciplinary collaborations to provide comprehensive integrated care for patients on the autism spectrum?

Patient-Centered Outcomes

1. How can cognitive behavioral therapy be used to treat sleeping disorders, such as insomnia among adult patients with ASD?
2. How common are associated features such as difficulties with sleep, eating, and movement among adults with ASD?

3. How can a HCP distinguish the effect of these difficulties on behavior when a patient with ASD is not responding to a medical treatment plan?
4. What is the optimal way to provide cancer risk assessment (i.e., primary prevention) to adults on the autism spectrum?
5. How does healthcare provider knowledge of the core characteristics and associated features of ASD affect the outcomes of care?
6. What are the long-term physical effects of polypharmacy among patients with ASD?
7. Can novel therapeutic aids (i.e., service pets) facilitate the completion of complex medical procedures for people with ASD?

Policy and Economics

1. How does the cost of lifelong care for chronic medical conditions differ for people with ASD as compared to the general population?
2. How might the medical home be adapted to serve the adult population with ASD and multiple medical comorbidities?

Sensory Processing

1. What is the potential impact of the social and physical sensory environments on the provision of health care for individuals with ASD?
2. What potential screening methods might be helpful in evaluating an individual with ASD's sensory processing differences in various healthcare settings? Which might be standardized to implement across healthcare settings?
3. What (a) anticipatory, (b) physical, and (c) social strategies can be applied to the care of people with ASD with medical problems, to support integrated health care?

INDEX

CHARLES C THOMAS · PUBLISHER, LTD.

THE PROFESSIONAL HELPER
(2nd Ed.)
By Willie V. Bryan
2015, 354 pp. (7 x 10)
$53.95 (paper), $53.95 (ebook)

SOLVING THE PUZZLE OF YOUR ADD/ADHD CHILD
By Laura J. Stevens
2015, 266 pp. (7 x 10), 7 il., 13 tables.
$35.95 (spiral), $35.95 (ebook)

BEHAVIORAL GUIDE TO PERSONALITY DISORDERS (DSM-5)
By Douglas H. Ruben
2015, 272 pp. (7 x 10), 31 il., 1 table.
$42.95 (paper), $42.95 (ebook)

SERVICE AND THERAPY DOGS IN AMERICAN SOCIETY
By John J. Ensminger
2010, 340 pp. (7 x 10), 25 il., 1 table.
$49.95 (paper), $49.95 (ebook)

THE SOCIOLOGY OF DEVIANCE
(2nd Ed.)
By Robert J. Franzese
2015, 398 pp. (7 x 10), 21 il., 6 tables.
$64.95 (paper), $64.95 (ebook)

A GUIDEBOOK TO HUMAN SERVICE PROFESSIONS (2nd Ed.)
By William G. Emener,
Michael A. Richard & John J. Bosworth
2009, 286 pp. (7 x 10), 2 il., 4 tables.
$49.95 (paper), $49.95 (ebook)

MULTICULTURAL ASPECTS OF HUMAN BEHAVIOR (3rd Ed.)
By Willie V. Bryan
2014, 278 pp. (7 x 10)
$45.95 (paper), $45.95 (ebook)

THE HANDBOOK OF CHILD LIFE
By Richard H. Thompson
2009, 378 pp. (7 x 10), 5 il., 15 tables.
$59.95 (paper), $59.95 (ebook)

HELPING SKILLS FOR HUMAN SERVICE WORKERS (3rd Ed.)
By Kenneth France & Kim Weikel
2014, 384 pp. (7 x 10), 6 il.
$59.95 (paper), $59.95 (ebook)

FINANCIAL MANAGEMENT FOR NONPROFIT HUMAN SERVICE ORGANIZATIONS (2nd Ed.)
By Raymond Sanchez Mayers
2004, 354 pp. (7 x 10), 19 il., 46 tables.
$61.95 (paper), $61.95 (ebook)

PARENTAL ALIENATION
By Demosthenes Lorandos,
William Bernet & S. Richard Sauber
2013, 550 pp. (7 x 10), 2 il.
$89.95 (hard), $89.95 (ebook)

THE RENAL PATIENT'S GUIDE TO GOOD EATING (2nd Ed.)
By Judith A. Curtis
2003, 226 pp. (7 x 10), 30 il.
$39.95 (spiral), $39.95 (ebook)

BASIC TRAINING FOR RESIDENTIAL CHILDCARE WORKERS
By Beverly Boone
2011, 224 pp. (7 x 10)
$36.95 (paper), $36.95 (ebook)

CASE MANAGEMENT IN SOCIAL WORK (2nd Ed.)
By Julius R. Ballew & George Mink
1996, 334 pp. (7 x 10), 23 il.
$53.95 (paper), $53.95 (ebook)

THE PARENTAL ALIENATION SYNDROME
By Linda J. Gottlieb
2012, 302 pp. (7 x 10)
$64.95 (hard), $44.95 (paper), $44.95 (ebook)

CHILD LIFE IN HOSPITALS
By Richard H. Thompson & Gene Stanford
1981, 284 pp. (6 x 9), 1 table.
$45.95 (paper), $45.95 (ebook)

Find us on
Facebook
FACEBOOK.COM/CCTPUBLISHER   **TO ORDER:** 1-800-258-8980 • books@cctthomas.com • www.cctthomas.com